MR-Guided Interventions

Editors

CLARE M.C. TEMPANY
TINA KAPUR

MAGNETIC RESONANCE IMAGING CLINICS OF NORTH AMERICA

www.mri.theclinics.com

Consulting Editors
SURESH K. MUKHERJI
LYNNE S. STEINBACH

November 2015 • Volume 23 • Number 4

ELSEVIER

1600 John F. Kennedy Boulevard • Suite 1800 • Philadelphia, Pennsylvania, 19103-2899

http://www.mri.theclinics.com

MRI CLINICS OF NORTH AMERICA Volume 23, Number 4
November 2015 ISSN 1064-9689, ISBN 13: 978-0-323-41338-1

Editor: John Vassallo (j.vassallo@elsevier.com)
Developmental Editor: Meredith Clinton

Magnetic Resonance Imaging Clinics of North America (ISSN 1064-9689) is published quarterly by Elsevier Inc., 360 Park Avenue South, New York, NY 10010-1710. Months of issue are February, May, August, and November. Business and Editorial Offices: 1600 John F. Kennedy Blvd., Ste. 1800, Philadelphia, PA 19103-2899. Customer Service Office: 3251 Riverport Lane, Maryland Heights, MO 63043. Periodicals postage paid at New York, NY and additional mailing offices. Subscription prices are $375.00 per year (domestic individuals), $581.00 per year (domestic institutions), $190.00 per year (domestic students/residents), $420.00 per year (Canadian individuals), $755.00 per year (Canadian institutions), $545.00 per year (international individuals), $755.00 per year (international institutions), and $275.00 per year (international and Canadian students/residents). International air speed delivery is included in all *Clinics* subscription prices. All prices are subject to change without notice. **POSTMASTER:** Send address changes to *Magnetic Resonance Imaging Clinics*, Elsevier Health Sciences Division, Subscription Customer Service, 3251 Riverport Lane, Maryland Heights, MO 63043. Customer Service (orders, claims, online, change of address): Elsevier Health Sciences Division, Subscription **Customer Service, 3251 Riverport Lane, Maryland Heights, MO 63043. Tel:1-800-654-2452 (U.S. and Canada); 314-447-8871 (outside U.S. and Canada). Fax: 314-447-8029. E-mail: journalscustomer service-usa@elsevier.com (for print support); journalsonlinesupport-usa@elsevier.com (for online support).**

Reprints. For copies of 100 or more of articles in this publication, please contact the Commercial Reprints Department, Elsevier Inc., 360 Park Avenue South, New York, NY 10010-1710. Tel.: 212-633-3874; Fax: 212-633-3820; E-mail: reprints@elsevier.com.

Magnetic Resonance Imaging Clinics of North America is covered in the *RSNA Index of Imaging Literature, MEDLINE/PubMed (Index Medicus),* and *EMBASE/Excerpta Medica.*

Printed in the United States of America.

Contributors

CONSULTING EDITORS

SURESH K. MUKHERJI, MD, MBA, FACR
Professor and Chairman; W.F. Patenge
Endowed Chair, Department of Radiology,
Michigan State University, East Lansing,
Michigan

LYNNE S. STEINBACH, MD, FACR
Professor of Radiology and Orthopaedic
Surgery, Department of Radiology and
Biomedical Imaging, University of California
San Francisco, San Francisco, California

EDITORS

CLARE M.C. TEMPANY, MD
Professor of Radiology, Harvard Medical
School; Ferenc Jolesz Chair of Radiology
Research, Director National Center for Image
Guided Therapy, Department of Radiology,
Brigham and Women's Hospital, Boston,
Massachusetts

TINA KAPUR, PhD
Assistant Professor of Radiology, Harvard
Medical School; Executive Director National
Center for Image Guided Therapy, Department
of Radiology, Brigham & Women's Hospital,
Boston, Massachusetts

AUTHORS

HENA AHMED, BS
Department of Neurosurgery, Brigham and
Women's Hospital, Harvard Medical School,
Boston, Massachusetts

ALLAN J. BELZBERG, MD
Associate Professor of Neurosurgery,
Department of Neurosurgery, The Johns
Hopkins University School of Medicine,
Baltimore, Maryland

MICHAEL A. BOWEN, NP
Adult Nurse Practitioner, Abdominal Imagine
and Intervention Division, Department of
Radiology and Imaging Sciences, Emory
University Hospitals, Atlanta, Georgia

ADRIENNE E. CAMPBELL-WASHBURN, PhD
Cardiovascular and Pulmonary Branch,
Division of Intramural Research, National
Heart, Lung, and Blood Institute, National
Institutes of Health, Bethesda, Maryland

JOHN A. CARRINO, MD, MPH
Professor of Radiology, Department of
Radiology and Imaging, Hospital for Special
Surgery, New York, New York

H. BALLENTINE CARTER, MD
The James Buchanan Brady Urological
Institute, The Johns Hopkins University,
Baltimore, Maryland

THANISSARA CHANSAKUL, MD
Division of Neuroradiology, Brigham and
Women's Hospital, Boston, Massachusetts

ANTONIO L. DAMATO, PhD
Department of Radiation Oncology, Brigham
and Women's Hospital, Boston,
Massachusetts

ARNOLD LEE DELLON, MD, PhD
Professor of Plastic Surgery and Neurosurgery,
Department of Plastic Surgery, Peripheral
Nerve Surgery, The Johns Hopkins University
School of Medicine, Baltimore, Maryland

S. SAEID DIANAT, MD
Department of Radiology, University of
Minnesota, Minneapolis, Minnesota

JOY EBERHARDT
Sr Medical Secretary, Interventional MRI
Program, Department of Radiology and
Imaging Sciences, Emory University Hospitals,
Atlanta, Georgia

ANTHONY Z. FARANESH, PhD
Cardiovascular and Pulmonary Branch,
Division of Intramural Research, National
Heart, Lung, and Blood Institute, National
Institutes of Health, Bethesda, Maryland

WESLEY FIELD, BS
Department of Neurosurgery, Brigham and
Women's Hospital, Harvard Medical School,
Boston, Massachusetts

JAN FRITZ, MD
Assistant Professor of Radiology and
Radiological Science, Russell H. Morgan
Department of Radiology and Radiological
Science, Johns Hopkins Medical Institutions,
Baltimore, Maryland

EVA C. GOMBOS, MD
Assistant Professor of Radiology, Harvard
Medical School; Division of Breast Imaging,
Department of Radiology, Brigham and
Women's Hospital, Boston, Massachusetts

KRZYSZTOF R. GORNY, PhD
Department of Radiology, Mayo Clinic,
Rochester, Minnesota

MICHAEL S. HANSEN, PhD
Cardiovascular and Pulmonary Branch,
Division of Intramural Research, National
Heart, Lung, and Blood Institute, National
Institutes of Health, Bethesda, Maryland

MICHAEL T. HAYES, MD
Department of Neurology, South Shore
Hospital, Weymouth, Massachusetts

STEVEN W. HETTS, MD
Department of Radiology and Biomedical
Imaging, University of California San Francisco,
San Francisco, California

NATHAN C. HIMES, MD
Division of Neuroradiology, Brigham and
Women's Hospital, Boston, Massachusetts

JAYENDER JAGADEESAN, PhD
Surgical Planning Laboratory, Brigham and
Women's Hospital, Boston, Massachusetts

DANIEL F. KACHER, MS
Surgical Planning Laboratory, Brigham
and Women's Hospital, Boston,
Massachusetts

AKIRA KAWASHIMA, MD, PhD
Department of Radiology, Mayo Clinic,
Rochester, Minnesota

THIELE KOBUS, PhD
Department of Radiology, Brigham and
Women's Hospital, Harvard Medical School,
Boston, Massachusetts; Department of
Radiology and Nuclear Medicine, Radboud
University Medical Center, Nijmegen,
Netherlands

ROBERT J. LEDERMAN, MD
Cardiovascular and Pulmonary Branch,
Division of Intramural Research, National
Heart, Lung, and Blood Institute, National
Institutes of Health, Bethesda, Maryland

THOMAS C. LEE, MD
Division of Neuroradiology, Brigham and
Women's Hospital, Boston, Massachusetts

PRASHEEL LILLANEY, PhD
Department of Radiology and Biomedical
Imaging, University of California San Francisco,
San Francisco, California

**WILLIAM OMAR CONTRERAS LOPEZ,
MD, PhD**
Division of Functional Neurosurgery, Institute
of Psychiatry, University of São Paulo School of
Medicine, São Paulo, Brazil

AARON LOSEY, MD
Department of Radiology and Biomedical
Imaging, University of California San Francisco,
San Francisco, California

KATARZYNA J. MACURA, MD, PhD, FACR
The Russell H. Morgan Department of
Radiology and Radiological Science, The
James Buchanan Brady Urological Institute,
The Johns Hopkins University, Baltimore,
Maryland

ALASTAIR J. MARTIN, PhD
Department of Radiology and Biomedical
Imaging, University of California San Francisco,
San Francisco, California

NATHAN McDANNOLD, PhD
Division of Neuroradiology, Department of
Radiology, Brigham and Women's Hospital,
Harvard Medical School, Boston,
Massachusetts

CAROLYN CIDIS MELTZER, MD, FACR
William P. Timmie Professor and Chair, Department of Radiology and Imaging Sciences, Associate Dean for Research, Emory University Hospitals and School of Medicine, Atlanta, Georgia

ANDREW S. MIKHAIL, PhD
Postdoctoral Fellow, Center for Interventional Oncology, Radiology and Imaging Sciences, Clinical Center, National Institutes of Health, Bethesda, Maryland

SRINIVASAN MUKUNDAN Jr, MD, PhD
Division of Neuroradiology, Department of Radiology, Brigham and Women's Hospital, Harvard Medical School, Boston, Massachusetts

LANCE A. MYNDERSE, MD
Department of Urology, Mayo Clinic, Rochester, Minnesota

SHERIF G. NOUR, MD, FRCR
Associate Professor of Radiology and Imaging Sciences; Director, Interventional MRI Program, Department of Radiology and Imaging Sciences, Emory University Hospitals and School of Medicine, Atlanta, Georgia

ARI PARTANEN, PhD
Senior Clinical Scientist, MR Therapy, Philips Healthcare, Andover, Massachusetts; Center for Interventional Oncology, Radiology and Imaging Sciences, Clinical Center, National Institutes of Health, Bethesda, Maryland

GREG PENNINGTON, BBA, MBA
Sr Manager, Clinical Operations, Department of Radiology and Imaging Sciences, Emory University Hospitals, Atlanta, Georgia

TRACY E. POWELL, MSN, NP
Adult Nurse Practitioner, Interventional MRI Program, Department of Radiology and Imaging Sciences, Emory University Hospitals, Atlanta, Georgia

DANIELLE M. RICHMAN, MD, MS
Department of Radiology, Brigham and Women's Hospital, Boston, Massachusetts

EHUD J. SCHMIDT, PhD
Associate Professor of Radiology, Harvard Medical School; Radiology Department, Brigham and Women's Hospital, Boston, Massachusetts

FABIO SETTECASE, MD, MSc
Department of Radiology and Biomedical Imaging, University of California San Francisco, San Francisco, California

TRAVIS S. TIERNEY, MD, PhD
Department of Neurosurgery, Brigham and Women's Hospital, Harvard Medical School, Boston, Massachusetts

ARADHANA M. VENKATESAN, MD
Associate Professor, Term Tenure Track, Section of Abdominal Imaging, Department of Diagnostic Radiology, M.D. Anderson Cancer Center, Houston, Texas

AKILA N. VISWANATHAN, MD, MPH
Department of Radiation Oncology, Brigham and Women's Hospital, Boston, Massachusetts

WEI WANG, PhD
Radiology, Brigham and Women's Hospital, Harvard Medical School, Boston, Massachusetts

ERIC H. WILLIAMS, MD
Assistant Professor of Plastic Surgery, Department of Plastic, Reconstructive, and Maxillofacial Surgery, The Johns Hopkins University School of Medicine, Baltimore, Maryland

BRADFORD J. WOOD, MD
Director, Center for Interventional Oncology and Chief, Interventional Radiology, Clinical Center, National Institutes of Health, Bethesda, Maryland

DAVID A. WOODRUM, MD, PhD
Department of Radiology, Mayo Clinic, Rochester, Minnesota

PAVEL YARMOLENKO, PhD
Assistant Professor, The Sheikh Zayed Institute for Pediatric Surgical Innovation, Children's National Medical Center, Washington, DC

Contents

Evolution of Movement Disorders Surgery Leading to Contemporary Focused Ultrasound Therapy for Tremor   515

Hena Ahmed, Wesley Field, Michael T. Hayes, William Omar Contreras Lopez, Nathan McDannold, Srinivasan Mukundan Jr, and Travis S. Tierney

> Progressively less invasive neurosurgical approaches for the treatment of movement disorders have evolved, beginning with open craniotomy for placement of lesions within pyramidal structures followed by refined stereotactic ablation of extrapyramidal targets that encouraged nondestructive electrode stimulation of deep brain structures. A noninvasive approach using transcranial high-energy focused ultrasound has emerged for the treatment of intractable tremor. The ability to target discreet intracranial sites millimeters in size through the intact skull using focused acoustic energy marks an important milestone in movement disorders surgery. This article describes the evolution of magnetic resonance-guided focused ultrasound for ventrolateral thalamotomy for tremor.

Magnetic Resonance Imaging–Guided Spine Interventions   523

Nathan C. Himes, Thanissara Chansakul, and Thomas C. Lee

> Magnetic resonance (MR) imaging–guided interventions for treatment of low back pain and for diagnosis and treatment of soft tissue and bony spinal lesions have been shown to be feasible, effective, and safe. Advantages of this technique include the absence of ionizing radiation, the high tissue contrast, and multiplanar imaging options. Recent advancements in MR imaging systems allow improved image qualities and real-time guidance. One exciting application is MR imaging–guided cryotherapy of spinal lesions, including treating such lesions as benign osteoid osteomas and malignant metastatic disease in patients who are not good surgical candidates. This particular technique shows promise for local tumor control and pain relief in appropriate patients.

3-Tesla High-Field Magnetic Resonance Neurography for Guiding Nerve Blocks and Its Role in Pain Management   533

Jan Fritz, Arnold Lee Dellon, Eric H. Williams, Allan J. Belzberg, and John A. Carrino

> Interventional magnetic resonance (MR) neurography is a minimally invasive technique that affords targeting of small nerves in challenging areas of the human body for highly accurate nerve blocks and perineural injections. This cross-sectional technique uniquely combines high tissue contrast and high-spatial-resolution anatomic detail, which enables the precise identification and selective targeting of peripheral nerves, accurate needle guidance and navigation of the needle tip within the immediate vicinity of a nerve, as well as direct visualization of the injected drug for the assessment of appropriate drug distribution and documentation of the absence of spread to confounding nearby nerves.

Contrast-enhanced breast magnetic resonance (MR) imaging is increasingly being used to diagnose breast cancer and to perform biopsy procedures. The American Cancer Society has advised women at high risk for breast cancer to have breast MR imaging screening as an adjunct to screening mammography. This article places special emphasis on biopsy and operative planning involving MR imaging, and reviews use of breast MR imaging in monitoring response to neoadjuvant chemotherapy. Described are peer-reviewed data on currently accepted MR imaging–guided procedures for addressing benign and malignant breast diseases, including intraoperative imaging.

Performing intraoperative cardiovascular procedures inside a magnetic resonance (MR) imaging scanner can potentially provide substantial advantage in clinical outcomes by reducing the risk and increasing the success rate relative to the way such procedures are performed today, in which the primary surgical guidance is provided by X-ray fluoroscopy, by electromagnetically tracked intraoperative devices, and by ultrasound. Both noninvasive and invasive cardiologists are becoming increasingly familiar with the capabilities of MR imaging for providing anatomic and physiologic information that is unequaled by other modalities. As a result, researchers began performing animal (preclinical) interventions in the cardiovascular system in the early 1990s.

Several advantages of magnetic resonance (MR) imaging compared with other imaging modalities have provided the rationale for increased attention to MR-guided interventions, including its excellent soft tissue contrast, its capability to show both anatomic and functional information, and no use of ionizing radiation. An important aspect of MR-guided intervention is to provide visualization and navigation of interventional devices relative to the surrounding tissues. This article focuses on the methods for MR-guided active tracking in catheter-based interventions. Practical issues about implementation of active catheter tracking in a clinical setting are discussed and several current application examples are highlighted.

⊙ Videos on the XMR suite at UCSF Medical Center and magnetic resonance imaging–guided electrophysiological ablation accompany this article

The use of magnetic resonance (MR) guidance for endovascular intervention is appealing because of its lack of ionizing radiation, high-contrast visualization of vessel walls and adjacent soft tissues, multiplanar capabilities, and potential to incorporate functional information such as flow, fluid dynamics, perfusion, and cardiac motion. This review highlights state-of-the-art imaging techniques and hardware used for passive tracking of endovascular devices in interventional MR imaging, including negative contrast, passive contrast, nonproton multispectral, and direct current techniques. The advantages and disadvantages of passive tracking relative to active tracking are also summarized.

The advent of focal therapies theoretically offers new treatment options for patients with localized prostate cancer. The goal of prostate cancer treatment is effective long-term cure with minimal impact on health-related quality of life. Multiparametric magnetic resonance imaging (MRI) of the prostate is being increasingly used for diagnosis, image-guided targeted biopsy, guidance for targeted focal and regional therapy, and monitoring the effectiveness of treatments for prostate cancer of all stages. In this article, the use of prostate MRI in the burgeoning domain of thermal ablative therapy for localized and recurrent prostate cancer is reviewed.

The optimal strategy for prostate cancer diagnosis is to avoid overdiagnosis, defined as diagnosis of clinically insignificant disease, and undersampling of the gland, which leads to missing clinically significant disease. Targeted prostate biopsy is a potential solution for decreasing the rate of both overdiagnosis and undersampling of prostate cancer. We focus here on different techniques for targeting prostate lesions identified on multiparametric magnetic resonance (MR) imaging and review different clinical settings in which MR imaging–targeted prostate biopsies are performed.

Gynecologic brachytherapy consists of positioning radioactive sources in catheters implanted inside a tumor. Magnetic resonance (MR) imaging provides tumor visibility and is ideal for image-guided insertions and treatment planning. It is important at first insertion and during treatment of large residual tumors potentially needing interstitial needles. Clear visibility of the tumor and the catheters is necessary for MR–guided brachytherapy. T2 sequences are ideal for tumor visibility but catheter visualization may be difficult. Active tracking and alternative sequences to improve catheter visibility have been explored. The use of digital applicator models, dummy markers, and CT-MR fusion is reviewed.

The use of clinical imaging modalities for the guidance of targeted drug delivery systems, known as image-guided drug delivery (IGDD), has emerged as a promising strategy for enhancing antitumor efficacy. Magnetic resonance (MR) imaging is particularly well suited for IGDD applications because of its ability to acquire images and quantitative measurements with high spatiotemporal resolution. The goal of IGDD strategies is to improve treatment outcomes by facilitating planning, real-time guidance, and personalization of pharmacologic interventions. This article reviews basic principles of targeted drug delivery and highlights the current status, emerging applications, and future paradigms of MR-guided drug delivery.

In this review, several clinical applications of magnetic resonance (MR)-guided focused ultrasound (FUS) are updated. MR-guided FUS is used clinically for thermal ablation of uterine fibroids and bone metastases. Thousands of patients have successfully been treated. Transcranial MR-guided FUS has received CE certification for ablation of deep, central locations in the brain. Thermal ablation of specific parts of the thalamus can result in relief of the symptoms in a number of neurological disorders. Several approaches have been proposed for ablation of prostate and breast cancer and clinical trials should show the potential of MR-guided FUS for these and other applications.

 This article includes a video of real-time imaging in an interactive environment

Interventional Magnetic resonance (MR) uses rapid imaging to guide diagnostic and therapeutic procedures. One of the attractions of MR-guidance is the abundance of inherent contrast mechanisms available. Dynamic procedural guidance with real-time imaging has pushed the limits of MR technology, demanding rapid acquisition and reconstruction paired with interactive control and device visualization. This article reviews the technical aspects of real-time MR sequences that enable MR-guided interventions.

In this article, we share our experience in establishing a clinic-based practice for Magnetic resonance (MR) imaging-guided interventions. Clinic resources and operational logistics are described and our institutional cost analysis for supporting the clinic activity is provided. We highlight the overall value of the clinic model in transitioning the field of interventional MR imaging from the "proof-of-concept" to the "working model" era and engage in a detailed discussion of our experience with the positive impact of the clinic on streamlining the procedural workflow, increasing awareness of the technology, expanding referral bases, and boosting the satisfaction of both patients and referring services.

MAGNETIC RESONANCE IMAGING CLINICS OF NORTH AMERICA

VISIT THE CLINICS ONLINE!
Access your subscription at:
www.theclinics.com

PROGRAM OBJECTIVE

The goal of *Magnetic Resonance Imaging Clinics of North America* is to keep practicing physicians up to date with current clinical practice by providing timely articles reviewing the state of the art in patient care.

TARGET AUDIENCE

All practicing physicians and healthcare professionals who provide patient care utilizing findings from Magnetic Resonance Imaging.

LEARNING OBJECTIVES

Upon completion of this activity, participants will be able to:
1. Review techniques in MR guided catheter tracking.
2. Discuss the roll of MR in drug delivery and pain management.
3. Recognize the applications of MR and ultrasound therapy for tremors, cancers, and other illnesses.

ACCREDITATION

The Elsevier Office of Continuing Medical Education (EOCME) is accredited by the Accreditation Council for Continuing Medical Education (ACCME) to provide continuing medical education for physicians.

The EOCME designates this enduring material for a maximum of 15 *AMA PRA Category 1 Credit*(s)™. Physicians should claim only the credit commensurate with the extent of their participation in the activity.

All other health care professionals requesting continuing education credit for this enduring material will be issued a certificate of participation.

DISCLOSURE OF CONFLICTS OF INTEREST

The EOCME assesses conflict of interest with its instructors, faculty, planners, and other individuals who are in a position to control the content of CME activities. All relevant conflicts of interest that are identified are thoroughly vetted by EOCME for fair balance, scientific objectivity, and patient care recommendations. EOCME is committed to providing its learners with CME activities that promote improvements or quality in healthcare and not a specific proprietary business or a commercial interest.

The planning committee, staff, authors and editors listed below have identified no financial relationships or relationships to products or devices they or their spouse/life partner have with commercial interest related to the content of this CME activity:

Hena Ahmed, BS; Allan Belzberg, MD; Michael A. Bowen, NP; Adrienne E. Campbell-Washburn, PhD; H. Ballentine Carter, MD; Thanissara Chansakul, MD; William Omar Contreras Lopez, MD, PhD; Antonio L. Damato, PhD; Seyed Saeid Dianat, MD; Joy Eberhardt; Anthony Z. Faranesh, PhD; Wesley Field, BS; Anjali Fortna; Eva C. Gombos, MD; Krzysztof R. Gorny, PhD; Michael S. Hansen, PhD; Michael T. Hayes, MD; Nathan C. Himes, MD; Jayender Jagadeesan, PhD; Daniel F. Kacher, MS; Tina Kapur, PhD; Akira Kawashima, MD, PhD; Thiele Kobus, PhD; Robert J. Lederman, MD; Thomas C. Lee, MD; Arnold Lee Dellon, MD, PhD; Prasheel Lillaney, PhD; Aaron Losey, MD; Katarzyna J. Macura, MD, PhD, FACR; Alastair J. Martin, PhD; Nathan McDannold, PhD; Carolyn C. Meltzer, MD, FACR; Andrew S. Mikhail, PhD; Suresh K. Mukherji, MD, MBA, FACR; Srinivasan Mukundan Jr, MD, PhD; Lance A. Mynderse, MD; Sherif G. Nour, MD, FRCR; Gregory Pennington, MBA, BBA; Tracy E. Powell, MSN, NP; Danielle M. Richman, MD, MS; Erin Scheckenbach; Fabio Settecase, MD, MSc; Karthik Subramaniam; Travis S. Tierney, MD, PhD; John Vassallo; Akila N. Viswanathan, MD, MPH; Wei Wang, PhD; Eric Williams, MD; Bradford J. Wood, MD; David A. Woodrum, MD, PhD; Pavel Yarmolenko, PhD.

The planning committee, staff, authors and editors listed below have identified financial relationships or relationships to products or devices they or their spouse/life partner have with commercial interest related to the content of this CME activity:

John A. Carrino, **MD, MPH** is a consultant/advisor for General Electric; Pfizer, Inc.; BioClinica; and Halyard Health, Inc.

Jan Fritz, **MD** is a consultant/advisor for, with research support from, Siemens AG.

Steven W. Hetts, **MD** is a consultant/advisor for Stryker Corporation, has stock ownership in Medina Medical, Inc., has research support from Siemens AG and MicroVention, Inc., has an employment affiliation with University of California San Francisco, and receives royalties/patents from Penumbra, Inc. His spouse/partner has employment affiliation with Stanford University.

Ari Partanen, **PhD** has an employment affiliation with Koninklijke Philips N.V.

Ehud Schmidt, **PhD** has research support from St Jude Medical, Inc.; Siemens AG; Physical Sciences, Inc, receives royalties/patents from St Jude Medical, Inc.; MRI Interventions, Inc.; and Physical Sciences, Inc.

Clare M.C. Tempany, **MD** is a consultant/advisor for Profound Medical Corp, has stock ownership in Spring Bank Pharmaceuticals and Medgenics, Inc., and is the editor of the *Journal of Viral Hepatitis*. Her spouse is a consultant/advisor for Merck & Co., Inc.; Gilead; Echosens; GlaxoSmithKline; Vertex Pharmaceuticals Incorporated; Novartis AG; Boehringer Ingelheim GmbH; Ligand Pharmaceuticals Incorporated; Spring Bank Pharmaceuticals; Medgenics, Inc.; Kadmon Corporation, LLC; Janssen Global Services, LLC; AbbVie, Inc.; and Achillion Pharmaceuticals, Inc., and has research support from AbbVie, Inc.; Bristol-Myers Squibb Company; Gilead; Merck & Co., Inc; and Vertex Pharmaceuticals Incorporated.

Aradhana M. Venkatesan, **MD** has research support from Koninklijke Philips N.V. via the National Institutes of Health.

UNAPPROVED/OFF-LABEL USE DISCLOSURE

The EOCME requires CME faculty to disclose to the participants:

1. When products or procedures being discussed are off-label, unlabelled, experimental, and/or investigational (not US Food and Drug Administration [FDA] approved); and
2. Any limitations on the information presented, such as data that are preliminary or that represent ongoing research, interim analyses, and/or unsupported opinions. Faculty may discuss information about pharmaceutical agents that is outside of FDA-approved labelling. This information is intended solely for CME and is not intended to promote off-label use of these medications. If you have any questions, contact the medical affairs department of the manufacturer for the most recent prescribing information.

TO ENROLL

To enroll in the *Magnetic Resonance Imaging Clinics of North America* Continuing Medical Education program, call customer service at 1-800-654-2452 or sign up online at http://www.theclinics.com/home/cme. The CME program is available to subscribers for an additional annual fee of USD 250.

METHOD OF PARTICIPATION

In order to claim credit, participants must complete the following:

1. Complete enrolment as indicated above.
2. Read the activity.
3. Complete the CME Test and Evaluation. Participants must achieve a score of 70% on the test. All CME Tests and Evaluations must be completed online.

CME INQUIRIES/SPECIAL NEEDS

For all CME inquiries or special needs, please contact elsevierCME@elsevier.com.

Dedication

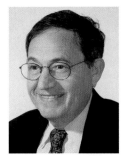

Ferenc A. Jolesz (1946-2014)

We dedicate this issue of *Magnetic Resonance Imaging Clinics of North America* to the late Dr Ferenc A. Jolesz (1946-2014). We, and all our contributing authors, have been and continue to be inspired by Dr Jolesz's vision. As the internationally recognized father of modern-day image-guided therapy, his vision of bringing imaging, in all its forms, into operating and procedures rooms, allowing for precise personalized therapy delivery, has been adopted by many all over the world. He was the founding director of the NIH National Center for Image-Guided Therapy, and the vision and inspiration behind the development and realization of the Advanced Multimodality Image Guided Operating suite at Brigham and Women's Hospital and Harvard Medical School in Boston.

We are indebted to him for inspiring us all.

Clare M.C. Tempany, MD
Department of Radiology
Brigham and Women's Hospital
Harvard Medical School
75 Francis Street
L1-050, ASB1
Boston, MA 02115, USA

Tina Kapur, PhD
Department of Radiology
Brigham and Women's Hospital
Harvard Medical School
75 Francis Street
L1-050, ASB1
Boston, MA 02115, USA

E-mail addresses:
ctempany@bwh.harvard.edu (C.M.C. Tempany)
tkapur@bwh.harvard.edu (T. Kapur)

Magn Reson Imaging Clin N Am 23 (2015) xv
http://dx.doi.org/10.1016/j.mric.2015.08.015
1064-9689/15/$ – see front matter © 2015 Published by Elsevier Inc.

mri.theclinics.com

Foreword

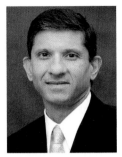

Suresh K. Mukherji, MD, MBA, FACR
Consulting Editor

This is truly a unique issue of *Magnetic Resonance Imaging Clinics of North America*. MR-guided interventions are an important area of clinical practice and future innovations. Dr Tempany and her group at the Brigham and Women's Hospital are on the forefront of this important and fascinating field. This is an area where Radiology is the driving force of innovation in other subspecialties. The articles include the applications of MR-guided innovations in brain, spine, women's health, genitourinary, cardiovascular system, and treatment monitoring. I want to personally thank Drs Tempany and Kapur for creating such a wonderful issue and thank all of the article authors for their outstanding contributions.

On a personal note, I was very touched by the dedication of this issue to Dr Ferenc Jolesz. Dr Jolesz is internationally recognized as the father of modern-day image-guided therapy. I did my Radiology residency at the Brigham and Women's Hospital from 1988 to 1992 and was inspired by his vision of bringing imaging into operating and procedures rooms. One of my first projects was working under Ferenc using an old lithotripsy machine to treat implanted tumors in mice. I will never forget his zeal and enthusiasm for his work and his colleagues. He was clearly an inspiration to me and to all those who worked with him, and for this, I am so very grateful.

Suresh K. Mukherji, MD, MBA, FACR
Department of Radiology
Michigan State University
846 Service Road
East Lansing, MI 48824, USA

E-mail address:
mukherji@rad.msu.edu

Magn Reson Imaging Clin N Am 23 (2015) xvii
http://dx.doi.org/10.1016/j.mric.2015.08.014

Preface
Magnetic Resonance-Guided Interventions: The State of the Art

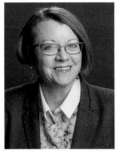 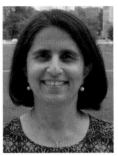

Clare M.C. Tempany, MD   Tina Kapur, PhD
Editors

This issue of *Magnetic Resonance Imaging Clinics of North America* brings together a wide range of expert opinions in the field of MR-guided therapy. The specific goal is to reflect the state of the art in the use of MR imaging to guide interventional radiology and surgery, and to allow us an opportunity to demonstrate the extraordinary advances being made in clinical care. The first set of three articles covers the use of MR imaging in guiding highly precise interventions in the brain and spine—focused acoustic energy through the intact-skull to treat tremors, cryotherapy of spinal lesions in very young patients, and nerve blocks and perineural injections in challenging areas. The next set of four articles covers the use of MR imaging in guiding interventions in the thoracic area—the more established use in breast biopsy, and emerging use in surgery planning and therapy monitoring, recent advances in techniques and hardware for tracking of catheters and endovascular devices, as well as the daunting challenges in building MR-compatible supporting devices for cardiac interventions. The third set of three articles covers the use of MR guidance for detection and treatments of cancers of the pelvis—targeted biopsy and focal and whole gland thermal ablative treatments for prostate cancer, and radiation therapy of gynecologic cancers. The last set of four articles covers technological aspects of interventional MR imaging—drug delivery, high-intensity focused ultrasound therapy, and the different demands on MR imaging for interventional compared with diagnostic use. The last article in the issue includes words of experience from a mature interventional MR imaging clinic-based practice on streamlining the procedural workflow, increasing awareness of the technology, expanding referral bases, and boosting the satisfaction of both patients and referring services.

We thank the contributing authors for sharing their knowledge in each of the articles, as well as the editors, Nina Geller, at Brigham and Women's Hospital, and Meredith Clinton, at Elsevier, for helping create this issue.

Clare M.C. Tempany, MD
Department of Radiology
Brigham and Women's Hospital
Harvard Medical School
75 Francis Street
L1-050, ASB1
Boston, MA 02115, USA

Tina Kapur, PhD
Department of Radiology
Brigham and Women's Hospital
Harvard Medical School
75 Francis Street
L1-050, ASB1
Boston, MA 02115, USA

E-mail addresses:
ctempany@bwh.harvard.edu (C.M.C. Tempany)
tkapur@bwh.harvard.edu (T. Kapur)

Magn Reson Imaging Clin N Am 23 (2015) xix
http://dx.doi.org/10.1016/j.mric.2015.08.013
1064-9689/15/$ – see front matter © 2015 Published by Elsevier Inc.

Evolution of Movement Disorders Surgery Leading to Contemporary Focused Ultrasound Therapy for Tremor

Hena Ahmed, BS[a], Wesley Field, BS[a], Michael T. Hayes, MD[b],
William Omar Contreras Lopez, MD, PhD[c],
Nathan McDannold, PhD[d], Srinivasan Mukundan Jr, MD, PhD[d],
Travis S. Tierney, MD, PhD[a],*

KEYWORDS

- Essential tremor • Focused ultrasound • Movement disorders • Pallidotomy • Thalamotomy
- Thermography

KEY POINTS

- Historically, patients with tremor of various causes, including essential tremor (ET), parkinsonian rest tremor, and action tremor, have been treated with stimulation or lesions placed in the ventrolateral thalamus.
- The most effective antitremor target in the brain may be the ventrointermedius (Vim) nucleus of the thalamus, a small subnucleus of the ventrolateral thalamus.
- It is now possible to create a lesion in the Vim nucleus using magnetic resonance (MR) imaging–guided high-energy focused ultrasound in a patient who is awake without a skin incision or craniotomy.

HISTORY OF MOVEMENT DISORDERS SURGERY

Gildenberg[1] describes five major epochs in the evolution of modern movement disorders surgery: (1) the presterotactic era before 1947, (2) the early stereotactic revolution between 1947 and 1969, (3) the latent period after the introduction of levodopa in the 1970s and 1980s, (4) the stereotactic revival of ablative surgery in the 1990s, and (5) the current modern period of deep brain stimulation. At present, with the advent of high-energy transcranial focused ultrasound, movement disorders surgery may be about to enter a sixth epoch. This article

The authors have nothing to disclose.
Dedication: This article is dedicated to the memory of Ferenc A. Jolesz, MD, the B. Leonard Holman Professor of Radiology, Department of Radiology, Harvard Medical School.
[a] Department of Neurosurgery, Brigham and Women's Hospital, Harvard Medical School, 75 Francis Street, Boston, MA, USA; [b] Department of Neurology, South Shore Hospital, 55 Fogg Road, Weymouth, MA 02190, USA; [c] Division of Functional Neurosurgery, Institute of Psychiatry, University of São Paulo School of Medicine, Av. Dr. Arnaldo, 455 - Cerqueira César São Paulo, Brazil; [d] Division of Neuroradiology, Department of Radiology, Brigham and Women's Hospital, Harvard Medical School, 75 Francis Street, Boston, MA, USA
* Corresponding author.
E-mail address: tstierney@partners.org

Magn Reson Imaging Clin N Am 23 (2015) 515–522
http://dx.doi.org/10.1016/j.mric.2015.05.008

traces the historical progression of movement disorders surgery from early open craniotomy to the so-called incisionless image-guided ultrasound surgery that is now being developed to treat ET. It also describes relevant history of focused ultrasound and a few general principles that have allowed neurosurgeons to treat intractable tremor with acoustic ablation.

The Prestereotactic Era

An early experimental understanding of motor systems began in the late 1800s, when Fritsch and Hitzig[2] conducted the first investigations into mammalian motor circuitry by applying local electrical stimulation to the cortical surface in dogs. Based on this pioneering work, Horsley, in 1909, resected a portion of the contralateral precentral gyrus in a 15-year-old boy for the treatment of postcarlatina hemiathetosis but acknowledged in later reports that these procedures often resulted in severe paralysis and paresis.[3,4] Hoping to alleviate tremor without weakness, Horsley and Clarke[3] attempted to target specific structures outside primary motor centers, for example, the deep cerebellar nuclei and other subcortical structures. They used the first skull-mounted stereotactic frame using external landmarks to guide slender probes and initiated the first use of discrete electrolytic lesions. The goal of these elegant preclinical investigations in the monkey was to find areas in the brain where small lesions could be accurately placed to control unwanted movements but not abolish movement altogether. This pioneering work in intracranial stereotaxy had to wait until the 1940s to finally be applied to human surgery (see later discussion).

Although Horsley and Clarke[3] laid the groundwork for an understanding of nonprimary motor areas in the brain, other investigators were beginning to study extracranial approaches to abnormal movements. As early as 1908, Foerster[5] reported posterior rhizotomy for control of spasticity and rigidity, leading others to try sympathetic ramisection and various ganglionectomies for similar indications throughout the 1920s and 1930s.[6,7] During this same period, surgical interest in open craniotomy for ablation of primary cortical structures continued despite permanent loss of function and high mortality. For example, Bucy and colleagues[8–10] continued to report their series treating athetosis and parkinsonism with ablation of both the supplementary and primary motor cortices despite accruing evidence from Meyers[11–13] and others that lesions confined strictly to the extrapyramidal system controlled tremor without weakness. Meyers reported excellent tremor control in

a patient with hemiparkinsonism by resection of the contralateral caudate head through a transventricular approach, confirming that the basal ganglia is a viable extrapyramidal target for tremor. For other patients, Meyers also explored sectioning of the anterior internal capsule, ansa lenticularis (ansotomy), and internal pallidum. Despite the success of these transventricular extrapyramidal operations, postoperative mortality was never reduced less than 10%, deterring others from adopting similar free-hand transventricular approaches.[14] Nevertheless, Meyers' contributions clearly showed that basal ganglia lesions could effectively treat tremor without causing paralysis or coma. These decisive observations set the stage for future stereotactic surgical methods in targeting extrapyramidal subcortical structures for the treatment of refractory movement disorders.[14,15]

The Early Stereotactic Revolution

It was not until after 1947, when Spiegel and colleagues[16] described a procedure to ablate discrete targets in the human brain using a modification of the Horsley-Clarke frame, that the era of stereotactic surgery clinically emerged. The major advantage of their approach was the use of indirect internal landmarks based on ventricular encephalography to identify particular sites in the brain, making it possible to introduce a probe through a small burr hole to the intended target without the need for direct open visualization. The first stereotactic operation was for the treatment of Huntington chorea in which alcohol injections were made into the pallidum and dorsomedian nucleus. Frame-based stereotaxy opened new doors for further exploration of other subcortical targets and ushered in a remarkably innovative period during which a variety of lesioning methods were explored, including chemical, cryo, thermal, physical, and ionizing energy methods.[17] Stereotaxy improved surgical safety, dramatically reducing the 10% to 15% mortality rates previously reported for open approaches to less than 1% by 1950.[18]

Target discovery was the major development of movement disorder surgery during this early exploratory period, and stereotactians focused predominantly on alleviating tremor and rigidity associated with Parkinson's disease. Based on Meyers' observations, several groups in the United States developed operations that lesioned the pallidum and/or its associated efferent tracts.[19–21] Other groups working in France[22,23] and Germany[24,25] found that lesion of the motor thalamus, the downstream target of the pallidum, produced complete arrest for virtually any type of tremor, including rest, intention, and postural types. Hassler and Riechert[24,26] refined the subnuclei nomenclature and boundaries of this part of the ventrolateral thalamus and, together with others, defined and demonstrated the small subnucleus they called the Vim nucleus (Vim) as the most effective antitremor target in the brain. This part of the thalamus links the deep cerebellar nuclei to the motor cortex and still remains the most common target used for the treatment of ET (see later discussion). The demonstrated safety of the stereotactic approach coupled with the discovery of symptom-specific targets set the stage for a short-lived heyday of stereotaxy during a golden period in the 1960s. Surgeons worldwide readily adopted the stereotactic methods as reflected in the large numbers of patients treated. By 1965, approximately 25,000 operations had been performed, and Spiegel[27,28] estimates that this number increased to approximately 37, 000 by 1969, the same year that Cotzias introduced levodopa.[29]

The Latent Period After the Introduction of Levodopa

During the early 1970s, levodopa advanced as the primary treatment method for disease, and the number of patients referred for surgery declined precipitously. This development, coupled with growing public discussions over psychiatric surgery,[30] led many surgeons to stereotactic interventions altogether by the early 1980s. Only a handful of centers maintained their stereotactic capability through this gloomy period,[31] treating a small number of refractory parkinsonian cases and other types of tremors. However, within a few years of its introduction, the enthusiasm for levodopa therapy was checked by the development of chronic drug-induced side effects. Severe peak-dose dyskinesia and end-dose freezing began to be widely reported in patients with long-term administration of levodopa.[32] Oddly, these so-called on-off effects would be the salvation of modern movement disorders surgery a few years later.

The Stereotactic Revival

In 1992, Laitinen[33,34] showed that the classic posteroventral pallidotomy not only controlled the cardinal motor manifestation of disease but most extraordinarily also abolished the effects of prolonged levodopa exposure.[35] The finding that an old ablative procedure treated not only the disease but also the problems associate with the side effects of the medicine to treat the disease was something of a renaissance moment for movement disorders surgery. Laitinen's findings rekindled the movement disorders neurologist's interest in surgery. At present, the major indication and common time for a surgical referral in patients with Parkinson's disease occurs at the onset of uncontrolled and unpredictable effects.[36] In addition to Parkinson's disease, neurologists increasingly began to refer patients with dystonia[37,38] and the more-difficult-to-treat tremors including poststroke, multiple sclerosis, and ET.[39,40] This clinical revival of ablative stereotaxy came when deep brain stimulation (DBS) was beginning to gain recognition and, probably to a large extent, was one of the major drivers leading the remarkable success of the modern DBS.[41]

Modern Period of Deep Brain Stimulation

In general, contemporary targets for DBS for both movement disorders[42] and psychiatric indications[43] were derived from the same targets historically used for ablations. However, this recent period has also seen the discovery of novel targets for movement disorders surgery for Parkinson disease in the form of the subthalamic nucleus[44,45] and the pedunculopontine reticular formation.[46,47] Although the DBS mechanisms are incompletely understood, high-frequency stimulation (>100 Hz) manifests functionally in the same way as a lesion. Neurosurgeons have, for some time, used intraoperative high-frequency stimulation at the intended target to predict whether a lesion would be effective.[48] The primary practical advantage of DBS over ablative procedures is usually said to be the ability to refine the physiologic postoperative response by changing electrical stimulation parameters. DBS is adjustable and reversible, whereas lesions are not. On the other hand, a well-placed lesion avoids implantation of hardware, concomitant risks of infection, and breakage that are associated with DBS.[49]

Several studies with class I level evidence confirmed the long-term control of the cardinal manifestations of essential and parkinsonian tremor,[36] and in 1997 and 2001, the US Food and Drug Administration approved DBS in the United States for ET and parkinsonian tremor, respectively. Despite its high cost, DBS has now virtually replaced lesion surgery as the dominant stereotactic surgical method in most movement disorders centers; this is in part because of better outcomes when examined head-to-head[50,51] and also because its seems that traditional radiofrequency lesion surgery carries a higher rate of complications.[52]

Despite several modern refinements in image guidance and target refinement, both conventional lesion surgery and DBS essentially rely on the same basic stereotactic principles introduced in the late 1940s. In particular, both require passage of probes through the skull and intervening brain to the desired target, and even though rates of complication in modern series are low, it may be possible to achieve substantially similar outcomes using completely noninvasive technology. High-energy transcranial focused ultrasound has emerged for the treatment of tremor, and a few proof-of-concept studies ablating the Vim nucleus for ET have been encouraging.

DEVELOPMENT OF INTRACRANIAL FOCUSED ULTRASOUND SURGERY

MR-guided focused ultrasound (MRgFUS) aims to (1) efficiently transmit ultrasound through the intact skull without excessive bone heating, (2) monitor tissue thermal changes, (3) use imaging to verify lesion location, and (4) confirm treatment efficacy through intraoperative clinical testing in an awake patient. Before its application in humans, MRgFUS was extensively safety tested in animal models, including rabbit[53] and primate.[54,55] MRgFUS accomplishes ultrasound delivery through an array of piezoelectric transducers (ie, a helmet containing approximately 1000 individual transducer elements). The transducers deliver a focused epicenter of high-frequency acoustic energy to a small volume of target tissue while avoiding significant bone heating by dispersing the incident acoustic energy over a large cranial surface. In addition, chilled degassed water runs between the transducer helmet and skull surface, actively cooling the scalp. The transducer array is paired to computed tomography (CT) software that corrects for variability in cortical bone thickness and acoustic impedance that can lead to focused ultrasound (FUS) wave distortion.[56] This computational ability is the key conceptual element allowing precise transcranial acoustic energy delivery. Small lesions are usually created for ablating most nuclear targets for movement disorders and chronic pain syndromes. However, larger volumes, such as tumors, require longer treatment times and multiple overlapping lesions.

MRgFUS incorporates tissue thermometry monitoring to precisely assess lesion shape and temperature increase. Several MR parameters are sensitive to changes in temperature, including T_1 and T_2 relaxation times, proton resonance shift, and diffusion.[57] The proton resonance shift method is the clinical standard for thermal monitoring and regulation. MR thermometry also detects pulses. Low-intensity FUS heats focal zone tissue to a few degrees less than ablation thresholds, acting as a control for planned focal sites.

MRgFUS offers the unique advantage of real-time lesion localization using standard MR imaging T_1 and T_2 sequences.

The first human work in the development of MRgFUS was a clinical attempt by McDannold and colleagues[58] to treat brain tumors at the authors' institution. In this study, CT:betw dates, 3 patients were treated for recurrent glioblastoma, with deep-seated and centrally located foci. A system equipped with 670 kHz frequency transducers in a 1.5-T GE (Fairfield, CT) MR imaging scanner was used. Focal area and skull bone heating were measured independently, although not all heating at every focal lesion site was measured. No undesired focal thermal elevations were detected. However, this study was halted after a fourth patient who was treated with a lower-frequency version of the device died because of intracranial hemorrhage of unknown cause. In the last year, this trial has resumed with the 650-kHz MRgFUS system.[59]

The second study using MRgFUS in humans was designed to produce small, well-circumscribed lesions in the normal brain. Central thalamotomies to treat chronic neuropathic pain were performed by Jeanmonod and colleagues[60] at the University Children's Hospital in Zurich.[61] CT:betw dates, 11 patients received thermally ablative lesions in the central lateral thalamus at maximum temperatures of 51°C to 64°C during short sonications. T_2 and diffusion-weighted imaging was used to visualize induced lesions 2 days postoperatively. The study notes that lesions were not detected in the first 2 patients. After the procedure, patients were assessed for pain using a visual analog scale (VAS) rating of pain intensity and detailed questionnaire (9 patients). Six patients reported immediate pain relief after the procedure. Mean pain relief after 2 days was 71% (9 patients), after 3 months was 49% (3 patients), and after 1 year was 60% (8 patients). VAS pain intensity mean scores were 60 at 3-month follow-up and 34 at 1-year follow-up. One patient experienced bleeding in the target region (8–10 mm diameter), leading to dysmetria and dysarthria that resolved within 1 year. No other significant adverse effects were reported.

Intracranial Focused Ultrasound: Proof of Concept Treating Essential Tremor

In 2009, the makers of the intracranial focused ultrasound system (InSightec, Inc, Tirat Carmel, Israel) partnered with Elias and colleagues[62] at the University of Virginia to plan for pilot clinical studies in the United States for an intracranial ultrasound procedure. ET was selected as the first treatment condition on which to focus because the clinical outcome (tremor severity) could be quantified objectively and because the historical success in treating the condition surgically had been well established.

ET is the most common movement disorder, affecting up to an estimated 4% of the general population.[63] Although the cause remains largely unknown, about half of all cases are familial, and transmission is most consistent with an autosomal dominant mechanism. No specific gene defect has yet been reported, but certain chromosomes have been implicated by linkage studies.[64,65] The tremor is postural, characterized by rhythmic oscillations (8–12 Hz) between opposing muscle groups and is exacerbated by movement.[66] ET progresses slowly over time and can lead to significant disability.[67] Although medical treatments are available to most patients, an estimated 25% to 30% of these patients cannot tolerate medication or become refractory to recommended treatment doses.[68] First-line oral medications typically include beta-blockers such as propranolol or anticonvulsants, particularly primidone. When the tremor progresses despite adequate oral therapy, surgical ablation or DBS of the Vim nucleus is indicated.

Three open-label clinical trials have illustrated the safety and efficacy of transcranial MRgFUS thalamotomy for refractive ET. Elias[62] evaluated 15 patients with severe, medication-refractory ET for unilateral treatment targeting the Vim nucleus of the thalamus. Patients were assessed postprocedure for the safety and efficacy of tremor suppression using the Clinical Rating Scale for Tremor and the Quality of Life in Essential Tremor Questionnaire. All 15 patients reported significant improvement in their dominant hand tremor symptoms and quality of life scores 1-year post-thalamotomy. Adverse effects of the treatment included transient cerebellar, motor, and speech abnormalities. Four patients reported persistent minor paresthesias after 12 months. T_2 and diffusion-weighted images were used to visualize acute lesions. Perilesional vasogenic edema was detected after 24 hours and 1 week but resolved within 1 month. At 3-month follow-up, punctate thalamic lesions were detectable in all cases and there was no evidence of hemorrhage on susceptible weighted images.

In Canada, Lipsman and colleagues[69] performed a separate proof-of-concept study in a small cohort of 4 patients with severe refractory ET. The study reported that initial clinical improvements in tremor appear at 50°C sonication, with tremor improvement after each cycle. The number of sonications delivered until tremor disappearance ranged from 12 to 29 over the course of 5

to 6 hours. At 1-month follow-up, reduction in the dominant arm tremor was 89% and reduction in motor-task impairment was 46%; at 3-month follow-up, these were 81% and 40%, respectively. Two patients reported paresthesia development during the procedure, and another patient had paresthesia in the tips of the thumb and index finger at 3-month follow-up. One patient developed deep vein thrombosis in the lower limb approximately 1 week after therapy. No other adverse effects were reported.

At the Yonsei University College of Medicine in Seoul, Chang and colleagues[70] reported successful treatment of ET using MRgFUS. The study was conducted in 11 patients with medication refractory ET. Of the 11 patients, 8 completed treatments; 3 patients did not because of insufficient temperature levels. Treated patients reported immediate improvement in tremor symptoms, which lasted through the 6-month follow-up point. A few patients reported bouts of dizziness during treatment; 1 patient reported delayed postoperative balance. No patients reported permanent adverse events.

SUMMARY

Transcranial MRgFUS represents a significant milestone in the history of stereotactic ablative surgery and the development of ultrasound technology. MRgFUS has been evaluated in preclinical animal models and clinical studies and was determined to be safe and effective for Vim thalamotomy for up to 1 year in patients with ET. If the perceived safety profile of the procedure is realized following expanded clinical trials with longer follow-up, surgeons and clinicians may increasingly prefer MRgFUS as the initial treatment modality for patients with ET. Nevertheless, there are concerns that bilateral treatment may produce dysarthria, and no center has yet addressed the problem of continued tremor progression on the untreated side.

In addition to being noninvasive, MRgFUS has several other appealing features, including an instantaneous treatment effect that is free of ionizing radiation. In theory, the treatment could be repeated multiple times. Perhaps the most valuable aspect of the procedure is that MR guidance can provide real-time feedback to guide lesion position and size. Future directions using MRgFUS in movement disorders surgery will probably include explorations of other targets such as the pallidum and the subthalamic nucleus and its surrounding fiber tracts to treat levodopa-induced dyskinesias and the primary dystonias. There are a large number of potential intracranial applications of the technology in addition to those of movement disorders. For instance, vascular, neuro-oncologic, and psychiatric indications are just now beginning to be explored. This elegant noninvasive technology will probably secure regulatory approval and clinical acceptance through strong evidence-based efforts gained in treating refractory ET. Ongoing refinements in computational and acoustic technology should allow high-energy lesions or low-energy neuromodulation to be targeted to virtually any point in the neuroaxis, further opening wide vistas for human brain exploration.

REFERENCES

1. Gildenberg PL. History of surgery for movement disorders. Neurosurg Clin N Am 1998;9(2):283–94.
2. Fritsch G, Hitzig E. Über die elektrische erregbarkeit des grosshirns. Arch Anat Physiol Swiss Med 1870; 37:300–32.
3. Horsley V, Clarke RH. The structure and functions of the cerebellum examined by a new method. Brain 1908;31:45–124.
4. Horsley V. The Linacre Lecture on the function of the so-called motor area of the brain. BMJ 1909;21:125–32.
5. Foerster O. Über eine neue operativ Methode der behandlung spastischer Lahmungen durch Resektion hinterer Ruchkenmarkswurzeln. Z Orthop Chir 1908;22:203–23.
6. Hunter JL. Influence of sympathetic nervous system in genesis of rigidity of striated muscle in spastic paralysis. Surg Gynecol Obstet 1924;39:721–43.
7. Rees CE. Observations following sympathetic ganglionectomy in case of postencephalitic parkinsonian syndrome. Am J Surg 1933;21:411–5.
8. Bucy PC, Buchanan DN. Athetosis. Brain 1932;55: 479–92.
9. Bucy PC, Case TJ. Tremor physiologic mechanism and abolition by surgical means. Arch Neurol Psychiatry 1939;41:721–46.
10. Bucy PC. The surgical treatment of abnormal involuntary movements. J Neurosurg Nurs 1970;2:31–9.
11. Meyers R. Surgical procedure for postencephalitic tremor, with notes on the physiology of premotor fibers. Arch Neurol Psychiatry 1940;44:455–9.
12. Meyers R. The modification of alternating tremors, rigidity and festination by surgery of the basal ganglia. Res Publ Assoc Res Nerve Ment Dis 1942;21(6):2–665.
13. Meyers R. Surgical experiments in the therapy of certain "extrapyramidal diseases". Acta Psychiatr Neurol Suppl 1951;26:1–42.
14. Meyers R. Historical background and personal experiences in the surgical relief of hyperkinesia and hypertonus. In: Fields W, editor. Pathogenesis and treatment of parkinsonism. Springfield (IL): Chas C Thomas; 1958. p. 229–70.
15. Meyers R. Dandy's striatal theory of the "center of consciousness": surgical evidence and logical analysis indicating its improbability. Arch Neurol Psychiatry 1951;65:659–71.
16. Spiegel EA, Wycis HT, Marks M, et al. Stereotaxic apparatus for operations on the human brain. Science 1947;106:349–50.
17. Gildenberg PL. Studies in stereoencephalotomy, VIII: comparison of the variability of subcortical lesions produced by various procedures (radio-frequency coagulation, electrolysis, alcohol injection). Confin Neurol 1957;17:299–309.
18. Riechert T. Long-term follow-up of results of stereotaxic treatment of extrapyramidal disorders. Confin Neurol 1962;22:356–63.
19. Spiegel EA, Wycis HT. Pallido-thalamotomy in chorea. Arch Neurol Psychiatry 1950;64:495–6.
20. Spiegel EA, Wycis HT, Szekely EG, et al. Campotomy in various extrapyramidal disorders. J Neurosurg 1963;20:871–81.
21. Cooper IS. Chemopallidectomy: an investigative technique in geriatric parkinsonians. Science 1955; 121:217.
22. Talairach J, De Ajuriaguerra J, David M. Etudes stéréotaxiques et structures encephaliques profondes chez l'homme. Presse Med 1952;28:605–9.
23. Albe-Fessard D, Arfel G, Guiot G, et al. Identification and precide delimitation of certain subcortical structures in man by electrophysiology. Its importance in stereotaxic surgery of dyskinesia. C R Hebd Seances Acad Sci (Paris) 1961;253:2412–4.
24. Hassler R, Riechert T. Indikationen und Lokalisations method der gezielten Hirnoperationen. Nervenarzt 1954;25:441–7.
25. Hassler R, Hess WR. Experimentelle und anatomische Befunde Über die Drehbewegungen und die nervösen Apparate. Arch Psychiatr Nervenkr 1954; 192:488–526.
26. Hassler R. Architectronic organization of the thalamic nuclei. In: Schaltenbrand G, Walker AE, editors. Stereotaxy of the human brain. Stuttgart (NY): Georg Thieme Verlag; 1982. p. 140–80.
27. Spiegel EA. History of human stereotaxy (stereoencephalotomy). In: Schaltenbrand G, Walker AE, editors. Stereotaxy of the human brain: anatomical, physiological and clinical applications. Stuttgart (NY): Georg Thieme Verlag; 1982. p. 3–10.
28. Spiegel EA. Methodological problems in stereoencephalotomy. Confin Neurol 1965;26:125–32.
29. Cotzias GC, Papavasiliou PS, Gellene R. Modification of parkinsonism—chronic treatment with L-DOPA. N Engl J Med 1969;280:337–45.
30. Valenstein ES. Brain control: a critical examination of brain stimulation and psychosurgery. New York: John Wiley & Sons, Inc; 1973.

31. Bakay RA. History of functional neurosurgery. In: Winn HR, editor. Youmans neurological surgery. Philadelphia: Saunders; 2004. p. 2653–69.

32. Marsden CD, Parkes JD. "On-off" effects in patients with Parkinson's disease on chronic levodopa therapy. Lancet 1976;1(7954):292–6.

33. Laitinen LV, Bergenheim AT, Hariz MI. Ventroposterolateral pallidotomy can abolish all parkinsonian symptoms. Stereotact Funct Neurosurg 1992;58:14–21.

34. Laitinen LV, Bergenheim AT, Hariz MI. Leksell's posteroventral pallidotomy in the treatment of Parkinson's disease. J Neurosurg 1992;76:53–61.

35. Svennilson E, Torvik A, Lowe R, et al. Treatment of parkinsonism by stereotactic thermolesions in the pallidal region: a clinical evaluation of 81 cases. Acta Psychiatr Neurol Scand 1960;35:358–77.

36. Tierney TS, Lozano AM. Functional neurosurgery of movement disorders. In: Iansek R, Morris M, editors. Rehabilitation in movement disorders. Cambridge (United Kingdom): Cambridge University Press; 2013. p. 36–43. Available at: https://books.google.com/books?hl=en&lr=&id=kb8HIUb_XDQC&oi=fnd&pg=PA36&dq=Tierney+TS,+Lozano+AM+functional+2013&ots=ZQ9DowKQKg&sig=PPY82LRaEZM4B8923uelGH5lD8U#v=onepage&q&f=false.

37. Yamashiro K, Tasker RR. Stereotactic thalamotomy for dystonic patients. Stereotact Funct Neurosurg 1993;60(1–3):81–5.

38. Lozano AM, Kumar R, Gross RE, et al. Globus pallidus internus pallidotomy for generalized dystonia. Mov Disord 1997;12(6):865–70.

39. Shahzadi S, Tasker RR, Lozano A. Thalamotomy for essential and cerebellar tremor. Stereotact Funct Neurosurg 1995;65(1–4):11–7.

40. Goldman MS, Kelly PJ. Symptomatic and functional outcome of stereotactic ventralis lateralis thalamotomy for intention tremor. J Neurosurg 1992;77(2):223–9.

41. DeLong MR, Benabid AL. Discovery of high-frequency deep brain stimulation for treatment of Parkinson disease: 2014 Lasker Award. JAMA 2014;312(11):1093–4.

42. Wichmann T, Delong MR. Deep brain stimulation for neurologic and neuropsychiatric disorders. Neuron 2006;52(1):197–204.

43. Tierney TS, Abd-El-Barr MM, Stanford AD, et al. Deep brain stimulation and ablation for obsessive compulsive disorder. Int J Neurosci 2014;124(6):394–402.

44. Bergman H, Wichmann T, DeLong MR. Reversal of experimental parkinsonism by lesions of the subthalamic nucleus. Science 1990;249(4975):1436–8.

45. Pollak P, Benabid AL, Gross C, et al. Effects of the stimulation of the subthalamic nucleus in Parkinson disease. Rev Neurol (Paris) 1993;149(3):175–6.

46. Munro-Davies LE, Winter J, Aziz TZ, et al. The role of the pedunculopontine region in basal-ganglia mechanisms of akinesia. Exp Brain Res 1999;129(4):511–7.

47. Mazzone P, Lozano A, Stanzione P, et al. Implantation of human pedunculopontine nucleus: a safe and clinically relevant target in Parkinson's disease. Neuroreport 2005;16(17):1877–81.

48. Fodstad H, Hariz M. Electricity in the treatment of nervous system disease. Acta Neurochir Suppl 2007;97(Pt 1):11–9.

49. Richter EO, Hamani C, Lozano AM. Efficacy and complications of deep brain stimulation for movement disorders. In: Bakay, Roy AE, editors. Movement disorder surgery: the essentials. Thieme; 2011. p. 227–36. Available at: https://books.google.com/books?hl=en&lr=&id=J37-K_mb4X8C&oi=fnd&pg=PR3&dq=richter+movement+disorder+chapter+16&ots=Bo-KbtPkBN&sig=OiXJSYNIX2-e-ELa3aeFeGp93oE#v=onepage&q&f=false.

50. Tasker RR. Deep brain stimulation is preferable to thalamotomy for tremor suppression. Surg Neurol 1998;49(2):145–53.

51. Tasker RR, Munz M, Junn FS, et al. Deep brain stimulation and thalamotomy for tremor compared. Acta Neurochir Suppl 1997;68:49–53.

52. Pahwa R, Lyons KE, Wilkinson SB, et al. Comparison of thalamotomy to deep brain stimulation of the thalamus in essential tremor. Mov Disord 2001;16(1):140–3.

53. Hynynen K, Clement GT, McDannold N, et al. 500-Element ultrasound phased array system for noninvasive focal surgery of the brain: a preliminary rabbit study with ex vivo human skulls. Magn Reson Med 2004;52:100–7.

54. Hynynen K, McDannold N, Clement G, et al. Pre-clinical testing of a phased array ultrasound system for MRI-guided noninvasive surgery of the brain—a primate study. Eur J Radiol 2006;59:149–56.

55. McDannold N, Moss M, Killiany R, et al. MRI-guided focused ultrasound surgery in the brain: tests in a primate model. Magn Reson Med 2003;49:1188–91.

56. Clement GT, Hynynen K. A non-invasive method for focusing ultrasound through the human skull. Phys Med Biol 2002;47(8):1219–36.

57. Rieke V, Pauly KB. MR thermometry. J Magn Reson Imaging 2008;27:376–90.

58. McDannold N, Clement GT, Black P, et al. Transcranial magnetic resonance imaging-guided focused ultrasound surgery of brain tumors: initial findings in 3 patients. Neurosurgery 2010;66:323–32.

59. Coluccia D, Fandino J, Schwyzer L, et al. First noninvasive thermal ablation of a brain tumor with MR-guided focused ultrasound. J Ther Ultrasound 2014;2:17.

60. Jeanmonod D, Werner B, Morel A, et al. Transcranial magnetic resonance imaging-guided focused ultrasound: noninvasive central lateral thalamotomy for chronic neuropathic pain. Neurosurg Focus 2012;32:E1.

61. Martin E, Jeanmonod D, Morel A, et al. High-intensity focused ultrasound for noninvasive functional neurosurgery. Ann Neurol 2009;66:858–61.

62. Elias WJ, Huss D, Voss T, et al. A pilot study of focused ultrasound thalamotomy for essential tremor. N Engl J Med 2013;369:640–8.

63. Louis ED, Ottman R, Hauser WA. How common is the most common adult movement disorder? Estimates of the prevalence of essential tremor throughout the world. Mov Disord 1998;13:5–10.

64. Higgins JJ, Pho LT, Nee LE. A gene (ETM) for essential tremor maps to chromosome 2p22-p25. Mov Disord 1997;12:859–64.

65. Gulcher JR, Jonsson P, Kong A, et al. Mapping of a familial essential tremor gene, FET1, to chromosome 3q13. Nat Genet 1997;17:84–7.

66. Elias WJ, Shah BB. Tremor. JAMA 2014;311:948–54.

67. Fahn S, Marsden CD, Calne DB. Classification and investigation of dystonias. In: Marsden CD, Fahn S, editors. Movement disorders, 2. London: Butterworths; 1987. p. 332.e58.

68. Koller WC, Vetere-Overfield B. Acute and chronic effects of propranolol and primidone in essential tremor. Neurology 1989;39:1587–8.

69. Lipsman N, Schwartz ML, Huang Y, et al. MR-guided focused ultrasound thalamotomy for essential tremor: a proof-of-concept study. Lancet Neurol 2013;12:462–8.

70. Chang WS, Jung HH, Kweon EJ, et al. Unilateral magnetic resonance guided focused ultrasound thalamotomy for essential tremor: practices and clinicoradiological outcomes. J Neurol Neurosurg Psychiatry 2015;86(3): 257–64.

Magnetic Resonance Imaging–Guided Spine Interventions

Nathan C. Himes, MD, Thanissara Chansakul, MD, Thomas C. Lee, MD*

KEYWORDS

- MR imaging–guided spine intervention • Low back pain • Cryotherapy • Epidural steroid injection
- Spinal nerve root block

KEY POINTS

- The availability of MR imaging–guided spine interventions for back pain is currently limited, but interest and expertise are growing.
- MR imaging–guided interventions for back pain can be beneficial because of superior visualization of soft tissues and fluid, and absence of exposure to ionizing radiation.
- MR imaging–guided interventions for diagnosis and treatment of soft tissue and bony spinal lesions are safe and effective because of their superior visualization of soft tissues and fluid enabling avoidance of injury to adjacent critical structures and absence of exposure to ionizing radiation.
- The availability of MR imaging–guided spine interventions for diagnosis and treatment of spinal lesions currently continues to be limited because of the equipment costs and lack of universal expertise.
- These costs will probably play an increasing role in the future for treatment of solid organ masses.

DEFINITION OF PROBLEM AND CLINICAL PRESENTATION

The information available regarding procedural strategies for MR imaging–guided spine interventions is currently limited compared with that of more conventional radiation-based image-guidance techniques, such as fluoroscopy; however, interest and expertise are growing. With ongoing advancements in MR imaging techniques, new applications and opportunities are emerging, including those for treatment of low back disorders.

Low back disorders are widely prevalent. Low back pain is the leading cause of occupational disability worldwide, with lifetime adult prevalence varying from 50% to 80%.[1] Percutaneous image-guided spinal injections with corticosteroids and anesthetics are established therapeutic methods for low back pain. These procedures are traditionally performed with proved safety and accuracy under fluoroscopy or computed tomography (CT).[2–4] Real-time CT guidance affords improved targeting because it allows cross-sectional visualization of critical anatomy, facilitates freehand real-time needle placement, and has the potential for more accurate placement into facet joints.[4–6] However, there is an unavoidable risk of ionizing radiation associated with these techniques. This is a concern, particularly when these procedures are performed on young individuals of fertile age and serial therapeutic procedures are required.

MR imaging is an emerging modality in the guidance of various minimally invasive therapeutic interventions for low back pain because of the absence of ionizing radiation, the high soft tissue and fluid contrast, and multiplanar imaging options it provides. Newly developed MR imaging systems have been used in a variety of spine procedures for back pain including nerve root injection, facet joint injection, epidural injection, and facet joint

The authors have nothing to disclose.
Division of Neuroradiology, Brigham and Women's Hospital, 75 Francis Street, PBB-339, Boston, MA 02115, USA
* Corresponding author.
E-mail address: tchlee@partners.org

Magn Reson Imaging Clin N Am 23 (2015) 523–532
http://dx.doi.org/10.1016/j.mric.2015.05.007
1064-9689/15/$ – see front matter © 2015 Elsevier Inc. All rights reserved.

neurotomy using cryotherapy. MR imaging–guided spine interventions are also available for the treatment and diagnosis of pathologic conditions, including biopsy and treatment of primary spinal tumors and metastatic disease.

Because MR imaging is superior to other imaging techniques in depicting soft tissue and bone lesions in the spine, it is sometimes advantageous to use MR imaging when performing percutaneous biopsies. It allows for the accurate targeting of the lesion to be biopsied and clearly depicts critical structures that need to be carefully navigated to reach the target. In addition, MR imaging often provides superior depiction of the internal composition of lesions, allowing for targeted site-specific biopsies of heterogeneous lesions.[7] Therefore, MR imaging can be used full circle with the detection of the initial lesion, planning and guidance for the biopsy of the lesion, and monitoring of treatment response following biopsy. MR imaging–guided biopsy does, however, require specialized biopsy equipment that is compatible with the MR imaging environment and that has limited susceptibility artifact.[8]

New applications of MR imaging–guided spine interventions are emerging, especially in the treatment of patients that are considered poor surgical candidates. Approximately one-half of the patients with metastatic disease have poorly controlled pain.[9,10] Frequently, these patients have exhausted conventional therapies; therefore, percutaneous treatments have emerged to reduce pain, allow for local tumor control, and improve quality of life. MR imaging–guided interventions reduce morbidity compared with that of surgery and other conventional techniques, such as radiation therapy, by using a percutaneous approach with only one to a few tiny skin punctures needed to insert the biopsy needles or treatment probes.

One emerging treatment option is MR imaging–guided cryotherapy for the treatment of bone and soft tissue metastases and some primary tumors. Because the MR imaging signal is temperature sensitive, MR imaging can be used to monitor thermal ablation that during cryotherapy is visualized as an area of decreased signal intensity surrounded by a rim of hyperintensity on T2-weighted images, often referred to as an "iceball."[11] The shape and size of the cryotherapy iceball is easily monitored and can be tailored in real time using multiple planes on MR imaging. MR imaging, well known as far superior to other imaging techniques for the depiction of soft tissue structures, can enable superior visualization of the critical structures, often near lesions in the spine, including spinal nerve roots, vasculature, and spinal cord with surrounding cerebral spinal fluid (CSF), which can be well-visualized in comparison with the iceball treatment zone. Tumors typically have increased signal intensity on T2-weighted images, whereas iceballs cause a signal void; therefore, the coverage of the treatment zone in relation to the extent of tumor is normally easily depicted. MR imaging is ideal for tailoring the iceball treatment zone to cover as much of the lesion as possible without damaging nearby critical soft tissues. Because of these advantages, MR imaging–guided percutaneous cryotherapy for both soft tissue and bone spinal metastatic disease and primary tumors has been shown to be safe and feasible in anatomic locations adjacent to critical structures.[12]

Although there are inherent advantages of MR imaging as a guidance modality, there are also several disadvantages.[7] There are fewer choices of MR imaging–compatible equipment and these often cost more than conventional equipment. MR imaging–guided procedures have the potential for being more time consuming and, therefore, more costly overall. However, faster imaging sequences with single images obtained on the order of 1 second and the advancement of actual real-time monitoring systems of the needle position are helping to significantly reduce the time required for MR imaging–guided biopsies. In addition, there is a myriad of patient-specific contraindications to the MR imaging environment, including the presence of pacemakers or other non–MR imaging compatible medical devices or foreign bodies.

ANATOMY

MR imaging is often much better at depicting lesions and surrounding normal anatomic structures because of its superior contrast resolution and often superior spatial resolution compared with CT. Vessels are typically easily identified on most MR pulse sequences as are other critical structures, including nerve roots, thecal sac, CSF, and the spinal cord. Especially with biopsies of the spine, needle tip positions in the extradural, intradural/extramedullary, and intramedullary spaces can be readily identified on MR imaging sequences. Multiplanar two-dimensional MR imaging sequences and three-dimensional MR imaging sequences with multiplanar reformats provide high spatial resolution depiction of the anatomy in any desired imaging plane.

Similar to fluoroscopy- and CT-guided spine injections, the targets of MR imaging–guided spine injections include nerve roots, facet joints, and epidural space. Selective nerve root injections are performed with percutaneous transforaminal drug delivery into the spinal nerve sheath. Facet joint injection is performed with percutaneous injection of the drug into the lumbar facet joint space. Epidural injection is performed with percutaneous translaminar injection of the drug into the epidural space through a posterior intervertebral approach.[3] Nontarget injection, including intravascular injection and injection into the subarachnoid space, is avoided with either real-time monitoring using fast MR imaging sequences or with aspiration before drug delivery.

IMAGING PROTOCOLS AND IMAGING FINDINGS

There has been a variety of MR imaging systems and configurations used for MR imaging–guided spinal interventions with greater emphasis now on the use of higher 3.0-T field strength systems. Higher-resolution spinal imaging and sequences with increased imaging speed are widely available on 3.0-T magnets. Wider-bore magnets (or typically lower field strength open-bore systems) allow for manipulation of the interventional equipment without moving the patient. After the initial high-resolution standard MR imaging sequences are obtained for lesion identification and planning, fast acquisition T1- or T2-weighted sequences are used for quick monitoring of needle advancement to the lesion of interest. If needed, specialized sequences that oversample the center of k-space (BLADE or PROPELLOR sequences) can be used to reduce patient motion artifact. In patients with spinal hardware, advanced MR imaging techniques, such as slice encoding for metal artifact correct and multiacquisition variable-resonance image combination, can be used to minimize metallic artifacts.[13]

MR imaging–guided spine interventions for low back pain have been performed in a few different MR imaging systems. In the past, MR imaging–guided spine interventions were performed in dedicated open low-field-strength MR imaging systems.[14–16] The low-field systems, however, had limited capability in providing real-time fluoroscopic guidance. More recently, a wide-bore high-field MR imaging system[5] and an open high-field system with vertical field orientation[17] have been used in spine interventions for low back pain. These novel high-field systems yield real-time or near real-time guidance and improved contrast-to-noise ratio.[5,17]

Fritz and colleagues[5] described the use of a 1.5-T open MR imaging system (Magnetom Espree, Siemens, Medical Solutions, Malvern, PA) with patients in prone position for different procedures including nerve root injection and facet joint injection (**Figs. 1** and **2**). For the diagnostic

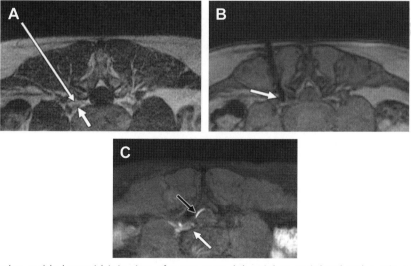

Fig. 1. MR imaging–guided steroid injection of nerve root. (*A*) Axial T1-weighted turbo spin echo MR image shows planned needle path (*long arrow*) to left L4 nerve root (*short arrow*). (*B*) Fast low angle shot (FLASH) two-dimensional MR imaging allows real-time visualization during placement of needle (*arrow*) to nerve root. (*C*) Axial fat-saturated T1-weighted turbo spin echo MR image after injection of 3 mL of steroid and gadolinium-based contrast mixture shows injectant (*white arrow*) in circumneural sheath of spinal nerves and in epidural space (*black arrow*). (*From* Fritz J, Thomas C, Clasen S, et al. Freehand real-time MRI-guided lumbar spinal injection procedures at 1.5 T: feasibility, accuracy, and safety. AJR Am J Roentgenol 2009;192:W163; with permission.)

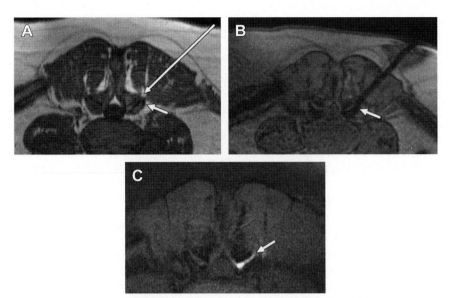

Fig. 2. MR imaging–guided injection of steroid into lumbar facet joint. (*A*) Axial T1-weighted turbo spin echo MR image shows planned needle path (*long arrow*) for steroid injection of the right L4-L5 facet joint (*short arrow*). (*B*) FLASH two-dimensional MR imaging allows real-time visualization during advancement of needle (*arrow*) to facet joint. (*C*) Axial fat-saturated T1-weighted turbo spin echo MR image acquired after injection of 0.8 mL of steroid and gadolinium-based contrast mixture demonstrates injectant (*arrow*) in joint space. (*From* Fritz J, Thomas C, Clasen S, et al. Freehand real-time MRI-guided lumbar spinal injection procedures at 1.5 T: feasibility, accuracy, and safety. AJR Am J Roentgenol 2009;192:W164; with permission.)

imaging phase of the procedure, this group used a body matrix coil with parallel imaging technology. The coil was then exchanged for a flexible loop coil for the interventional phase. Each procedure started with axial T1-weighted turbo spin echo imaging for planning of a needle path for direct access to target structures. For MR fluoroscopic determination of skin entry site, continuously acquired and displayed single-slice T1/T2*-weighted fast low angle shot (FLASH) two-dimensional MR imaging or T2-weighted fast imaging with steady-state precession was used as a syringe filled with saline solution or gadolinium-enhanced saline solution was moved over the skin. Following antiseptic preparation of the skin, draping, and induction of local anesthesia, the T1/T2*-weighted FLASH two-dimensional MR imaging sequence was used to navigate the puncture needle to the target structure with real-time MR imaging guidance. Injectants used in this study contained gadolinium-based contrast material. Following drug injection, T1-weighted imaging with fat suppression was performed for visualization of fluid distribution.

Fritz and colleagues[5] also described the use of a 1.5-T open MR imaging system in guiding nonselective epidural injection in which injections were performed with the patient inside the bore and monitoring was continuously acquired and displayed as single-slice T1-weighted fast imaging with steady-state precession images (**Fig. 3**).

Streitparth and colleagues[17] described the use of a 1.0-T open high-field MR imaging system (Panorama HFO, Philips, Best, Netherlands) for nerve root and facet injections. The system used was comprised of two horizontally opposed superconducting magnetic pole shoes with a distance of 40 cm between them creating a vertical static magnetic field. The patient was placed in the lateral position. A multipurpose loop coil was fixed to the back of the patient in an orthogonal position to B_0. The intervention began with determination of the skin entry point using the finger-pointing technique. For localization of the target anatomy and subsequent near real-time needle guidance, proton density-weighted turbo spin echo imaging was exploited. Immediately before and after injection, heavily T2-weighted fat-saturated Spectral Presaturation with Inversion Recovery (SPIR) images were acquired to confirm injectant distribution.

Both of these groups demonstrated accuracy, safety, and efficiency of the aforementioned MR imaging–guided techniques for treatment of low back pain with no major complications reported. The duration of the procedure may be slightly longer, but the absence of radiation with these techniques makes them appealing, particularly for young patients or patients who require

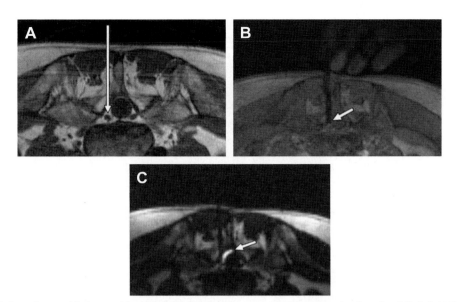

Fig. 3. MR imaging–guided steroid epidural injection for nonspecific lower back pain. (*A*) Axial T1-weighted turbo spin echo MR image shows planned needle path (*arrow*) into epidural space. (*B*) FLASH two-dimensional MR imaging allows real-time visualization during needle (*arrow*) advancement into epidural space. (*C*) Axial T1-weighted real-time fast imaging with steady-state precession shows distribution of steroid and gadolinium-based contrast mixture (*arrow*) in epidural space. (*From* Fritz J, Thomas C, Clasen S, et al. Freehand real-time MRI-guided lumbar spinal injection procedures at 1.5 T: feasibility, accuracy, and safety. AJR Am J Roentgenol 2009;192:W165; with permission.)

repetitive therapy. The real-time and near real-time sequences used by both groups provide adequate anatomic delineation and acceptable, limited extent of needle-related artifact.

Another emerging application of MR imaging–guided treatment of chronic low back pain in a carefully selected group of patients is MR imaging–guided percutaneous cryotherapy of the facet joint. Cryodenervation was recently introduced as an alternative method for facet joint denervation for patients in whom lumbar zygapophyseal joints are a significant source of back pain.[18] The lumbar facet joints are treated unilaterally or bilaterally when pain is distinctly localized and improves with facet drug injection. The therapeutic approach is based on using near real-time MR imaging guidance of the cryogenic probe toward the target lumbar facet joint. MR imaging allows accurate visualization of the growth of the cryogenic iceball and improves the accuracy of the treatment because the effect on the facet joint and surrounding tissues can be continuously monitored. However, currently, there are limited published studies on MR imaging–guided cryodenervation.

In addition to the MR imaging–guided spinal interventions for benign pathology described previously, we also present a variety of MR imaging–guided procedures involved in the diagnosis and treatment of pathologic conditions of the spine: fine-needle aspiration of an intrathecal nodule at the L1-L2 level, C1-C2 puncture with injection of intrathecal gadolinium to evaluate for spinal CSF leak, and cryoablation of L4-L5 posterior element metastatic disease.

INTRATHECAL NODULE BIOPSY

A 47-year-old woman presented with progressive cognitive deficits, diplopia, CN III palsy, and was noted to have scattered foci of leptomeningeal enhancement within the brain. Multiple lumbar punctures with CSF collection and an open neurosurgical biopsy of the dura overlying the frontal lobe were unrevealing, and therefore, a request was made for percutaneous biopsy of an approximately 1 cm focus of nodular enhancement at the conus medullaris (**Fig. 4**). Given this location, an MR imaging–guided percutaneous fine-needle aspiration was performed.

A flexible ring coil was placed over the lower back along with three gadolinium markers within the coil for initial imaging and selection of the skin entry point. A 16-gauge MR imaging–compatible introducer needle was advanced to the edge of the thecal sac at the level of the conus medullaris using a T1-weighted, three-dimensional gradient echo sequence, allowing for rapid acquisitions with high spatial resolution over the region

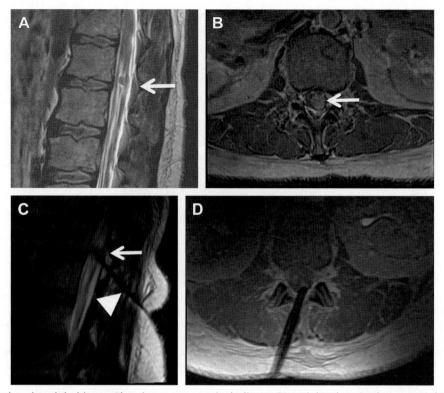

Fig. 4. Intrathecal nodule biopsy. Planning sequences including a T2-weighted sagittal sequence (*A*) and a T1-weighted postcontrast axial sequence (*B*) demonstrated a T2 hypointense, enhancing 1-cm nodule (*arrow*) involving the conus medullaris at the level of the inferior endplate of L1. A turbo spin echo sagittal T2-weighted sequence (*C*) shows the introducer needle (*arrowhead*) with coaxial biopsy needle entering into the intrathecal nodule (*arrow*). An axial T1-weighted three-dimensional gradient echo sequence (*D*) demonstrates introduction of the biopsy needle in coaxial fashion through the introducer needle targeting the intrathecal nodule.

of interest. Three 22-gauge MR imaging–compatible spinal needles were used serially in a coaxial fashion through the introducer needle to enter the thecal sac and obtain fine-needle aspiration biopsies from the conus nodule and obtain CSF for flow cytometry. Biopsy needle placement within the conus nodule was also confirmed using the rapid acquisition T1-weighted, three-dimensional gradient echo sequences. There were no complications on postbiopsy imaging. Flow cytometry from the samples obtained during the MR imaging–guided procedure were consistent with B-cell lymphoma.

C1-C2 PUNCTURE WITH INTRATHECAL GADOLINIUM INJECTION

A 41-year-old man presented with longstanding low-intracranial pressure headaches, exacerbated on standing, status post multiple epidural blood patches for presumed CSF leak that was not apparent on conventional CT myelogram. Given

the patient's prior history of C6 corpectomy and small calcified disk protrusion at T1-T2, a lower cervical/upper thoracic level CSF leak was suspected. MR imaging–guided intrathecal gadolinium injection with C1-C2 puncture was considered the best option for detection of a small, heretofore undetected leak because it allows for the immediate imaging postinjection of intrathecal gadolinium and multiple rapid dynamic contrast-enhanced acquisitions following injection to evaluate for abnormal accumulation of extradural accumulation of gadolinium to identify the level of the CSF leak. Although this is an off-label use of gadolinium, MR myelography has been described in the literature[19] and institutional review board approval was obtained for administration in this case.

With the patient in a left lateral decubitus position in the MR imaging scanner, a 22-gauge MR imaging–compatible spinal needle was advanced into the CSF space at the C1-C2 level using intermittent turbo spin echo T2-weighted sequences (**Fig. 5**).

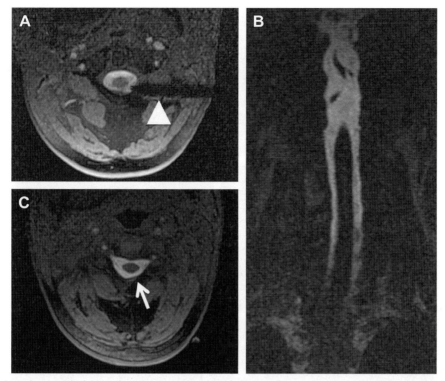

Fig. 5. MR imaging–guided intrathecal injection of gadolinium for evaluation of CSF leak. (*A*) An axial T2-weighted sequence shows the signal void from the spinal needle (*arrowhead*) entering into the CSF space at the C1-C2 level. Multiplanar rapid acquisition dynamic contrast-enhanced T1-weighted sequences were obtained every 1 minute postinjection to evaluate for CSF leak. (*B*) Coronal acquisition in one of the later phases. (*C*) A subtle extradural collection of gadolinium is seen along the dorsal aspect of the thecal sac at the T1-T2 level (*arrow*).

When CSF was returned, confirming the appropriate position, 0.5 mL of Magnevist (0.5 mol/L) diluted with 10 mL of sterile saline was injected. This was followed by the acquisition of multiple dynamic contrast-enhanced heavily T1-weighted sequences with the field of view covering the cervical and upper thoracic spine obtained every minute for 12 minutes following injection. These findings revealed an apparent subtle leak of contrast at the T1-T2 level. Subsequently, a CT-guided epidural blood patch targeted the T1-T2 level with partial relief of the patient's symptoms.

CRYOABLATION OF SPINAL METASTATIC DISEASE

A 68-year-old man with a history of metastatic prostate cancer and diffuse large B-cell lymphoma was found to have a new mass eroding the right L4 lamina and right L4-L5 facet joint. To prevent spinal canal compromise and instability at this level, MR imaging–guided cryoablation was considered the most appropriate treatment in this nonsurgical candidate.

After the patient was placed under general anesthesia, he was positioned prone on the MR imaging table. Preliminary imaging was obtained to confirm the target and to determine the approach. Initially, a 16-gauge MR imaging–compatible introducer was placed along the right paraspinal area at the L4-L5 level under MR imaging guidance. Fine-needle aspiration biopsies using 22-gauge MR imaging–compatible Chiba needles were obtained in a coaxial fashion under MR imaging guidance to ensure targeting of the lesion. Core biopsy samples were obtained coaxially using an 18-gauge MR imaging–compatible core biopsy needle.

Using MR imaging guidance (**Fig. 6**), two 17-gauge cryoprobes were placed into either side of the mass. With frequent MR imaging monitoring, using turbo spin echo T2-weighted sequences to ensure the iceballs encompassed the mass but did not involve the CSF, alternating cycles of freezing and thawing were performed as follows: 15-minute freeze, followed by 10-minute passive thawing, followed by 15-minute freeze, then 3-minute active thawing. The second cycle of

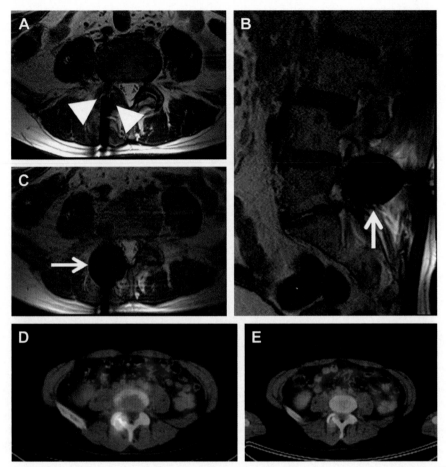

Fig. 6. Cryoablation of metastatic spinal disease. Axial turbo spin echo T2-weighted sequence (*A*) shows the placement of two cryoprobes (*arrowheads*) at either side of the lesion at the right L4 lamina bordering the right L4-L5 facet joint. During a maximal freeze period, the iceball (*arrows*) can be seen in relation to the surrounding structures and adjacent CSF and cauda equina nerve roots (*B*, *C*), ensuring coverage of the lesion without subsequent freezing of these adjacent structures. Fused axial image of the PET-CT study before the cryoablation (*D*) shows the lesion to be highly fluorodeoxyglucose avid, with follow-up PET 6 months following the procedure (*E*) showing near complete resolution of the fluorodeoxyglucose avidity at the treatment site.

freezing was performed at 100%, then decreased to 40% at 7 minutes, then 20% at 10 minutes. Following the active thaw, the cryoprobes were removed without complication. On subsequent follow-up, the patient reported improvement in his pain without evidence of complication. The subsequent follow-up PET/CT studies showed there was complete resolution of fluorodeoxyglucose activity of the lesion and no further thinning of the lamina or epidural extension.

PEARLS, PITFALLS, AND VARIANTS

MR imaging fluoroscopic imaging used during needle placement needs to provide good imaging contrast and produce sharp and symmetric needle artifacts to achieve improved accuracy and safety.

Different imaging protocols exist, including gradient echo and turbo spin echo sequences. Adequate needle visualization is important for preventing complications, including bleeding, dural puncture, spinal anesthesia, neural trauma, hematoma formation, and steroid side effects.[20]

Detection of intravascular location of the needle is crucial to avoid nontarget drug injection and ensure drug delivery to the target. Aspiration should be performed before drug injection to detect intravascular needle location. Continuous monitoring of injection with real-time MR imaging may improve sensitivity in detecting vascular uptake.[21,22]

Monitoring of drug distribution following injection is commonly performed to ensure target injection and detect injection into nontargeted structures. This is performed with fat-saturated T1-weighted imaging if the injectant contains gadolinium-based contrast material or with T2-weighted sequence if contrast material is not used.

MR imaging–guided spinal interventions are also available for the diagnosis and treatment of different spinal pathologies, including primary and metastatic soft tissue and bony lesions of the spine. Because of the superior contrast resolution and spatial resolution offered by MR imaging, it is often ideal as a guidance modality to avoid critical structures adjacent to the targeted lesion.

MR imaging–guided cryotherapy of soft tissue and bony metastatic disease has the ability to obtain local tumor control and pain relief in patients who have often exhausted other treatment options. Cryotherapy is far less likely to harm major blood vessels and CSF because of the warm flow within these structures; has inherent pain alleviation effects immediately postprocedure unlike other ablation techniques, such as radiofrequency ablation; and provides a sharply demarcated zone of treatment.

INFORMATION THE REFERRING PHYSICIAN NEEDS TO KNOW

The availability of MR imaging–guided spine interventions for back pain is currently limited, but interest and expertise are growing. With ongoing advancements in MR imaging techniques, new applications emerge. MR imaging–guided injections of the nerve root, facet joint, and epidural space have been successfully performed.

MR imaging–guided interventions for back pain can be beneficial because of superior visualization of soft tissues and fluid, and absence of exposure to ionizing radiation. MR imaging–guided interventions for diagnosis and treatment of soft tissue and bony spinal lesions are safe and effective because they provide superior visualization of soft tissues and fluid, can avoid injury to adjacent critical structures, and provide absence of exposure to ionizing radiation.

The current availability of MR imaging–guided spine interventions for diagnosis and treatment of spinal lesions continues to be limited because of the equipment costs and lack of universal expertise. However, in the near future, it will probably play an increasing role as it currently does in treatment of solid organ masses. In particular, cryoablation for local tumor control and pain relief in spinal metastatic disease seems to be one of the more appropriate applications.

SUMMARY

MR imaging–guided interventions for treatment of low back pain and for diagnosis and treatment of soft tissue and bony spinal lesions have been shown to be feasible, effective, and safe. Several advantages of this emerging technique include the absence of ionizing radiation, the high tissue contrast, and multiplanar imaging options. Recent advancements in MR imaging systems allow improved image quality and real-time guidance. MR imaging–guided cryotherapy of spinal metastatic disease shows special promise for local tumor control and pain relief in appropriately chosen patients.

REFERENCES

1. Andersson GB. Epidemiology of low back pain. Acta Orthop Scand Suppl 1998;281:28–31.
2. Derby R, Kine G, Saal JA, et al. Response to steroid and duration of radicular pain as predictors of surgical outcome. Spine 1992;17:S176–83.
3. Fritz J, Niemeyer T, Clasen S, et al. Management of chronic low back pain: rationales, principles, and targets of imaging-guided spinal injections. Radiographics 2007;27:1751–71.
4. Meleka S, Patra A, Minkoff E, et al. Value of CT fluoroscopy for lumbar facet blocks. AJNR Am J Neuroradiol 2005;26:1001–3.
5. Fritz J, Thomas C, Clasen S, et al. Freehand real-time MRI-guided lumbar spinal injection procedures at 1.5 T: feasibility, accuracy, and safety. AJR Am J Roentgenol 2009;192:W161–7.
6. Wagner AL. Selective lumbar nerve root blocks with CT fluoroscopic guidance: technique, results, procedure time, and radiation dose. AJNR Am J Neuroradiol 2004;25:1592–4.
7. Carrino JA, Khurana B, Ready JE, et al. Magnetic resonance imaging-guided percutaneous biopsy of musculoskeletal lesions. J Bone Joint Surg Am 2007;89:2179–87.
8. Kettenbach J, Kacher DF, Koskinen SK, et al. Interventional and intraoperative magnetic resonance imaging. Annu Rev Biomed Eng 2000;2:661–90.
9. Cleeland CS, Gonin R, Hatfield AK, et al. Pain and its treatment in outpatients with metastatic cancer. N Engl J Med 1994;330:592–6.
10. Daut RL, Cleeland CS. The prevalence and severity of pain in cancer. Cancer 1982;50:1913–8.
11. Silverman SG, Tuncali K, Adams DF, et al. MR imaging-guided percutaneous cryotherapy of liver tumors: initial experience. Radiology 2000;217:657–64.
12. Tuncali K, Morrison PR, Winalski CS, et al. MRI-guided percutaneous cryotherapy for soft-tissue and bone metastases: initial experience. AJR Am J Roentgenol 2007;189:232–9.
13. Lee YH, Lim D, Kim E, et al. Usefulness of slice encoding for metal artifact correction (SEMAC) for

reducing metallic artifacts in 3-T MRI. Magn Reson Imaging 2013;31:703–6.

14. Fritz J, Clasen S, Boss A, et al. Real-time MR fluoroscopy-navigated lumbar facet joint injections: feasibility and technical properties. Eur Radiol 2008;18:1513–8.

15. Ojala R, Vahala E, Karppinen J, et al. Nerve root infiltration of the first sacral root with MRI guidance. J Magn Reson Imaging 2000;12:556–61.

16. Sequeiros RB, Ojala RO, Klemola R, et al. MRI-guided periradicular nerve root infiltration therapy in low-field (0.23-T) MRI system using optical instrument tracking. Eur Radiol 2002;12:1331–7.

17. Streitparth F, Walter T, Wonneberger U, et al. Image-guided spinal injection procedures in open high-field MRI with vertical field orientation: feasibility and technical features. Eur Radiol 2010;20: 395–403.

18. Barlocher CB, Krauss JK, Seiler RW. Kryorhizotomy: an alternative technique for lumbar medial branch rhizotomy in lumbar facet syndrome. J Neurosurg 2003;98:14–20.

19. Chazen JL, Talbott JF, Lantos JE, et al. MR myelography for identification of spinal CSF leak in spontaneous intracranial hypotension. AJNR Am J Neuroradiol 2014;35:2007–12.

20. Falco FJ, Manchikanti L, Datta S, et al. An update of the effectiveness of therapeutic lumbar facet joint interventions. Pain Physician 2012;15:E909–53.

21. Smuck M, Fuller BJ, Yoder B, et al. Incidence of simultaneous epidural and vascular injection during lumbosacral transforaminal epidural injections. Spine J 2007;7:79–82.

22. Sullivan WJ, Willick SE, Chira-Adisai W, et al. Incidence of intravascular uptake in lumbar spinal injection procedures. Spine 2000;25:481–6.

3-Tesla High-Field Magnetic Resonance Neurography for Guiding Nerve Blocks and Its Role in Pain Management

Jan Fritz, MD[a],*, Arnold Lee Dellon, MD, PhD[b],
Eric H. Williams, MD[c], Allan J. Belzberg, MD[d],
John A. Carrino, MD, MPH[e]

KEYWORDS

- Interventional MR neurography • Pudendal nerve block • Posterior femoral cutaneous nerve block
- Obturator nerve block • Lateral femoral cutaneous nerve block

KEY POINTS

- Interventional magnetic resonance (MR) neurography uniquely combines highest tissue contrast and high-spatial-resolution MR neurography with interventional MR.
- Interventional MR neurography affords accurate nerve blocks and perineural injections through direct visualization of nerve targets, accurate needle tip visualization, and objective assessment of the distribution of the injectant.
- Interventional MR neurography benefits patients and operators through the absence of procedure-related ionizing radiation.
- MR neurography-guided nerve blocks carry a high degree of validity because targets, needle tip, and distribution of injectants are visualized with high accuracy.
- Selective MR neurography-guided nerve blocks are especially helpful to identify neuropathies of the pudendal nerve, posterior femoral cutaneous nerve, lateral femoral cutaneous nerve, and obturator nerve.

INTRODUCTION

Interventional magnetic resonance (MR) neurography[1] is a combination of high-contrast and high-spatial-resolution MR neurography[2,3] and interventional MR imaging.[4-6] MR neurography has the distinct ability to map the course of a nerve in its entirety from the spinal cord origin to the periphery and localize an abnormal appearance to a

Dr J. Fritz has received a research grant from Siemens AG and is also a research consultant for Siemens AG. Dr A.L. Dellon, Dr E.H. Williams, Dr A.J. Belzberg, and Dr J.A. Carrino have nothing to disclose.
[a] Russell H. Morgan Department of Radiology and Radiological Science, The Johns Hopkins University School of Medicine, 601 North Wolfe Street, JHOC 3142, Baltimore, MD 21218, USA; [b] Department of Plastic and Reconstructive Surgery, The Johns Hopkins University School of Medicine, 601 North Caroline Street, Baltimore, MD 21287, USA; [c] Department of Plastic, Reconstructive, and Maxillofacial Surgery, The Johns Hopkins University School of Medicine, 600 North Wolfe Street, Baltimore, MD 21287, USA; [d] Department of Neurosurgery, The Johns Hopkins University School of Medicine, 600 North Wolfe Street, Baltimore, MD 21287, USA; [e] Department of Radiology and Imaging, Hospital for Special Surgery, 535 East 70th Street, New York, NY 10021, USA
* Corresponding author.
E-mail address: jfritz9@jhmi.edu

Magn Reson Imaging Clin N Am 23 (2015) 533–545
http://dx.doi.org/10.1016/j.mric.2015.05.010
1064-9689/15/$ – see front matter © 2015 Elsevier Inc. All rights reserved.

specific site. With interventional MR imaging, the nerve target and surrounding anatomic structures, as well as the location and spread of the injected drug, can be directly visualized. With use of proper technique, MR neurography-guided nerve blocks offer exquisite technical accuracy that provides the interventionalist with the means for an objective assessment of the technical adequacy of blocks and validity of pain responses.

In addition to history and physical examination, diagnostic MR neurography is used to rule out neoplastic neuropathies, identify abnormal nerves, and localize the site of impairment. On diagnostic MR neurography, signs of nonneoplastic neuropathy include enlargement of a nerve, abnormal T2 prolongation, effacement of the fascicular-like internal structure, irregularity and thickening of the mesoneurium, perineurium, and epineurium, impaired axonal flow, and perineural soft tissue scarring.

In concert with history, a skilled physical examination, targeted conductive nerve studies, and high-spatial-resolution diagnostic MR neurography, perineural injections are used to identify a pain-mediating nerve and treat neuropathic pain (**Table 1**).[1] Diagnostic nerve blocks with a local anesthetic are used to prove or disprove that a particular nerve is a substantial contributor to the patient's pain syndrome.[7,8] A nerve block may be used to confirm an MR neurographically abnormal-appearing nerve as the pain generator, to identify the pain-mediating nerves in the setting of multiple MR neurographically abnormal-appearing nerves, and to identify a pain-mediating nerve in the case of a normal-appearing MR neurography examination. Perineurally delivered

corticosteroids may result in an interruption of inflammatory pathways on a cellular level and sustained pain relief.[9–11]

MR neurography guidance is especially suited for deeply situated and small targets and for injectants that require accurate drug delivery, such as Botulinum neurotoxin.[1,12] Interventional MR neurography rivals computed tomography because it provides superior contrast resolution and avoids potentially harmful ionizing radiation exposure.[13,14] MR imaging guidance exemplarily complies with the ALARA (as low as reasonably achievable) practice mandate and is especially valuable in adolescents, young women of childbearing age, and pregnant women.[6,14–16] Cumulative radiation doses can be avoided if serial nerve block protocols are used.[17] It represents a preferred technique in cases where computed tomography, ultrasound, and radiograph fluoroscopy guidance is challenging or failed.

Factors that influence the availability of interventional MR neurography are local expertise, technical equipment, availability, cost related to the local health care environment, and time constraints and therefore may be currently limited to specialized centers. However, clinical 3 T wide-bore scanners have gained broad acceptance and equip many sites to perform MR neurography-guided procedures.

In this article, the technical background of interventional MR neurography is discussed, concepts and designs of nerve block regimens are reviewed, MR neurography-guided injection techniques are described, and targets and procedures for the diagnosis and therapy of nerve pain related to

Table 1
Indications for MR neurography-guided injections in the pelvis

Diagnostic Nerve-Related Injection	Therapeutic Nerve-Related Injections
Clinically suspected neuropathy	Adjunct to conservative treatment
Discordance between clinical findings and imaging (false negative or false positive results)	Inoperable condition
Presurgical testing (eg, neurolysis, neurotomy, and tumor resection in multiple lesions)	Bridging of prolonged recovery following surgery
Unsatisfactory postsurgical results and recurrence	Induction of atrophy of a muscle causing nerve compression
Allergy to iodinated contrast agents	Unsatisfactory postsurgical results and recurrence
Small piriformis muscle not adequately visualized or targeted with other techniques	Contraindication or adverse effects to systemic pain medications/steroids and allergy to iodinated contrast agents

Adapted from Fritz J, Chhabra A, Wang KC, et al. Magnetic resonance neurography-guided nerve blocks for the diagnosis and treatment of chronic pelvic pain syndrome. Neuroimaging Clin N Am 2014;24:211–34; with permission.

the pudendal nerve, posterior femoral cutaneous nerve, lateral femoral cutaneous nerve, and obturator nerve are illustrated.

TECHNIQUE AND EQUIPMENT

Similar to the progression of interventional MR imaging from low-field strength to 1.5 T,[5] the transition of interventional MR neurography from 1.5 T to 3 T yields similar benefits.[1,6,14,15] Because of a near-linear relationship between the static magnetic field and spin polarization, 3 T field strength results in an approximately 1.8 to 2 times increase of the detectable MR signal, when compared with 1.5 T field strength. The higher MR signal afforded by a 3 T MR imaging system can be used for higher spatial image resolution and improved visualization of small nerves or for increased temporal resolution and faster MR imaging acquisition. In addition to the increase in signal-to-noise ratios, 3 T MR imaging also has the potential to generate increased contrast to noise ratios and better conspicuity of abnormal nerve. Because of an inverse square root relationship between the time needed for image acquisition and signal, images can be obtained up to 4 times faster at 3 T when compared with 1.5 T. Owing to the direct proportionality of the number of image acquisitions, the reduction of the number of excitations from 2 to 1 will decrease the length of time of image acquisition by 50%, thereby maintaining a net increase in signal-to-noise ratio of 40%. Wide-bore magnet designs can offer similarly sufficient patient access than dedicated open MR imaging systems.[5,9,18] If the isocenter of the bore can be reached, table movement can be minimized and needle maneuvering can be performed while the patient is in the bore of the magnet.[5,6,15]

The static magnetic field, radiofrequency pulses, and the gradient magnetic field contribute to special conditions of an interventional MR imaging environment.[1] Similar to diagnostic MR imaging, an effective screening procedure for patients, operators, and other individuals entering the MR suite is crucial in order to guard the safety of MR interventions and to avoid accidents.[19] In addition to general contraindications of MR imaging, pacemakers require careful consideration.[20]

Devices that cannot be used safely in an MR environment may experience considerable traction forces that may be strong enough to accelerate an otherwise considered safe device to cause serious impact injuries or cause temperature increases of metallic and conductive objects, which can be high enough to cause burn injuries to patients and operators.[21,22] A conventional stainless steel injection needle, for instance, may not be used safely for interventional MR neurography.[5] A variety of MR-compatible needles and accessories are commercially available for different field strengths.

In order to ensure accurate and safe procedures at 3 T, several factors that may adversely affect device visualization and patient safety need to be considered. Specifically at 3 T, the increased precession frequency of protons requires radiofrequency excitation pulses with shorter wavelength and higher energy, resulting in higher energy transfers and depositions into the human body. Spin excitation may be performed with body coil techniques rather than surface transmit coils in order to limit local heating and in normal mode with a power deposition not to exceed 2 W/kg.

The power deposition of radiofrequency pulses increases with field strength, the square of the flip angle, and the number of radiofrequency pulses in a given time. The use of conventional fast spin-echo pulse sequences may require adjustment to different radiofrequency pulse types, shorter radiofrequency pulse durations, decreased flip angles, fewer slices, and different repetition times.

Gradient echo sequences have favorable specific absorption rate properties because of often small flip angles and lack of 180° refocusing pulses. However, the exaggerating effect of gradient echo sequences on local field inhomogeneities and susceptibility-related artifacts of even MR-conditional needles at lower field strengths may interfere with MR imaging guided injection procedures at 3 T field strength.

Despite modifications of pulse sequence protocols to limit energy deposition, heating of a metallic injection needle remains a possibility at 3 T. In addition to the radiofrequency-related increase in energy deposition, heating of injection needles may occur through electromagnetic resonance effects, for which an injection needle may become susceptible during interventional MR imaging at 3 T static field strength. The magnitude of this effect depends on the physical length of the injection needle and the radiofrequency wavelength. The injection needle may serve as an antenna for the electromagnetic field of the radiofrequency pulses and the induction of a current. The maximum effect theoretically occurs when the length of the needle matches half the length of the radiofrequency wave, which may be considered the critical length. At 0.2 T, the critical length is approximately 188 cm and decreases to approximately 23 cm at 1.5 T. When compared with 1.5-T static magnetic field strength, at 3 T, the radiofrequency wavelength shortens by 50% with an approximate radiofrequency wavelength of 26 cm in water. An injection needle of 13 cm length or longer placed in water-containing tissue might, therefore, act as a suitable antenna for a 126-MHz radiofrequency pulse. Needles exceeding lengths of 10 cm need to be used with caution and may require further pulse sequence adaptations.

The constant and reliable visualization of the injection needle is a prerequisite for effective and safe percutaneous MR-guided drug delivery. For MR neurography-guided injections, passive needle visualization technique is accurate, safe, and simple because no additional equipment or postprocessing of MR images is needed.[23] The needle artifact is created by the lack of mobile protons of the metallic needle, localized spin dephasing, local gradient disturbances, and signal displacement in frequency-encoding directions.[24] Optimized spin-echo pulse sequences can result in the display of the true needle position with an error margin of 1 mm at 1.5 T.[25]

The needle artifact reaches a magnitude with needle orientations at 90° orientation to the static magnetic field, which is the case for procedures performed in the true transverse plane in a system with a horizontally oriented bore magnet. At 3 T, this technique is prone to an increased size of the resultant susceptibility-related needle artifact. In order to compensate for those effects, MR-compatible needles are typically manufactured from alloys of relatively low magnetic susceptibilities, such as titanium, nickel, cobalt, molybdenum, and chromium.

The type of pulse sequence and parameters, such as echo time, voxel size, readout, and radiofrequency bandwidth, further influence the needle artifact and enable the operator to optimize the appearance of the needle artifact. Although dephasing is less pronounced with turbo spin-echo sequences, short echo times can further decrease the needle artifact. Increasing the readout bandwidth minimizes signal displacement in in-plane frequency encoding direction and limits the size of the needle artifact. Maximizing the slice encoding gradient strengths minimizes through-plane displacement and the resulting needle artifact, which can be achieved through a smaller field-of-view and thin slice thickness. Needle optimization steps often come at the expense of a decreasing signal-to-noise ratio, which may require compensation by additional excitations.

Reliable visualization of the distribution of the injected agent and detection of spread to nearby structures is necessary to judge the technical success of a nerve block and the validity of a non-confounded pain response.[7] Injectants can be visualized based on their naturally long T2 constants. In case the needle is still in place, most injectants can be visualized by their high contrast-to-noise ratio to surrounding tissues with T2-weighted pulse sequences using echo times in excess of 100 ms.[5,16,26–28] If fat

suppression is desired, inversion recovery is the technique of choice because spectral fat saturation will fail because of the altered local static magnetic field strength around the needle tip. This technique can be of specific advantage in patients with hypersensitivity to iodine, for whom iodine-based contrast agents as used, such as computed tomography and radiographic fluoroscopy, are contraindicated.[29,30]

The combined use of surface and table element coils in a sandwich configuration allows parallel imaging acquisition with an acceleration factor of at least 2. A 5-step workflow algorithm may be used (**Table 2**).[1] A large multichannel surface coil is advantageous for the acquisition of initial focused MR neurography images, whereas for needle placement, a smaller multichannel surface coil allows better access to the interventional site and sterile coverage.

Versatile MR imaging pulse sequences for MR imaging-guided injection procedures at 3 T are listed in **Table 3**. An initial high-spatial-resolution MR neurography sequence (see **Table 3**, sequence 1) with an in-plane resolution of approximately 0.6 × 0.6 mm is used for visualization of the target nerve and planning of a safe needle path. Accurate needle visualization can be achieved with the use of high receiver bandwidth conventional turbo spin echo (see **Table 3**, sequence 2) and half-Fourier acquisition single-shot turbo spin echo (see **Table 3**, sequence 3)

Table 2
Workflow for 3 T MR neurography-guided injections

Step	Action
1	Focused MR neurography for visualization of the target and planning of the needle path
2	Determination of a suitable skin entry point using skin markers
3	Needle placement using intermittent MR imaging guidance
4	Confirmation of the final needle tip position
5	Optional sterile saline or sterile D5 water test injection followed by drug injection with monitoring of adequate distribution by the intermittent acquisition of fluid-sensitive MR images

Adapted from Fritz J, Chhabra A, Wang KC, et al. Magnetic resonance neurography-guided nerve blocks for the diagnosis and treatment of chronic pelvic pain syndrome. Neuroimaging Clin N Am 2014;24:211–34; with permission.

Table 3
Three-Tesla MR imaging protocol for MR neurography-guided nerve blocks and injections

Number	1	2	3	4	5
Sequence type	Two-dimensional turbo spin echo	Two-dimensional turbo spin echo	Half-Fourier acquisition single-shot turbo spin-echo	Half-Fourier acquisition single-shot turbo spin-echo	Half-Fourier acquisition single-shot turbo spin-echo
Weighting	Intermediate	Intermediate	T2	T2	T2
Orientation	Axial	Axial and sagittal	Axial and sagittal	Axial and sagittal	Axial and sagittal
Repetition time (ms)	7110	2500	2290	3440	3660
Echo time (ms)	28	24	89	120	90
Inversion time (ms)	—	—	—	—	220
Echo train length	25	24	159	162	157
Slice thickness (mm)/gap (mm)	2/0	2/0	4/0	3/0	4/0
Number of slices	51	5	1	3	3
Number of excitations	1	1	1	2	3
Field of view (mm)	350 × 280	350 × 280	350 × 280	350 × 280	350 × 280
Base resolution (pixel)	576	512	384	384	384
Phase resolution (%)	75	75	75	75	75
Receiver bandwidth (Hz)	300	490	480	305	205
Acquisition time	4 min 20 s	14 s	2 s	12 s	23 s

sequences, which differ in spatial resolution, edge sharpness, and acquisition speed. The distribution of the delivered injectant is in most cases efficiently visualized with a fast non-fat-saturated T2-weighted half-Fourier acquisition single-shot turbo spin echo sequence (see **Table 3**, sequence 4). The addition of an inversion pulse for fat suppression causes a marked increase in fluid conspicuity (see **Table 3**, sequence 5).

PRINCIPLES OF DIAGNOSTIC AND THERAPEUTIC NERVE BLOCKS

The function of diagnostic and therapeutic nerve blocks and injections is based on the theories of pain causation.[8] The selective perineural injection of a local anesthetic results in temporary cessation of nerve activity.[31] Pain conducted through the blocked nerve will temporarily cease.

Diagnostic injections may be ideally performed with superficial, local anesthesia at the skin entry site, whereas deep local anesthesia requires careful consideration and cautious administration so as to not inadvertently block a nerve that could confound the pain response of the target nerve. Some cases will require general anesthesia due to severe claustrophobia or inability to lay flat for the extent of the procedure. The authors prefer propofol as the sole anesthetic agent in such cases, which is sufficient to achieve general anesthesia in most cases. With this approach, narcotics can be avoided, which may confound the production of a valid pain response.

A valid nerve block requires technically adequate delivery of the local anesthetic to the targeted nerve. This technically adequate delivery includes accurate determination of the actual course and location of the nerve accounting for individual difference and variant anatomy as well visualization of sufficient contact of the injectant with the target nerve and absence of spread to nearby nerves. Small volumes of up to 3 mL help to control local spread and avoid false positive results by unintended anesthesia of locally or coinnervating nerves. The use of high-spatial-resolution and high-contrast-resolution interventional MR neurography is an excellent technique to ensure nerve block validity.

The first assessment of characteristic skin anesthesia may be performed on the table with the needle still in place, followed by assessments at 30 and 60 minutes following the injection. Pain responses may be obtained while the patient is at rest and ideally while performing typically painful maneuvers, such as climbing stairs and sitting on hard chairs. Numerical pain rating scales allow for the quantification of pain intensity. A positive nerve block maybe defined by the patient's subjective impression of a meaningful improvement of symptoms or as quantitative pain relief of 50% or more in conjunction with documented numbness of the cutaneous distribution of the targeted nerve. After a meaningful pain relief, improvement of function, or both, the patient's typical symptoms recur after the local anesthetic has naturally worn off. A positive pain response of a valid nerve block indicates that the blocked nerve is a substantial contributor to the patient's pain syndrome, whereas a negative pain response indicates that the blocked nerve does not contribute to the pain. It may be important to note that there may be more than one pain generator, which adds complexity and typically requires additional selective nerve blocks.

The validity of a single nerve block result may be statistically increased with timely separated additional blocks.[1] Such blocks may consist of performing the block again in identical fashion (confirmatory blocks), with a local anesthetic of different duration of action (comparative blocks), with an agent that has no pharmacologic properties to block nerve conduction (placebo controlled blocks), intended targeting of a different nerve or anatomic structure (target controlled block), and combinations thereof.[7]

In confirmatory blocks, the second injection should mirror the test result of the initial injection. In comparative blocks, prolonged pain relief is expected following injection following the injection of the longer-acting local anesthetic drug. In placebo-controlled blocks, sterile saline or sterile D5 water may be injected perineurally and therefore no pain relief is expected. Placebo response or psychogenic mechanisms can result in a positive pain response. In target controlled blocks, a nearby nerve is targeted with the expectation to produce a different pattern of anesthesia. The needle approach should be similar to avoid detection by the patient. In the authors' experience, such protocols are especially valuable if nerve blocks are obtained to help to guide surgical management. If multiple nerves are suspected to produce pain, objective results usually require multiple nerve blocks in separate sessions.

MR neurography guidance ensures high accuracy of test results, which are based on their high face validity.[1] MR neurography guidance exemplarily fulfills the 2 major requirements for valid test results, which are the direct and unambiguous visualization of the target structure as well as distribution of the injected drug relative to the target structure; this avoids false negative test results that can occur through targeting of an unintended anatomic structure or lack of contact of the injectant with the target nerve as well as false positive results through unrecognized spread of the local anesthetic to and anesthesia of a nearby nerve that mimics the expected test result.

Invalid blocks have a high risk of defining the pain generator or pain-mediating nerves incorrectly, which can lead to an erroneous diagnosis, ineffective treatment, and increased cost.[1] The importance of the high validity and therefore accuracy of MR neurography nerve blocks is the authors' rationale for its use.

PROCEDURES
Perineural Pudendal Nerve Injections

The pudendal nerve is formed by the S2-S4 spinal nerves and exits the pelvis through the infrapiriform foramen, which is a structure of the greater sciatic foramen.[32] It is formed by the piriform muscle, greater sciatic notch, sacrotuberous ligament, and sacrospinous ligament. Because at this location, the pudendal nerve travels together with the inferior gluteal nerve, sciatic nerve, posterior femoral cutaneous nerve, and sympathetic nerves, a selective pudendal nerve block may not be possible at this location.

The pudendal nerve then travels together with the sciatic and posterior femoral cutaneous nerve in the subgluteal space, where eventually the pudendal nerve diverges medially and the sciatic and posterior femoral cutaneous nerves laterally. The pudendal nerve curves around the ischial spine between the sacrotuberous and sacrospinous ligaments to enter the pudendal canal (**Fig. 1**A). The pudendal nerve gives rise to one or more rectal branches or perineal branches and terminates into the dorsal nerve of the penis or clitoris. The perineal branch corresponds with the perineal branch of the posterior femoral cutaneous nerve.

The pudendal nerve provides sensory innervation to the inferomedial buttocks area, perirectal area, perineum, and posterior scrotum. Motor supply is given to the bulbospongiosus and ischiocavernosus muscles, which play a major role in ejaculation, orgasm, and control of the external anal sphincter.

Pudendal nerve entrapments can cause pelvic pain syndromes that have traditionally been referred to as pudendal neuralgia, but may be more accurately termed pelvic pain of pudendal nerve origin.[33] Diagnostic MR neurography and the Nantes criteria can help to diagnose pudendal

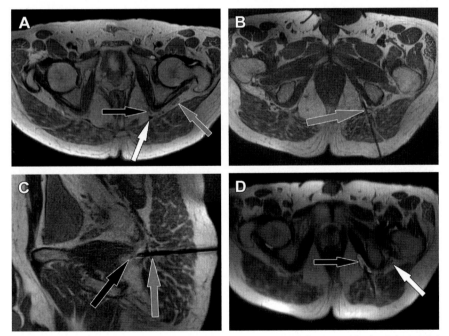

Fig. 1. Three-Tesla high-resolution MR neurography-guided pudendal nerve block. (*A*) Axial intermediate-weighted MR neurography image shows the pudendal nerve (*black arrow*) at the entrance level of the pudendal canal, deep to the sacrotuberous ligament (*white arrow*). The posterior femoral cutaneous nerve (*gray arrow*) courses approximately 4.5 cm laterally in the subgluteal space. (*B, C*) Axial (*B*) and sagittal (*C*) intermediate-weighted turbo spin-echo MR images demonstrate the needle tip (*gray arrow*) in the pudendal canal, just next to the pudendal nerve (*black arrow*). (*D*) Axial T2-weighted half-Fourier acquisition single-shot turbo spin-echo image demonstrates the injected local anesthetic (*black arrow*) filling the pudendal canal and surrounding the pudendal nerve without spread to the posterior femoral cutaneous nerve (*white arrow*).

neuralgia,[34] which consist of pain in the anatomic territory of the pudendal nerve, pain worsened by sitting, the patient is not awaken at night by the pain, no objective sensory loss on clinical examination, and positive diagnostic pudendal nerve block. Purely coccygeal, gluteal, or hypogastric pain, exclusively paroxysmal pain, exclusive pruritus, and the presence of imaging abnormalities able to explain the symptoms may serve as exclusion criteria. Electroneuromyography may contribute helpful information; however, it was found to have limited sensitivity and specificity in the diagnosis of pudendal nerve entrapment syndrome.[35]

Diagnostic pudendal nerve blocks represent a means of functional testing that is best interpreted in concert with history, skilled physical examination, and diagnostic MR neurography findings.[9,34] The pudendal nerve may be entrapped at various locations, extending from the infrapiriformis foramen to the distal pudendal canal.[9] The pudendal nerve may be blocked proximally to the entrapment site[9,36–39]; however, selective pudendal nerve blocks may not be possible in the infrapiriformis foramen and upper subgluteal space, because of the proximity of the posterior femoral cutaneous nerve, which shares sensory perineal innervation. A pudendal perineural injection at these locations is prone to false-positive testing because of an uncontrollable spread of the local anesthetic to the posterior femoral cutaneous nerve.

With an injection of 3 mL or less, exclusive perineural drug delivery to the pudendal nerve can reliably be achieved subjacent to the sacrotuberous ligament at the entrance level of the pudendal canal (see **Fig. 1**). High-spatial-resolution MR neurography guidance provides exquisite anatomic detail of this region. At this location, the posterior femoral cutaneous nerve has diverged into the lateral aspect of the subgluteal space (see **Fig. 1** A). With accurate needle cannulation of the entrance of the pudendal canal, the injected local anesthetic will flow into the pudendal canal and anesthetize the pudendal nerve, including rectal, perineal, and terminal branches, and backspill can be limited (see **Fig. 1** D). MR imaging is excellent to monitor the injected local anesthetic and to define the distribution of the local anesthetic inside the pudendal canal where the nerve resides. Following the injection, the patient may remain in the prone position, including transportation and recovery, for at least 30 minutes to avoid extrusion of the injectant out of the pudendal canal.

Intramuscular Piriformis Injection

The piriformis muscle originates from the anterior surface of the sacrum and smaller areas of the greater sciatic notch and sacrotuberous ligament[1,40] and divides the greater sciatic foramen into the suprapiriformis and infrapiriformis foramina. The anterior surface and inferior margin of the muscle may contact the nerves of the infrapiriform foramen, which are the inferior gluteal, pudendal, sciatic, posterior femoral cutaneous nerves, sympathetic fibers, and nerves to the obturator internus and quadratus femoris.[41] At this location, compression may occur. The piriformis muscle travels inferolaterally to insert with its tendon superiorly at the greater trochanter of the femur. At the level of the posteroinferior acetabulum, the piriformis muscle-tendon junction drapes over the cortex, which can create a narrowed passage for the sciatic and posterior femoral cutaneous nerves.

Piriformis syndrome describes a pain syndrome that is thought to be caused by compromise of structures traveling deep to the piriformis muscle tendon unit.[42] Depending on the affected structure, a different pattern can manifest, including a sciatica-like, pudendal neuralgia-like, and posterior femoral cutaneous neuropathy-like syndrome. The pathophysiology is unclear; however, compression by the piriformis muscle and inflammation has been postulated.[18,42,43]

Because of the variety of possible presentations, piriformis syndrome is not well defined.[44] An important part in the work-up is a diagnostic pelvis MR neurography examination to detect masses and aberrant anatomy of the sciatic nerve, including an intramuscular piriformis course. The significance of size and asymmetry of the piriformis muscles is unclear.[18,45]

The rationale for injections of Botulinum toxin into the piriformis muscle is based on suspected compression of the neurovascular structures deep to the piriformis muscle. As Botulinum neurotoxin A inhibits the presynaptic release of acetylcholine at the neuromuscular junction, a successful intramuscular injection induces paralysis and atrophy of the piriformis muscle.[46] The loss of piriformis function and volume can reverse an underlying nerve compression and relieve symptoms. In the authors' practice, the intramuscular injection of 100 Units of Botulinum neurotoxin A into the piriformis muscle leads to reliable atrophy of the piriformis muscle.[43,47] Botulinum toxin A was proved to have better efficacy over placebo and corticosteroid plus lidocaine injections.[43,47]

MR imaging guidance is especially valuable to accurately guide puncture and drug delivery into previously treated piriformis muscle of smaller volume (**Fig. 2**). The authors often combine the procedure with a therapeutic perineural injection of the

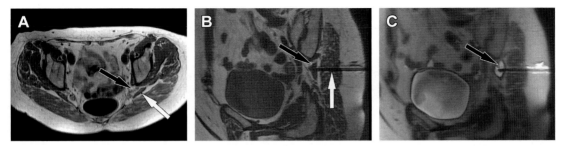

Fig. 2. Three-Tesla MR-guided injection of the left piriformis muscle in a patient with piriformis syndrome and piriformis atrophy due to a previous intermuscular Botulinum neurotoxin A injection. (*A*) Axial intermediate-weighted MR image shows the left piriformis muscle (*white arrow*) and subjacent nerves and vessels (*black arrow*). (*B*) Sagittal intermediate-weighted turbo spin-echo MR image demonstrates the needle tip (*white arrow*) in the atrophied piriformis muscle (*black arrow*). (*C*) Fluid-sensitive, sagittal half-Fourier acquisition single-shot turbo spin-echo image demonstrates the exclusive intramuscular accumulation (*black arrow*) of the injected Botulinum neurotoxin A agent.

infrapiriformis foramen to bridge the time needed for piriformis muscle atrophy to occur.

Posterior Femoral Cutaneous Nerve

The posterior femoral cutaneous nerve exits the pelvis together with the sciatic and pudendal nerve[48] through the infrapiriformis foramen. In intimate proximity to the sciatic nerve, both nerves travel deep to the piriformis muscle inferiorly and laterally in the subgluteal space. The posterior femoral cutaneous nerve gives rise to the inferior cluneal branches near the inferior margin of the gluteus maximus muscle, which supplies the inferior lateral buttock area. A very small branch innervates the ischial tuberosity, which is generally too small to be visualized on MR neurography. The perineal branch has been found to arise approximately 4 cm (range 3–5.5 cm) inferior to the ischial tuberosity, where the sacrotuberous ligament inserts; however, in the authors' experience, MR neurography visualization suggests a higher original in some cases.[49] The perineal branch of the posterior femoral cutaneous nerve innervates the most inner aspect of the inferior buttocks area toward the perianal region, lateral perineum, and proximal medial thigh as well as the posterolateral aspect of the scrotum and labium majus, and portions of the penis/clitoris. The final branch of the posterior femoral cutaneous nerve innervates the skin over the posterior thigh and eventually pierces through the fascia lata.

Neuropathies of the posterior femoral cutaneous nerve can be caused by compression and entrapment, repetitive trauma from cycling, impact injury, hamstring tendinosis, and tears and injection injury.[1] The clinical manifestations vary and depend on the level of injury and involved branches. Involvement of the cluneal branches cause a clunealgia-like picture with pain localizing

to the inferior lateral buttock area.[50] Involvement of the perineal branch causes posterior perineal pain[50] and often resembles pudendal neuralgia because there is coinnervation of the perineal area.[49] Neuropathy of the perineal branch of the posterior femoral cutaneous nerve is an important differential diagnosis of pudendal neuralgia. Involvement of distal posterior femoral cutaneous nerve presents characteristically as pain and paresthesia localizing to the posterior thigh.

As perineal pain syndrome can be caused by neuropathy of the perineal branch of the posterior femoral cutaneous nerve and the pudendal nerve, selective diagnostic nerve blocks play a pivotal role in their differentiation. Patients with a negative pain response to a technically adequately performed pudendal nerve block should receive a posterior femoral cutaneous nerve block. Similarly, in patients with a positive pain response to a pudendal nerve block, a posterior femoral cutaneous nerve block can be of value as a target-controlled block. A positive pain response will identify the posterior femoral cutaneous nerve as an additional contributor to the pain syndrome, whereas the negative pain response (true negative response) will further validate the positive pain response of the pudendal nerve block.[51,52]

A valid posterior femoral cutaneous nerve block requires perineural drug delivery and absence of spread to the pudendal nerve. With high-spatial-resolution MR neurography (**Fig. 3**A), both the pudendal and the posterior femoral cutaneous nerve can be reliably identified and selectively targeted.[2,32] Isolated blocks of the posterior femoral cutaneous nerve may only be possible at a lower level in the subgluteal space because there is sufficient distance to the medially located pudendal nerve. The posterior femoral cutaneous nerve can be blocked at level of the cluneal branches, branches to the ischial tuberosity (see **Fig. 3**), at

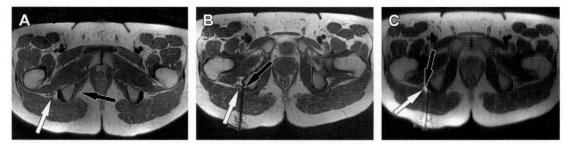

Fig. 3. Three-Tesla MR neurography-guided injection of the right posterior femoral cutaneous nerve. (*A*) Axial intermediate-weighted MR neurography image shows the right posterior femoral cutaneous nerve (*white arrow*) in the subgluteal space posterior to the sciatic nerve and the pudendal nerve medially in the pudendal canal (*black arrow*). (*B*) Axial intermediate-weighted turbo spin-echo MR image demonstrates the needle tip (*black arrow*) in the right subgluteal space next to the right posterior femoral cutaneous nerve (*white arrow*). (*C*) Axial T2-weighted half-Fourier acquisition single-shot turbo spin-echo image demonstrates the injected local anesthetic (*black arrow*) circumferentially surrounding the right posterior femoral cutaneous nerve (*white arrow*).

the level of the perineal branch and at the level of the most distal branch to the posterior thigh. As the posterior femoral cutaneous nerve travels side by side with the sciatic nerve through the subgluteus maximus space (see **Fig. 3**A), concomitant sciatic nerve anesthesia can occur. Concomitant sciatic nerve anesthesia may be prevented by the injection of only a small volume of local anesthetic or dilution of the local anesthetic concentration. Concomitant sciatic anesthesia usually does not represent a confounder for interpretation of the pain response because the sciatic sensory innervation largely involves the skin below the knee and motor innervation above the knee.

Lateral Femoral Cutaneous Nerve

The lateral femoral cutaneous nerve receives L2 and L3 spinal nerve contributions and innervates the anterolateral thigh above the knee.[32,48] The nerve travels over the iliacus muscle inferior to the iliohypogastric and ilioinguinal nerves.

Neuropathy of the lateral femoral cutaneous nerve often presents as pain and dysesthesia, which is commonly referred to as meralgia paresthetica.[53]

The lateral femoral cutaneous nerve can be subjected to irritation throughout its entire course[1]; however, entrapment or compression is thought to occur most commonly under the inguinal ligament where the nerve exits the pelvis.[54] At this site, the lateral femoral cutaneous nerve exits the pelvis 0.1 to 7.3 cm medial to the anterior superior iliac spine under the inguinal ligament,[55,56] and in up to 25%, the nerve courses lateral, superior, or through the inguinal ligament.[56–60] The rationale for intrapelvic blocks of the lateral femoral cutaneous nerve, proximal to the inguinal ligament, is based on the assumption that entrapment most commonly occurs at the level of the inguinal ligament and on the considerable degree of anatomic variation at and distal to the level of the inguinal ligament.

MR neurography guidance reliably visualizes the intrapelvic course and location of the lateral femoral cutaneous nerve (**Fig. 4**). Indications include

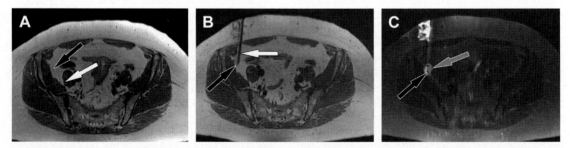

Fig. 4. Three-Tesla MR neurography-guided injection of the right lateral femoral cutaneous nerve. (*A*) Axial intermediate-weighted MR neurography image shows the right lateral femoral cutaneous nerve (*black arrow*) medial to the right iliacus muscle and the femoral nerve (*white arrow*) in contact with the lateral psoas muscle margin. (*B*) Axial intermediate-weighted turbo spin-echo MR image demonstrates the needle tip (*white arrow*) next to the right lateral femoral cutaneous nerve (*black arrow*). (*C*) Fluid-sensitive, fat-suppressed half-Fourier acquisition single-shot turbo spin-echo image demonstrates the injected local anesthetic (*gray arrow*) circumferentially surrounding the right lateral femoral cutaneous nerve (*black arrow*).

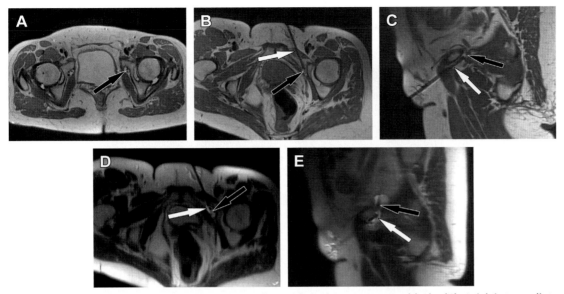

Fig. 5. Three-Tesla high-resolution MR neurography-guided obturator nerve block. (*A*) Axial intermediate-weighted MR neurography image shows the obturator nerve (*black arrow*) at the junction of the obturator tunnel and obturator foramen. (*B, C*) Double angulated axial oblique (*B*) and sagittal oblique (*C*) intermediate-weighted turbo spin-echo MR images demonstrate the needle tip (*white arrow*) in the obturator foramen, just next to the obturator nerve (*black arrow*). (*D, E*) Double angulated axial oblique (*D*) and sagittal oblique (*E*) T2-weighted half-Fourier acquisition single-shot turbo spin-echo images demonstrate the injected local anesthetic (*white arrow*) filling the obturator foramen and surrounding the obturator nerve (*black arrow*).

uncertainty of the diagnosis based on clinical presentation and diagnostic MR neurography findings and the attempt to predict the effectiveness of decompressive surgery.[61,62] When performing these blocks, care must be taken to ensure a sufficient distance to the femoral nerve because sensory femoral nerve anesthesia through unintended spread of the local anesthetic may cause anesthesia of the anterior femoral cutaneous nerve, which is a differential diagnosis of meralgia paresthetica.

Obturator Nerve

The obturator nerve receives L2, L3, and L4 contributions, travels anterior to the psoas muscle, along the lateral pelvic wall, through the fibro-osseous obturator tunnel and obturator foramen toward the thigh.[32,48,63] Sensory innervations include hip joint and the skin of the distal inner thigh.[48,63–65]

Obturator neuropathy may present as groin pain, hip pain, pain in the adductor region, as well as pain and paresthesia in the inner distal thigh.[66] This pain syndrome can be exercise related and therefore seen in athletes.[64] The entrapment is thought to occur at the level of the obturator foramen and proximal thigh, rather than in the obturator tunnel.[64] Therefore, blocks may be best performed in the obturator foramen (**Fig. 5**). If MR neurography demonstrates a more proximal entrapment site, the nerve may be blocked there.

Obturator nerve blocks in the obturator foramen often require a double angulated needle path in the lateromedial and inferosuperior direction (see **Fig. 5**). Because nonorthogonal needle paths are difficult to realize under computed tomography, reliable visualization of the obturator foramen with ultrasonography is challenging, and soft tissue structures such as the iliac vessels and the spermatic cord cannot be seen under fluoroscopy guidance, MR neurography guidance is an ideal modality.

SUMMARY

Interventional MR neurography is a powerful technique for highly selective blocks of small peripheral nerves in challenging locations that uniquely combines highest tissue contrast and high-spatial-resolution anatomic detail MR imaging for visualization of nerves, accurate needle navigation, and objective assessment of appropriate drug distribution.

REFERENCES

1. Fritz J, Chhabra A, Wang KC, et al. Magnetic resonance neurography-guided nerve blocks for the diagnosis and treatment of chronic pelvic pain syndrome. Neuroimaging Clin N Am 2014;24: 211–34.

2. Chhabra A, Lee PP, Bizzell C, et al. 3 Tesla MR neurography–technique, interpretation, and pitfalls. Skeletal Radiol 2011;40:1249–60.

3. Howe FA, Filler AG, Bell BA, et al. Magnetic resonance neurography. Magn Reson Med 1992;28:328–38.

4. Carrino JA, Blanco R. Magnetic resonance–guided musculoskeletal interventional radiology. Semin Musculoskelet Radiol 2006;10:159–74.

5. Fritz J, Pereira PL. MR-guided pain therapy: principles and clinical applications. Rofo 2007;179:914–24 [in German].

6. Fritz J, Thomas C, Clasen S, et al. Freehand real-time MRI-guided lumbar spinal injection procedures at 1.5 T: feasibility, accuracy, and safety. AJR Am J Roentgenol 2009;192:W161–7.

7. Fritz J, Niemeyer T, Clasen S, et al. Management of chronic low back pain: rationales, principles, and targets of imaging-guided spinal injections. Radiographics 2007;27:1751–71.

8. Bogduk N. International Spinal Injection Society guidelines for the performance of spinal injection procedures. Part 1: Zygapophysial joint blocks. Clin J Pain 1997;13:285–302.

9. Filler AG. Diagnosis and treatment of pudendal nerve entrapment syndrome subtypes: imaging, injections, and minimal access surgery. Neurosurg Focus 2009;26:E9.

10. Lee HM, Weinstein JN, Meller ST, et al. The role of steroids and their effects on phospholipase A2. An animal model of radiculopathy. Spine (Phila Pa 1976) 1998;23:1191–6.

11. Losel R, Wehling M. Nongenomic actions of steroid hormones. Nat Rev Mol Cell Biol 2003;4:46–56.

12. Fritz J, Bizzell C, Kathuria S, et al. High-resolution magnetic resonance-guided posterior femoral cutaneous nerve blocks. Skeletal Radiol 2013;42:579–86.

13. Brenner DJ, Hall EJ. Computed tomography–an increasing source of radiation exposure. N Engl J Med 2007;357:2277–84.

14. Fritz J, Thomas C, Tzaribachev N, et al. MRI-guided injection procedures of the temporomandibular joints in children and adults: technique, accuracy, and safety. AJR Am J Roentgenol 2009;193:1148–54.

15. Fritz J, Henes JC, Thomas C, et al. Diagnostic and interventional MRI of the sacroiliac joints using a 1.5-T open-bore magnet: a one-stop-shopping approach. AJR Am J Roentgenol 2008;191:1717–24.

16. Fritz J, Tzaribachev N, Thomas C, et al. Evaluation of MR imaging guided steroid injection of the sacroiliac joints for the treatment of children with refractory enthesitis-related arthritis. Eur Radiol 2011;21:1050–7.

17. Sodickson A, Baeyens PF, Andriole KP, et al. Recurrent CT, cumulative radiation exposure, and associated radiation-induced cancer risks from CT of adults. Radiology 2009;251:175–84.

18. Filler AG, Haynes J, Jordan SE, et al. Sciatica of non-disc origin and piriformis syndrome: diagnosis by magnetic resonance neurography and interventional magnetic resonance imaging with outcome study of resulting treatment. J Neurosurg Spine 2005;2:99–115.

19. Kanal E, Borgstede JP, Barkovich AJ, et al. American College of Radiology White Paper on MR Safety: 2004 update and revisions. AJR Am J Roentgenol 2004;182:1111–4.

20. Shellock FG, Kanal E. Guidelines and recommendations for MR imaging safety and patient management. III. Questionnaire for screening patients before MR procedures. The SMRI Safety Committee. J Magn Reson Imaging 1994;4:749–51.

21. Shellock FG, Crues JV. MR procedures: biologic effects, safety, and patient care. Radiology 2004;232:635–52.

22. Dempsey MF, Condon B, Hadley DM. Investigation of the factors responsible for burns during MRI. J Magn Reson Imaging 2001;13:627–31.

23. Lufkin R, Teresi L, Chiu L, et al. A technique for MR-guided needle placement. AJR Am J Roentgenol 1988;151:193–6.

24. Ludeke KM, Roschmann P, Tischler R. Susceptibility artefacts in NMR imaging. Magn Reson Imaging 1985;3:329–43.

25. Lewin JS, Duerk JL, Jain VR, et al. Needle localization in MR-guided biopsy and aspiration: effects of field strength, sequence design, and magnetic field orientation. AJR Am J Roentgenol 1996;166:1337–45.

26. Fritz J, Clasen S, Boss A, et al. Real-time MR fluoroscopy-navigated lumbar facet joint injections: feasibility and technical properties. Eur Radiol 2008;18:1513–8.

27. Sequeiros RB, Ojala RO, Klemola R, et al. MRI-guided periradicular nerve root infiltration therapy in low-field (0.23-T) MRI system using optical instrument tracking. Eur Radiol 2002;12:1331–7.

28. Ojala R, Vahala E, Karppinen J, et al. Nerve root infiltration of the first sacral root with MRI guidance. J Magn Reson Imaging 2000;12:556–61.

29. Safriel Y, Ali M, Hayt M, et al. Gadolinium use in spine procedures for patients with allergy to iodinated contrast–experience of 127 procedures. AJNR Am J Neuroradiol 2006;27:1194–7.

30. Shetty SK, Nelson EN, Lawrimore TM, et al. Use of gadolinium chelate to confirm epidural needle placement in patients with an iodinated contrast reaction. Skeletal Radiol 2007;36:301–7.

31. Butterworth JF, Strichartz GR. Molecular mechanisms of local anesthesia: a review. Anesthesiology 1990;72:711–34.

32. Chhabra A, Soldatos T, Andreisek G. Lumbosacral plexus. In: Chhabra A, Andreisek G, editors. Magnetic resonance neurography. New Delhi: Jaypee Brothers Medical Publishers; 2012. p. 161–81.

33. Dellon AL, Coady D, Harris D. Pelvic pain of puden-dal nerve origin: surgical outcomes and learning curve lessons. J Reconstr Microsurg 2015;31: 283–90.

34. Labat JJ, Riant T, Robert R, et al. Diagnostic criteria for pudendal neuralgia by pudendal nerve entrap-ment (Nantes criteria). Neurourol Urodyn 2008;27: 306–10.

35. Lefaucheur JP, Labat JJ, Amarenco G, et al. What is the place of electroneuromyographic studies in the diagnosis and management of pudendal neuralgia related to entrapment syndrome? Neurophysiol Clin 2007;37:223–8.

36. Filippiadis DK, Velonakis G, Mazioti A, et al. CT-guided percutaneous infiltration for the treatment of Alcock's neuralgia. Pain Physician 2011;14:211–5.

37. Romanzi L. Techniques of pudendal nerve block. J Sex Med 2010;7:1716–9.

38. Thoumas D, Leroi AM, Mauillon J, et al. Pudendal neuralgia: CT-guided pudendal nerve block tech-nique. Abdom Imaging 1999;24:309–12.

39. Rofaeel A, Peng P, Louis I, et al. Feasibility of real-time ultrasound for pudendal nerve block in patients with chronic perineal pain. Reg Anesth Pain Med 2008;33:139–45.

40. Smoll NR. Variations of the piriformis and sciatic nerve with clinical consequence: a review. Clin Anat 2010;23:8–17.

41. Rohen JW, Yokochi C, Ltjen-Drecoll E. Color atlas of anatomy a photographic study of the human body. 5th edition. Philadelphia: Lippincott Williams & Wil-kins; 2002.

42. Robinson D. Piriformis syndrome in relation to sciatic pain. Am J Surg 1947;73:355–8.

43. Fishman LM, Anderson C, Rosner B. BOTOX and physical therapy in the treatment of piriformis syn-drome. Am J Phys Med Rehabil 2002;81:936–42.

44. Halpin RJ, Ganju A. Piriformis syndrome: a real pain in the buttock? Neurosurgery 2009;65:A197–202.

45. Russell JM, Kransdorf MJ, Bancroft LW, et al. Mag-netic resonance imaging of the sacral plexus and piriformis muscles. Skeletal Radiol 2008;37:709–13.

46. Blasi J, Chapman ER, Link E, et al. Botulinum neuro-toxin A selectively cleaves the synaptic protein SNAP-25. Nature 1993;365:160–3.

47. Childers MK, Wilson DJ, Gnatz SM, et al. Botulinum toxin type A use in piriformis muscle syndrome: a pilot study. Am J Phys Med Rehabil 2002;81:751–9.

48. Gray H, Lewis WH. Anatomy of the human body. 20th edition. New York: Bartleby.com; 2000.

49. Tubbs RS, Miller J, Loukas M, et al. Surgical and anatomical landmarks for the perineal branch of the posterior femoral cutaneous nerve: implications in perineal pain syndromes. Laboratory investiga-tion. J Neurosurg 2009;111:332–5.

50. Dellon AL. Pain with sitting related to injury of the posterior femoral cutaneous nerve. Microsurgery 2015. [Epub ahead of print].

51. Darnis B, Robert R, Labat JJ, et al. Perineal pain and inferior cluneal nerves: anatomy and surgery. Surg Radiol Anat 2008;30:177–83.

52. Hughes PJ, Brown TC. An approach to posterior femoral cutaneous nerve block. Anaesth Intensive Care 1986;14:350–1.

53. Roth V. Meralgia paresthetica. Med Obozr Mosk 1895;43:678.

54. Alberti O, Wickboldt J, Becker R. Suprainguinal retroperitoneal approach for the successful surgical treatment of meralgia paresthetica. J Neurosurg 2009;110:768–74.

55. Grothaus MC, Holt M, Mekhail AO, et al. Lateral femoral cutaneous nerve: an anatomic study. Clin Orthop Relat Res 2005;(437):164–8.

56. Kosiyatrakul A, Nuansalee N, Luenam S, et al. The anatomical variation of the lateral femoral cutaneous nerve in relation to the anterior superior iliac spine and the iliac crest. Musculoskelet Surg 2010;94:17–20.

57. de Ridder VA, de LS, Popta JV. Anatomical varia-tions of the lateral femoral cutaneous nerve and the consequences for surgery. J Orthop Trauma 1999;13:207–11.

58. Aszmann OC, Dellon ES, Dellon AL. Anatomical course of the lateral femoral cutaneous nerve and its susceptibility to compression and injury. Plast Reconstr Surg 1997;100:600–4.

59. Murata Y, Takahashi K, Yamagata M, et al. The anat-omy of the lateral femoral cutaneous nerve, with special reference to the harvesting of iliac bone graft. J Bone Joint Surg Am 2000;82:746–7.

60. Ray B, D'Souza AS, Kumar B, et al. Variations in the course and microanatomical study of the lateral femoral cutaneous nerve and its clinical importance. Clin Anat 2010;23:978–84.

61. Lee CH, Dellon AL. Surgical management of groin pain of neural origin. J Am Coll Surg 2000;191:137–42.

62. Ducic I, Dellon AL, Taylor NS. Decompression of the lateral femoral cutaneous nerve in the treatment of meralgia paresthetica. J Reconstr Microsurg 2006; 22:113–8.

63. Kendir S, Akkaya T, Comert A, et al. The location of the obturator nerve: a three-dimensional description of the obturator canal. Surg Radiol Anat 2008;30: 495–501.

64. Bradshaw C, McCrory P. Obturator nerve entrap-ment. Clin J Sport Med 1997;7:217–9.

65. Birnbaum K, Prescher A, Hessler S, et al. The sen-sory innervation of the hip joint–an anatomical study. Surg Radiol Anat 1997;19:371–5.

66. Tipton JS. Obturator neuropathy. Curr Rev Muscu-loskelet Med 2008;1:234–7.

Magnetic Resonance Imaging–Guided Breast Interventions
Role in Biopsy Targeting and Lumpectomies

Eva C. Gombos, MD[a],*, Jayender Jagadeesan, PhD[b],
Danielle M. Richman, MD, MS[c], Daniel F. Kacher, MS[b]

KEYWORDS

- Breast cancer • Needle biopsy • MR imaging guidance • Lumpectomy • Extent of disease
- Tumor ablation • Neoadjuvant chemotherapy

KEY POINTS

- Breast MR imaging is the most sensitive imaging tool of detecting breast cancer and may reveal breast cancer that is occult to physical examination and by conventional imaging modalities (mammography and ultrasound).
- In cases in which a suspicious lesion is detected by MR imaging and no obvious correlative finding is found by other methods, MR imaging–guided tissue sampling is needed to determine the underlying histopathology.
- Studies have shown advantages of breast MR imaging for predicting recurrence-free survival and pathologic complete response over physical examination and conventional imaging.
- Regarding lumpectomy planning, anticipated benefits from higher sensitivity of preoperative MR imaging have not been clearly shown in large studies.

PROBLEM AND CLINICAL PRESENTATIONS
Use of Contrast-Enhanced Breast MR Imaging

Contrast-enhanced breast MR imaging is an important adjunctive modality for screening and diagnosis of breast cancer. MR imaging has been demonstrated as beneficial and used increasingly as an adjunct to mammography[1] in screening in a subset of women at high risk for developing breast cancer because of its high sensitivity and negative predictive value. MR imaging is being used to assess response for neoadjuvant chemotherapy treatment (NACT), detect otherwise occult breast cancer presenting as metastatic axillary or systemic disease, evaluate extent of disease in patients with newly diagnosed breast cancer, and assess contralateral breast. Additional clinical trials are needed to determine the significance of MR imaging–detected, otherwise occult disease.[2]

MR Imaging–Guided Tissue Sampling

In cases in which MR imaging alone detects a suspicious lesion (ie, no correlative finding with other methods), MR imaging–guided tissue sampling

Disclosures: Dr E.C. Gombos discloses that she is receiving royalties for a book published by Amirsys, Inc. Dr J. Jagadeesan discloses that this project was supported by the National Center for Research Resources and the National Institute of Biomedical Imaging and Bioengineering of the National Institutes of Health through Grant Numbers P41EB015898 and P41RR019703. Dr D.M. Richman and Dr D.F. Kacher have nothing to disclose.
[a] Division of Breast Imaging, Department of Radiology, Brigham and Women's Hospital, 75 Francis Street, Boston, MA 02115, USA; [b] Surgical Planning Laboratory, Brigham and Women's Hospital, 75 Francis Street, Boston, MA 02115, USA; [c] Department of Radiology, Brigham and Women's Hospital, 75 Francis Street, Boston, MA 02115, USA
* Corresponding author.
E-mail address: egombos@partners.org

Magn Reson Imaging Clin N Am 23 (2015) 547–561
http://dx.doi.org/10.1016/j.mric.2015.05.004
1064-9689/15/$ – see front matter © 2015 Elsevier Inc. All rights reserved.

is needed to determine the underlying histopathology.

Margin Status at Breast-Conserving Therapy

The current positive or close margin rate at initial surgery requiring an additional operation with re-excision is estimated to range from 30% to 60%.[3,4] There is no ideal method for margin evaluation during surgery. However, there are trials in progress on the use of MR imaging guidance and MR imaging evaluation of the margins intraoperatively with the goal of reducing the need for additional operations.[5]

NEED FOR MR IMAGING–GUIDED PROCEDURES

Recommendations for performance of breast MR imaging are conditioned on a standard level of quality of MR imaging studies with high spatial resolution images. The American College of Radiology accreditation process includes the requirement for facilities to have the ability to provide MR imaging–guided biopsy when offering breast MR imaging.[6]

When a suspicious lesion has been detected by breast MR imaging, and biopsy for histologic diagnosis is suggested, the first step should be to evaluate the area by mammography and targeted ultrasound (US) for a possible correlate.[7] US guidance is preferred over MR imaging for biopsy if a sonographic correlate can be identified.[7] US is readily available and US-guided biopsies are quicker, more comfortable for the patient, do not require intravenous contrast, and are less expensive. A US correlate can be identified in approximately half of the cases.[7,8] If the findings of this approach are unrevealing or uncertain, an MR imaging–guided biopsy should be performed.[9–15]

BREAST MR IMAGING AND TECHNIQUES

There are widespread variations in breast MR imaging techniques, with different approaches to balance morphology, kinetic information, and use of fat saturation versus subtraction techniques. Obtaining good quality breast MR imaging is conditioned on many factors: use of a high-field-strength magnet and a dedicated breast coil, appropriate breast positioning, injection of gadolinium contrast material, high-spatial-resolution imaging without artifacts, and specified adequate timing of the dynamic sequences.

The following MR imaging equipment specifications and performance must meet all state and federal requirements, and the American College of Radiology practice parameters and technical standards guidelines including routine quality control should apply.[6] Field strength: a 1.5- or 3-T magnet has typically been used for breast MR imaging. Positioning: all routine clinical breast MR imaging examinations are performed with the patient in prone position with simultaneous bilateral imaging using a dedicated (bilateral) breast MR imaging coil containing two individual depressions for the left and right breast. Prone positioning helps to move the breasts away from the chest wall and minimizes respiratory and cardiac motion effects.[16] Resolution, contrast, and artifacts: the slice thickness should be 3 mm or less; in-plane pixel resolution should be 1 mm or less so as to reduce the problem of volume averaging and to detect and characterize small abnormalities. Chemical fat suppression is helpful as a method for reducing the fat signal. Subtraction imaging for assessment of enhancement and fat suppression are recommended. Misregistration caused by patient motion can occur, and motion correction may aid in reducing artifacts encountered with image subtraction. Contrast: gadolinium intravenous contrast is needed in the evaluation of breast cancer. Dynamic kinetic information based on enhancement data at appropriate time intervals is extremely important for lesion classification.

CHALLENGES IN MR IMAGING–GUIDED BREAST BIOPSY TARGETING

Many of the challenges experienced with MR imaging–guided biopsy are similar to those encountered using stereotactic biopsy with patients prone on a dedicated table and are related to targeting (ie, difficulty with posterior targets or those that are superficial), positioning, and compression (eg, an accordion effect at clip deployment or problems with very dense breasts). Furthermore with MR imaging-guidance, the patient needs to be removed from the magnet to be repositioned for the biopsy to be performed, because there is somewhat limited access to the medial and posterior breast. Additional difficulties may arise, including contrast washout, lesion location-related problems, and/or limitations in confirming lesion sampling.[9,17]

Cancellation of the procedure is frequent (reported as between 8% and 13%).[18] Nonvisualization of the suspicious finding may be caused by change in tissue enhancement because the patient is in different phase of her period and/or may be related to compression of breast tissue with decreased inflow of contrast material.

Signal-void artifact from needles, obturators, and wires used in the MR imaging setting and hemorrhage (hyperintense on T1 sequences) may obscure the target. Air entered or generated from needle placement frequently interferes with target visualization.

MR IMAGING–GUIDED BREAST CORE NEEDLE BIOPSY

A dedicated breast MR imaging coil and prone positioning on a moveable examination table is typically required with MR imaging conditional biopsy equipment. Usually a larger needle (11–14 gauge) and vacuum assistance are used for sampling, although smaller, spring-activated 14- to 18-gauge sizes are also available. Needle susceptibility artifact should be reduced by appropriate imaging protocol without compromising image quality and lesion detection.

The grid technique is widely implemented because of its ease of use. Other localizing methods include pillar and post, and free-hand techniques.[13,14] Protocols may differ among facilities. Usually, after localizing images, axial and sagittal T1-weighted, fat saturated images are obtained before and after injection of the contrast agent in the area of interest. The imaging protocol should minimize image acquisition time while maintaining lesion visualization. There is a short period following the administration of the intravenous contrast during which the area of interest can be visualized. Following identification, targeting the lesion includes identifying the correct opening within the grid for introducer and for needle insertion. Most systems offer an approach from the lateral, or from the medial direction. There is frequently tissue displacement during the needle insertion and repeated adjustments in needle positioning may be required (**Fig. 1**). Placing a marker clip at the biopsy site, typically followed by two mammographic views to document clip location, is recommended. Vacuum-assisted core biopsy tissue sampling with MR imaging–guided devices has been shown to be technically successful in 94% to 98% of cases and is an accepted alternative for histopathologic assessment to surgical biopsy.[9,10,17]

MR IMAGING–GUIDED WIRE LOCALIZATION

The first MR imaging–guided interventional procedure developed was needle localization before surgery. The procedure is occasionally performed when the extent of disease is not apparent by conventional imaging modalities, and therefore prelumpectomy localization is best done with MR imaging. Currently, MR imaging–guided core biopsy has replaced many MR imaging needle localizations. Excision is sometimes considered when core biopsy is not possible (eg, there is a posterior target location or an extremely small breast) or per patient's preference.[12]

The positioning and targeting for needle localization is the same as that for needle biopsy. After lesion identification and location determination, a guide needle is introduced to the appropriate depth. After imaging confirms appropriate location and depth, an MR imaging conditional localization hook wire is deployed through the needle. The guiding needle is similar to the Kopans needle used for mammographic localizations. The MR imaging wire is softer than conventional, non–MR imaging conditional wires and therefore deployment in hard fibrous tissue may occasionally be difficult and they have a tendency to break during surgery.[17] Following the localization procedure, a mammogram can visualize for the surgeon the site of the wire within breast tissue, and nipple and chest-wall positions.

PATHOLOGY CORRELATION OF MR IMAGING–GUIDED BIOPSIES

Evaluating concordance is important in all image-guided biopsies, and especially important for MR imaging–guided biopsies because sampling accuracy is subject to uncertainty. Concordance decisions begin in the planning phase with the radiologist defining the expected pathology result based on original images. Because there is no specimen image confirmation of the target (as in a stereotactic core biopsy specimen radiograph showing calcifications), or direct visualization of sampling (as in US-guided biopsies with real-time observation of sampling), accuracy is difficult to determine from core biopsy images. The procedure radiologist should review images to determine whether procedure images support lesion retrieval. The final decision about concordance versus discordance is made when the radiologist decides if pathology results agree with the expected outcome.

Based on the radiologist's degree of certainty regarding satisfactory tissue sampling, benign concordant histologic results may warrant short-term (6-month) follow-up MR imaging to confirm stability.[11] For discordant lesions, surgical excision is recommended. Imaging histologic discordance rate has been reported as approximately 7% to 9%.[9,18] Higher rates of imaging-histologic discordance and underestimation of atypical ductal hyperplasia and ductal carcinoma in situ (DCIS) have been reported with MR imaging–guided biopsies than with stereotactic mammographic biopsies.[19,20]

For cases that have been assessed as possibly missed or discordant, repeat biopsy or surgical

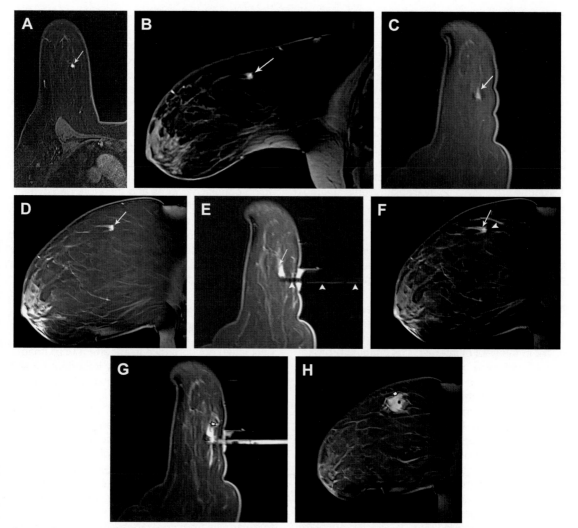

Fig. 1. MR imaging–guided core needle biopsy planning and procedure. Baseline MR imaging identifies a suspicious 7-mm mass in the upper inner right breast (axial and sagittal images, *A, B*), not seen clearly by other imaging modalities; a decision about MR imaging–guided biopsy was made. A high signal intensity fiducial marker is placed on a grid hole. Following localizing images, precontrast images and axial and sagittal postcontrast sequences (*C, D*) are obtained to reidentify the target. Needle insertion site is determined by measuring the target location relative to the fiducial's position. After placement of the obturator, axial and sagittal sequences are obtained to confirm proper depth and location before the biopsy (*E, F*). Further sagittal and axial images are performed following the biopsy to show hyperintense hematoma (developed in this case at the site) and to verify the deployment and location of the marker clip (signal void artifact) (*G, H*). *Arrowheads*, obturator; *long arrows*, targeted mass; *open arrow*, hematoma.

excision is recommended. MR imaging–guided core biopsy malignancy rates varying between 16% and 37% have been reported.[9,12,15,17,18]

Regarding pathology examination of excisional biopsy specimen of MR imaging–guided wire localization, MR imaging of a breast specimen with current clinical scanners is not useful for lesion detection because detection is based on visualization of enhancement with the injected contrast agent. Gross examination and specimen radiography do not identify most of the malignancies in MR imaging localized procedures. For that reason, optimal pathology processing of MR imaging–guided excisions requires microscopic examination of the entire specimen tissue.[21]

SURGICAL PLANNING WITH PREOPERATIVE MR IMAGING FOLLOWING NEOADJUVANT CHEMOTHERAPY

Systemic chemotherapy improves survival for patients with invasive breast cancer. It is the standard of care for node-positive patients and is used for many patients with high-risk node-negative disease with invasive breast cancer. During the past approximately 20 years, there has been an option to administer chemotherapy before surgery (NACT) rather than following surgery (adjuvant chemotherapy) for those women requiring systemic therapy. The main advantage of preoperative NACT is the reduction in primary tumor size and conversion from node-positive into node-negative status. NACT is used for treatment of locally advanced breast cancer to allow for surgery in cases in which skin or pectoral muscle is involved (Fig. 2). NACT is also used in early stage breast cancer to enable breast-conserving therapy (BCT) when originally mastectomy was planned, or to achieve better cosmetic outcomes because of smaller surgical resection volume. Despite less extensive surgery following NACT, several studies showed similar local recurrence rates with preoperative NACT compared with adjuvant chemotherapy, although some studies suggested a trend for higher locoregional recurrence.[22,23] The National Surgical Adjuvant Breast and Bowel Project B18 and other clinical trials comparing neoadjuvant with adjuvant chemotherapy found that there is no significant difference in overall or disease-free survival between patients receiving adjuvant or neoadjuvant chemotherapy; however, more women undergoing preoperative chemotherapy were eligible and received breast-conservation treatment.[22,24,25]

Accurate monitoring of NACT response is essential; imaging may demonstrate stable or progressive disease, or remission, and even complete response (Box 1). Pathologic complete response is defined as the absence of any residual invasive tumor cells in the original tumor bed; however, residual DCIS may be present (Fig. 3). Attaining pathologic complete response following NACT has been shown as a prognostic factor for overall better survival, and for disease-free survival.[23]

MR IMAGING–GUIDED BREAST ABLATION

The aim of ablative therapy is to achieve a well-defined area encompassing the tumor, irreversible cell damage, protein denaturation, and coagulation necrosis, while sparing overlying and surrounding tissues. The role of imaging is to aid the clinician in planning the probe placement for optimal coverage, targeting the lesion, and monitoring the deposition of energy. The advantages of MR imaging guidance in these tasks are three-dimensional visualization via multiplanar, multislice acquisition, high sensitivity, and delineation of breast lesions, and tissue thermal sensitivity. A therapeutic probe is percutaneously placed in the lesion to deliver cooling (cryoablation) or heating energy (radiofrequency ablation [RFA], laser interstitial thermal therapy [LITT]) so as to cause cell death. High-intensity focused US (HIFU) can achieve these goals without use of an invasive probe. Ablative techniques may be useful in

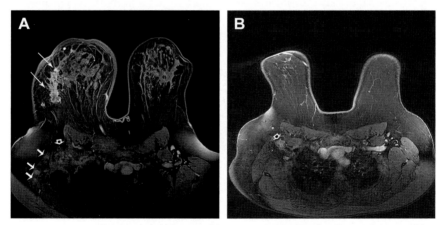

Fig. 2. Tumor response can render previously inoperable tumors operable, leading to increased breast conservation rate and smaller resection volumes. A 43-year-old woman with a new diagnosis of triple negative inflammatory right breast cancer. Baseline MR imaging shows an extensive, large, irregular mass (*long arrows*) and multiple ill-defined masses with rim-enhancement in the right lateral chest wall musculature (*short arrows*). Axillary adenopathy is present (*open arrow*) (*A*). The patient underwent neoadjuvant chemotherapy. Presurgical MR imaging 5 months later shows disappearance of the previous large mass and disappearance of the lateral chest wall masses. Remaining ill-defined axillary adenopathy is seen (*open arrow*) (*B*). The patient underwent right mastectomy with axillary dissection. There was no residual carcinoma on histopathology examination in the 8.5-cm fibrous tumor bed. Thirteen removed lymph nodes showed treatment effect but with no carcinoma. Summary: pathologic complete response (Miller-Payne grade 5 and residual cancer burden 0).

patients with benign lesions,[26] those who refuse surgery,[27] patients with stage 4 breast cancer who need palliative care,[28] or patients with recurrent disease.[29]

There are uncertainties that may prevent image-guided minimally invasive tumor ablation in patients with early stage breast cancer from becoming a viable alternative treatment of lumpectomy. It remains to conclusively show that clinical outcomes (clear margins, recurrence rate, morbidity, and mortality) are comparable with the standard of care, surgery followed by whole breast radiation. Careful inclusion criteria and control measures are critical elements.

MR Imaging–Guided Cryoablation

Percutaneous cryoablation using freezing temperatures is delivered by gas-cooled probes.[30] Although most breast ablation has been guided by US,[31] MR imaging is particularly well suited for monitoring the growth of the iceball. The iceball appears as a signal void because of the short T2* of the crystalized water and, unlike with US, the tissue beyond the iceball is not subject to shadowing.[32]

In a feasibility study, Morin and colleagues[33] reported on the MR imaging–guided cryoablation in 25 patients with breast carcinoma without complications. Four weeks after treatment, surgical excision was performed for histopathologic correlation. Total ablation was achieved in 13 of the 25 tumors treated. Pusztaszeri and colleagues[34] reported that in all 10 of the evaluated patients undergoing MR imaging–guided cryotherapy followed by surgical excision, the iceball engulfed the tumor, but only two patients had a complete response. The authors suggested that components of undetected DCIS in the larger tumors were far from the two probes used. Five patients suffered from skin necrosis, a complication that can be avoided by selection criteria of

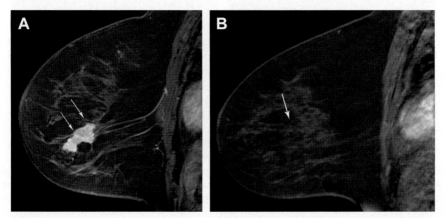

Fig. 3. MR imaging has been shown to be of value in predicting tumor size when there is no response or there is a complete response. A 54-year-old woman with an estrogen receptor (ER)/PR negative, ERBB2 (Her-2/neu) positive, high-grade invasive ductal carcinoma (IDC). (*A*) Baseline MR imaging shows the known mass (*arrows*). (*B*) Post-treatment MR imaging shows no residual mass or enhancement in the area of primary tumor, only artifact from prior treatment (*arrow*). Lumpectomy pathology showed a 1.6-cm fibrous area consistent with treated tumor bed with scattered small foci of DCIS. Findings remain compatible with a Miller-Payne grade 5 response.

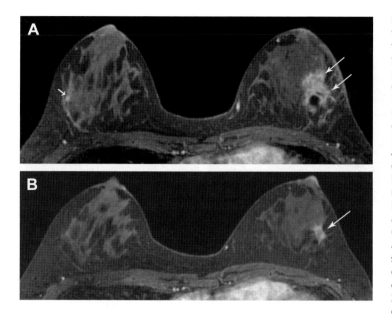

Fig. 4. Underestimation of residual tumor size by MR imaging (ER-positive cancers). A 37-year-old woman with no known risk factors and left palpable lump. Ultrasound-guided core needle biopsy showed grade II/III IDC, ER/PR(+), ERBB2 (Her-2/neu) (-). (*A*) MR imaging for extent of disease shows a 2.7-cm irregular, spiculated mass with rapid washout (*long arrows*). In addition, a 0.5-cm enhancing mass was seen only by MR imaging on the contralateral, right breast (*short arrow*). Right MR imaging–guided core biopsy showed a grade II/III IDC, ER/PR (+), ERBB2 (Her-2/neu) (-) IDC. (*B*) MR imaging at completion of NACT showed no residual lesion on the right and decreased size, minimal residual enhancement on the left (RECIST 37%, partial response) (*arrow*). Bilateral mastectomy pathology showed a 0.1-cm residual IDC on the right and no pathologic response on the left (the residual carcinoma was 90% cellular and appeared viable).

minimum distance between the lesion and the skin or managed with the use of warm saline on the skin or saline injection.[35] In these studies, the patient was supine. More recently, Tozaki and colleagues[36] treated a single patient with core needle biopsy proved invasive ductal carcinoma without an intraductal component using a non–MR imaging compatible cryotherapy system. MR imaging of a prone patient with a breast coil was used to define the target tissue. A US system safely integrated into the MR imaging room was used to place the probes. At the 9-week MR imaging evaluation, the lesion was not enhancing and was shown to be inside the cryozone. No viable cancer cells were noted on histology following a lumpectomy at 14 weeks.

MR Imaging Temperature Mapping in the Breast

A tool common to the ablative techniques that use elevated temperature is noninvasive MR imaging temperature mapping based on temperature-sensitive MR imaging parameters, such as the proton resonance frequency, the diffusion coefficient, T1 and T2 relaxation times, magnetization transfer, proton density, and temperature-sensitive contrast agents.[28] Through empirical experimentation, cell death can be correlated with thermal dose, which is derived from time-temperature curves.[37] Although proton resonance frequency shift is useful for measuring temperature in aqueous tissue, the chemical shift in fat is

almost constant with the temperatures used in thermal ablation. However, the T1 temperature dependence can be exploited in fat.[38,39]

MR Imaging–Guided Radiofrequency Ablation

RFA refers to the destruction of tissue via the application of electromagnetic fields created by interstitial electrode delivery of energy (0.4–8 MHz). A dispersive electrode on the thigh or back is used to complete the electrical circuit. Current density is induced in the tissue, causing resistive heating. RF energy deposition is a function of tissue conductivity and is difficult to predict and control. The formation of the thermal lesion may be inhomogeneous, especially in regions of the tissue boundaries. Susceptibility artifacts around the probe during MR imaging may prevent accurate temperature monitoring. No monopolar commercial solution is currently available to remedy the problem of electromagnetic interference emitting from the RF generator manifesting as noise in the MR images. Several research sites have implemented gating[40] or filtering solutions.

van den Bosch and colleagues[41] performed MR imaging–guided RFA on three patients followed immediately by surgical excision for histopathologic correlation (**Fig. 5**). US-guided large-core needle biopsy confirmed invasive ductal carcinoma in all three patients, with DCIS adjacent to the invasive lesion in the second and third patients. Patients were positioned prone in a 0.5-T vertically open MR imaging scanner. Measurements from a

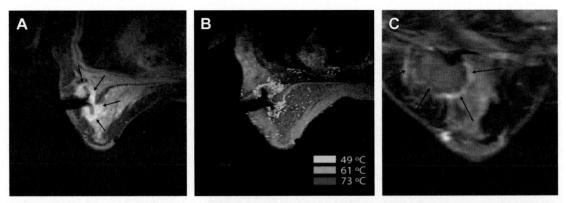

Fig. 5. MR imaging–guided RFA. (*A*) Contrast-enhanced three-point Dixon gradient-echo images with patient in prone position showing the fully deployed LeVeen needle electrode (signal void) centrally in the enhancing tumor mass (*arrows*) in the right breast. (*B*) Same axial positioning showing the magnetic resonance proton-resonance frequency (PRF) shift thermomap (*yellow* zone 49°C, *orange* 61°C, *red* 73°C) around the deployed RFA electrode centrally in the mass. (*C*) Postprocedure contrast-enhanced water-selective, spectral-spatial (AU11) fast spin echo image of the right breast demonstrates a small enhancing rim representing the border of the ablation zone corresponding to fresh scar tissue (*arrows*). (*From* van den Bosch M, Daniel B, Rieke V, et al. MRI-guided radiofrequency ablation of breast cancer: preliminary clinical experience. J Magn Reson Imaging 2008;27(1):206; with permission.)

fiberoptic temperature probe were used for comparisons with MR imaging temperature mapping. Histopathology confirmed successful (100%) tumor ablation in one patient, and partial tumor destruction (33% and 50%, respectively) in two patients. The lesion size was probably underestimated on the MR image in the latter two cases. It was noted that susceptibility artifact caused by the 6-mm diameter probe would create a challenge for temperature mapping in lesions less than 10 mm. A high success rate for the technique in other organs[42] may encourage industry to provide complete solutions for breast MR imaging–guided RFA.

MR Imaging–Guided Laser Interstitial Thermal Therapies

During LITT, light energy is delivered directly to tissue via percutaneous optical fiber, and creates a zone of thermal ablation. Optical fibers are inherently MR imaging conditional and can be extended such that the laser device can be situated outside the scanner room. Larger lesions can be treated with the use of either diffusing tips or a beam splitter and multiple fibers.[43]

LITT has been used successfully for the treatment of benign fibroadenomata[44,45] and breast cancer in several institutions.[46–48] Use of MR imaging systems at field strengths as low as 0.2 T have been reported for targeting and monitoring.[49] Mumtaz and colleagues[46] correlated preprocedural and postprocedural MR imaging with histopathology in a study of 20 women with proved breast cancer. The nonenhancing area of ablated

tissue correlated well with necrotic area seen histopathologically.

In the study by Harms and colleagues,[45] although no histopathology correlation was available, tumor sizes were observed to be reduced on follow-up imaging at 5 months. The same group also investigated MR imaging–guided LITT for treatment of breast cancer in 12 women with 22 breast lesions. Complete destruction was achieved in only three women; they had tumors with diameters of less than 3 cm. In the nine other patients, tumors larger than 3 cm were incompletely destroyed.[50]

MR Imaging–Guided High Intensity Focused Ultrasound

In MR imaging–guided HIFU, focal heating of target tissue is achieved via deposition of acoustic energy (1–2 MHz) generated by a piezoelectric transducer array that is acoustically coupled to the breast of a prone patient via a water bath. A temperature elevation to 55°C to 90°C is produced during a 10- to 20-second sonication.[51]

Preliminary data with MR imaging–guided HIFU have shown partial or complete coagulation of targeted benign fibroadenomas.[52] The first case report of HIFU used to treat cancer with a 1.5-T magnet was in a 56-year-old patient with a 22-mm invasive breast cancer.[53] Gianfelice and colleagues[54] used HIFU with a 1.5-T system to treat 24 patients who either refused surgery or were at increased risk for surgery. Each patient with no evidence of metastatic disease underwent one or two ablation procedures for a single lesion smaller than 25 mm. Of the 24 patients, 19 (79%) had negative percutaneous needle biopsy results following the procedures. One patient experienced a second-degree skin burn, and no other complications were reported.

A total of 45 of the 57 patients enrolled in treat and resect protocols at three centers[55–58] had 100% of the lesion included in the treatment field, but only 21 had complete ablation on histologic examination. Four patients experienced skin burns that were either healed or resected in the surgical approach to the lesion. All studies enrolled patients with a single invasive tumor smaller than 3.5 cm that was greater than 1 cm from the skin and chest wall and a 1.5-T MR imaging was used for guidance. Each patient underwent a standard lumpectomy within 5 weeks of ablation. Technical failures included the inability to target 100% of the tumor volume or failure to deliver 100% of the planned thermal energy to the targeted area.

Furusawa and Yasuda[59] treated 50 patients who did not subsequently have lumpectomy. The purpose of this phase III study was to determine the efficacy and safety of HIFU followed by radiotherapy as a local treatment of early breast cancer. The patients had a single biopsy-proved invasive tumor greater than 1 cm from the skin and chest wall. The average tumor size was 11.0 mm (6–15 mm). Forty-one of the patients had their lesions completely treated. There were no severe adverse events and no local recurrence. Hardware has now been developed by multiple vendors[60] and efforts are underway to develop temperature mapping techniques that can simultaneously monitor aqueous and fatty tissue.[61]

MR IMAGING: ROLE IN SURGICAL PLANNING
Evaluation of Extent of Disease

There are several objectives for MR imaging evaluation of the ipsilateral breast in patients with a recent cancer diagnosis: tumor and possible additional foci location within the breast and in relationship to chest wall, possible chest wall involvement, and detection of axillary nodes/masses or internal mammary chain nodes. Studies have shown that MR imaging has superior sensitivity to conventional imaging for detecting clinically occult cancer foci in women with breast cancer.[62,63] According to a 2008 meta-analysis, MR imaging detects additional ipsilateral disease in an average of 16% of women with a known breast cancer.[64]

MR imaging detection rates of finding more than one cancer focus are consistent with prior studies of breast cancer: Holland and colleagues[65] classical pathology studies on serial sectioning of mastectomy specimens in patients with presumed

single breast cancer sites identified additional disease further than 2 cm from the index tumor in 43% of the cases.

MR imaging studies have described multifocality (additional site of cancer within the same quadrant) in 4% to 9% of women, and multicentricity (additional site of cancer in different quadrant) in 7% to 10% of cases (Fig. 6).[62,66–68] Criticisms of breast MR imaging include that the additional disease found has no clinical impact because it will be treated with radiation therapy. The clinical significance of additional foci is not clear because local recurrence rates following BCT are low, at less than 10% in 10 years.[69] These data suggest that radiation with adjuvant therapy can control the additional tumor foci not detected clinically or by conventional imaging.

Two prospective randomized trials studied the use of breast MR imaging for extent of disease evaluation. In the COMICE (Comparative Effectiveness of MR Imaging in Breast Cancer) trial, with a relatively short-term follow-up, no significant difference in re-excision rates was found (19% in each arm) and there were comparable local recurrence rates.[70] In the MONET (MR Mammography of Nonpalpable Breast Tumors) trial, a higher reoperation rate was found for the MR imaging group (34%) than for the non–MR imaging group (12%).[71] The MONET study had a strong selection bias: 50% of compared cancer cases were mammographic calcifications and proved to be DCIS at excision. Both trials have been criticized for including use of a variety of equipment, technique, sequencing, and interpretation. Neither of these two studies included a strategy for managing data gained from MR imaging and consistently incorporating them into surgical planning.

The expectation from staging MR imaging was that more accurate staging of extent of disease would probably decrease the number of surgeries required to achieve clear margins and could potentially reduce local recurrence and improve survival. The impact of breast MR imaging on frequency of positive margins was analyzed by a meta-analysis, examining the effect of preoperative MR imaging compared with standard preoperative assessment on surgical outcomes. It was found that preoperative MR imaging did not have a positive effect on outcomes but patients with preoperative MR imaging had significantly increased mastectomy rates.[63]

Selection of Patients and Surgical Planning for Breast-Conserving Surgery

Breast-conserving surgery (BCS) is performed with the goal of removing breast malignancy and

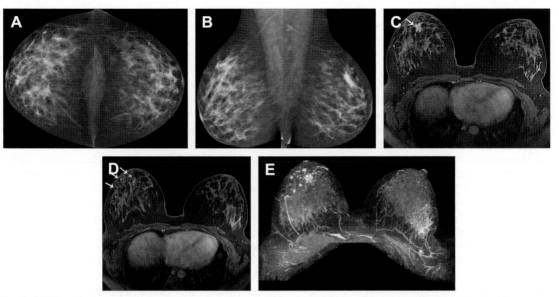

Fig. 6. MR imaging may detect occult and multifocal disease. A 39-year-old asymptomatic woman with a strong family history and known BRCA2 mutation presented for screening studies by mammography (*A, B*) and MR imaging (*C–E*) on the same day. Mammogram was interpreted as negative; however, MR imaging revealed a 2-cm lesion and multiple associated satellite lesions (*arrows*). Mastectomy confirmed multifocal disease.

adequate surrounding margin to preserve breast with good cosmesis. In appropriate candidates, survival rates are equivalent to those of mastectomy. It is considered when a satisfactory aesthetic result can be achieved with estimated low risk of in-breast recurrence. Mastectomy is preferred when a cosmetically acceptable outcome for the patient is unattainable by lumpectomy. Ineligibility for BCS includes multifocal and multicentric disease or the inability to achieve negative pathologic margins. Patients who are not able to receive or who reject radiation treatment (eg, previous radiation therapy in the area) are also excluded.

Preoperative needle localization and wire placement with image guidance for nonpalpable lesions and/or to define radiologic extent of disease is performed to aid lesion removal. Larger extent of disease may require bracketing. New localization techniques being used or tested include intraoperative US,[72] radioisotope seeds for lesion marking,[73] and nonradioactive electromagnetic wave technology.[74]

Up to 60% of patients undergoing BCS require re-excision, with the mainstream re-excision rates approximately 20% to 40%.[75–83] Intraoperative margin assessment with frozen section histopathology analysis and imprint cytology provides useful information on margin status. It is crucial to achieve clear margins because presence of close or positive margins is associated with increased locoregional recurrence and a decrease

in long-term survival.[80,84,85] Reoperations increase cost; delay completion of therapy; increase the potential for complications, including infection and diminished cosmetic outcomes; and have negative psychological impact on the patient.[83,86–88]

Intraoperative MR Imaging for Lumpectomy

The use of MR imaging scanners within the operating room has been shown to facilitate and refine the surgical approach, tumor localization, and detection of residual lesions in neurosurgery.[89] In breast surgery, only a few intraoperative MR imaging–guided lumpectomy studies have been performed. Gould and colleagues[90] used a 0.5-T vertically open scanner and reported close agreement between maximum dimensions of MR imaging size dimensions of benign breast lesions and pathology measurements. All postprocedure scans demonstrated complete resection.

Hirose and colleagues[91] at Brigham and Women's Hospital (BWH), using the same type of 0.5-T vertically open scanner, reported that all the tumors in the 20 patients with invasive breast cancers were localized with MR imaging at the MR imaging–guided lumpectomy. Although re-excision was prompted by MR imaging guidance only and obviated a second operation in four (20%) of the cases, the procedure was suspended. The suboptimal image quality at 0.5 T made reliable detection of a residual tumor a challenge. Dynamic imaging with fat saturation was not possible because of low field strength. For these reasons, BWH chose to change the program to a 3-T MR imaging scanner.

The Advanced Multimodal Image-Guided Operating Suite

The advanced multimodal image-guided operating (AMIGO) suite was the first operating suite equipped with three sterile procedure rooms (MR imaging, operating room, and PET-CT rooms). In the center of the MR imaging room is a high-field (3 T) wide-bore (70 cm) Siemens Verio MR imaging scanner (Siemens AG, Erlangen, Germany) that is ceiling mounted and has the ability to move in and out of the surgical field.

BWH successfully demonstrated the feasibility of lumpectomy and intraoperative MR imaging in the

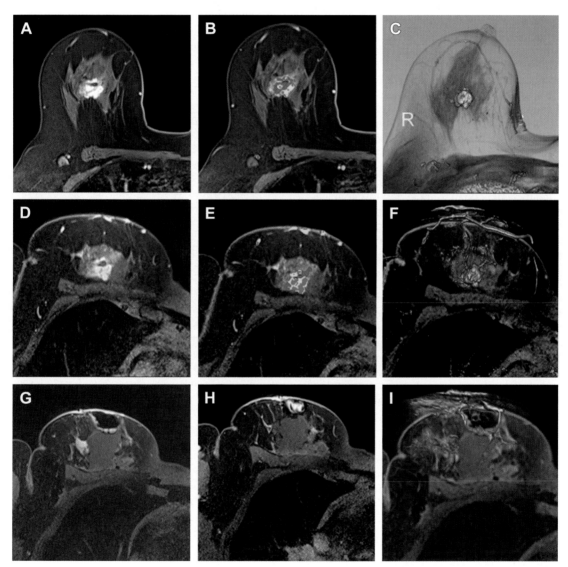

Fig. 7. The first lumpectomy procedure in the AMIGO suite. Diagnostic imaging: (A) first postcontrast image showing the rapidly enhancing tumor; (B) CADstream output showing regions of enhancement with subsequent washout (red), plateau (yellow), and persistent (blue) signal intensity; (C) three-dimensional volume-rendered image showing the tumor and the breast outline. Preprocedural imaging: (D) first postcontrast image showing the tumor in the supine position; (E) CADstream output obtained intraoperatively showing the segmented tumor; (F) three-dimensional volume-rendered image showing the tumor in the supine surgical position. Postprocedural imaging: (G) first postcontrast image showing the surgical cavity filled with saline immediately after BCS; (H) CADstream output showing no enhancing remnant tumor; (I) three-dimensional volume-rendered image showing the surgical cavity.

AMIGO suite.[5] On the day of surgery, the patient undergoes wire localization of the tumor with an MR imaging conditional wire. A sentinel lymph node biopsy and a standard lumpectomy are performed in the AMIGO suite, followed by saline placement in the cavity and temporary closure of the breast to limit MR imaging artifact by air-tissue susceptibility mismatch. MR imaging–visible fiducial markers are used to mark the superior and inferior margins of the surgical cavity. The MR scanner enters the operating room, and is positioned over the supine patient on the surgical table. The intraoperative MR imaging is done using a Siemens cardiac (32 channel) coil with foam cushion pads placed under the coil to prevent excessive pressure. The precontrast and postcontrast VIBE images are obtained with the intubated patient in breath hold with the anesthesiologist's assistance. The contract-enhanced sequences are obtained with additional delay times to account for the reduced perfusion immediately following surgery.

Seven patients with breast cancer were evaluated with prone diagnostic and supine preprocedural dynamic contrast-enhanced MR imaging as part of the phase I clinical trial investigating intraoperative MR imaging for BCT margin assessment in the AMIGO suite. Sixty-five geometric, structural, and heterogeneity metrics were computed including volume, surface area, compactness, maximum three-dimensional diameter, and sphericity. Distance of the tumor center from nipple, chest wall, and skin were computed. The initial results suggest that there is a substantial difference in tumor deformity based on the patient's position (prone vs supine). Tumors measure larger in volume and surface area, and closer to the nipple and chest wall on supine than on prone images, underscoring the importance of preoperative supine MR imaging, which simulates the intraoperative position of the breast.[92]

The AMIGO trial demonstrated that there is no significant enhancement from bleeding vessels in an operative field if adequate hemostasis is obtained. However, fiducials are needed for accurate orientation of the margins (**Fig. 7**).[93]

SUMMARY

Breast MR imaging is the most sensitive examination for breast cancer detection and has become a well-established screening method supplementing mammography in high-risk women. MR imaging has been suggested as an adjunctive for identifying the extent of breast carcinoma and for guiding treatment planning. Currently, MR imaging for preoperative evaluation of disease extent in newly diagnosed breast cancer is controversial.

REFERENCES

1. Saslow D, Boetes C, Burke W, et al. American Cancer Society guidelines for breast screening with MRI as an adjunct to mammography. CA Cancer J Clin 2007;57(2):75–89.
2. Solin LJ, Orel SG, Hwang WT, et al. Relationship of breast magnetic resonance imaging to outcome after breast-conservation treatment with radiation for women with early-stage invasive breast carcinoma or ductal carcinoma in situ. J Clin Oncol 2008; 26(3):386–91.
3. Waljee JF, Hu ES, Newman LA, et al. Predictors of re-excision among women undergoing breast-conserving surgery for cancer. Ann Surg Oncol 2008;15(5):1297–303.
4. Menes TS, Tartter PI, Bleiweiss I, et al. The consequence of multiple re-excisions to obtain clear lumpectomy margins in breast cancer patients. Ann Surg Oncol 2005;12(11):881–5.
5. Golshan M, Sagara Y, Wexelman B, et al. Pilot study to evaluate feasibility of image-guided breast-conserving therapy in the advanced multimodal image-guided operating (AMIGO) suite. Ann Surg Oncol 2014;21(10):3356–7.
6. ACR Practice Parameter for the Performance of Contrast-Enhanced Magnetic Resonance Imaging (MRI) of the Breast. 2014. Available at: http://www.acr.org/~/media/2a0eb28eb59041e2825179afb72ef624.pdf. Accessed March 20, 2015.
7. Meissnitzer M, Dershaw DD, Lee CH, et al. Targeted ultrasound of the breast in women with abnormal MRI findings for whom biopsy has been recommended. AJR Am J Roentgenol 2009;193(4):1025–9.
8. Abe H, Schmidt RA, Shah RN, et al. MR-directed ("second-look") ultrasound examination for breast lesions detected initially on MRI: MR and sonographic findings. AJR Am J Roentgenol 2010; 194(2):370–7.
9. Noroozian M, Gombos EC, Chikarmane S, et al. Factors that impact the duration of MRI-guided core needle biopsy. AJR Am J Roentgenol 2010;194(2): W150–7.
10. Schrading S, Simon B, Braun M, et al. MRI-guided breast biopsy: influence of choice of vacuum biopsy system on the mode of biopsy of MRI-only suspicious breast lesions. AJR Am J Roentgenol 2010; 194(6):1650–7.
11. Li J, Dershaw DD, Lee CH, et al. MRI follow-up after concordant, histologically benign diagnosis of breast lesions sampled by MRI-guided biopsy. AJR Am J Roentgenol 2009;193(3):850–5.
12. Han BK, Schnall MD, Orel SG, et al. Outcome of MRI-guided breast biopsy. AJR Am J Roentgenol 2008;191(6):1798–804.
13. Ghate SV, Rosen EL, Soo MS, et al. MRI-guided vacuum-assisted breast biopsy with a handheld

portable biopsy system. AJR Am J Roentgenol 2006;186(6):1733–6.

14. van den Bosch MA, Daniel BL, Pal S, et al. MRI-guided needle localization of suspicious breast lesions: results of a freehand technique. Eur Radiol 2006;16(8):1811–7.

15. Liberman L, Bracero N, Morris E, et al. MRI-guided 9-gauge vacuum-assisted breast biopsy: initial clinical experience. AJR Am J Roentgenol 2005;185(1): 183–93.

16. Yeh ED, Georgian-Smith D, Raza S, et al. Positioning in breast MR imaging to optimize image quality. Radiographics 2014;34(1):E1–17.

17. Lehman CD, Deperi ER, Peacock S, et al. Clinical experience with MRI-guided vacuum-assisted breast biopsy. AJR Am J Roentgenol 2005;184(6): 1782–7.

18. Lee JM, Kaplan JB, Murray MP, et al. Imaging histologic discordance at MRI-guided 9-gauge vacuum-assisted breast biopsy. AJR Am J Roentgenol 2007;189(4):852–9.

19. Lee JM, Kaplan JB, Murray MP, et al. Underestimation of DCIS at MRI-guided vacuum-assisted breast biopsy. AJR Am J Roentgenol 2007; 189(2):468–74.

20. Liberman L, Holland AE, Marjan D, et al. Underestimation of atypical ductal hyperplasia at MRI-guided 9-gauge vacuum-assisted breast biopsy. AJR Am J Roentgenol 2007;188(3):684–90.

21. Carlson JW, Birdwell RL, Gombos EC, et al. MRI-directed, wire-localized breast excisions: incidence of malignancy and recommendations for pathologic evaluation. Hum Pathol 2007;38(12):1754–9.

22. Mauri D, Pavlidis N, Ioannidis JP. Neoadjuvant versus adjuvant systemic treatment in breast cancer: a meta-analysis. J Natl Cancer Inst 2005; 97(3):188–94.

23. Chen AM, Meric-Bernstam F, Hunt KK, et al. Breast conservation after neoadjuvant chemotherapy: the MD Anderson Cancer Center experience. J Clin Oncol 2004;22(12):2303–12.

24. Fisher B, Bryant J, Wolmark N, et al. Effect of preoperative chemotherapy on the outcome of women with operable breast cancer. J Clin Oncol 1998; 16(8):2672–85.

25. Wolmark N, Wang J, Mamounas E, et al. Preoperative chemotherapy in patients with operable breast cancer: nine-year results from National Surgical Adjuvant Breast and Bowel Project B-18. J Natl Cancer Inst Monogr 2001;(30):96–102.

26. Niu L, Wu B, Xu K. Cryosurgery for breast fibroadenomas. Gland Surg 2012;1(2):128–31.

27. Littrup PJ, Jallad B, Chandiwala-Mody P, et al. Cryotherapy for breast cancer: a feasibility study without excision. J Vasc Interv Radiol 2009;20(10):1329–41.

28. Rieke V, Butts Pauly K. MR thermometry. J Magn Reson Imaging 2008;27(2):376–90.

29. Niu L, Mu F, Zhang C, et al. Cryotherapy protocols for metastatic breast cancer after failure of radical surgery. Cryobiology 2013;67(1):17–22.

30. Rabin Y, Coleman R, Mordohovich D, et al. A new cryosurgical device for controlled freezing. Cryobiology 1996;33(1):93–105.

31. Sabel MS. Cryoablation as a replacement for surgical resection in early stage breast cancer. Curr Breast Cancer Rep 2011;3(2):109–16.

32. Pfleiderer SO, Freesmeyer MG, Marx C, et al. Cryotherapy of breast cancer under ultrasound guidance: initial results and limitations. Eur Radiol 2002;12(12):3009–14.

33. Morin J, Traoré A, Dionne G, et al. Magnetic resonance-guided percutaneous cryosurgery of breast carcinoma: technique and early clinical results. Can J Surg 2004;47(5):347–51.

34. Pusztaszeri M, Vlastos G, Kinkel K, et al. Histopathological study of breast cancer and normal breast tissue after magnetic resonance-guided cryotherapy ablation. Cryobiology 2007;55(1):44–51.

35. Tuncali K, Morrison PR, Winalski CS, et al. MRI-guided percutaneous cryotherapy for soft-tissue and bone metastases: initial experience. AJR Am J Roentgenol 2007;189(1):232–9.

36. Tozaki M, Fukuma E, Suzuki T, et al. Ultrasound-guided cryoablation of invasive ductal carcinoma inside the MR room. Magn Reson Med Sci 2010;9(1): 31–6.

37. Thrall DE, Rosner GL, Azuma C, et al. Using units of CEM 43 degrees C T90, local hyperthermia thermal dose can be delivered as prescribed. Int J Hyperthermia 2000;16(5):415–28.

38. Hynynen K, McDannold N, Mulkern RV, et al. Temperature monitoring in fat with MRI. Magn Reson Med 2000;43(6):901–4.

39. Sprinkhuizen SM, Konings MK, van der Bom MJ, et al. Temperature-induced tissue susceptibility changes lead to significant temperature errors in PRFS-based MR thermometry during thermal interventions. Magn Reson Med 2010;64(5):1360–72.

40. Zhang Q, Chung YC, Lewin JS, et al. A method for simultaneous RF ablation and MRI. J Magn Reson Imaging 1998;8(1):110–4.

41. van den Bosch M, Daniel B, Rieke V, et al. MRI-guided radiofrequency ablation of breast cancer: preliminary clinical experience. J Magn Reson Imaging 2008;27(1):204–8.

42. Lewin JS, Nour SG, Connell CF, et al. Phase II clinical trial of interactive MR imaging-guided interstitial radiofrequency thermal ablation of primary kidney tumors: initial experience. Radiology 2004;232(3): 835–45.

43. van Hillegersberg R, van Staveren HJ, Kort WJ, et al. Interstitial Nd:YAG laser coagulation with a cylindrical diffusing fiber tip in experimental liver metastases. Lasers Surg Med 1994;14(2):124–38.

44. Lai LM, Hall-Craggs MA, Mumtaz H, et al. Interstitial laser photocoagulation for fibroadenomas of the breast. Breast 1999;8(2):89–94.

45. Harms S, Mumtaz H, Hronas T, et al. MRI directed interstitial thermal ablation of breast fibroadenomas. Hoboken (NJ): Wiley &Sons, Inc; 1999.

46. Mumtaz H, Hall-Craggs MA, Wotherspoon A, et al. Laser therapy for breast cancer: MR imaging and histopathologic correlation. Radiology 1996;200(3): 651–8.

47. Dowlatshahi K, Fan M, Gould VE, et al. Stereotactically guided laser therapy of occult breast tumors: work-in-progress report. Arch Surg 2000;135(11): 1345–52.

48. Dowlatshahi K, Francescatti DS, Bloom KJ. Laser therapy for small breast cancers. Am J Surg 2002; 184(4):359–63.

49. Vogl TJ, Mack MG, Straub R, et al. MR-guided laser-induced thermotherapy with a cooled power laser system: a case report of a patient with a recurrent carcinoid metastasis in the breast. Eur Radiol 2002;12(Suppl 3):S101–4.

50. Harms SE. Percutaneous ablation of breast lesions by radiologists and surgeons. Breast Dis 2001;13: 67–75.

51. Hynynen K, Freund WR, Cline HE, et al. A clinical, noninvasive, MR imaging-monitored ultrasound surgery method. Radiographics 1996;16(1):185–95.

52. Hynynen K, Pomeroy O, Smith DN, et al. MR imaging-guided focused ultrasound surgery of fibroadenomas in the breast: a feasibility study. Radiology 2001;219(1):176–85.

53. Huber PE, Jenne JW, Rastert R, et al. A new noninvasive approach in breast cancer therapy using magnetic resonance imaging-guided focused ultrasound surgery. Cancer Res 2001;61(23): 8441–7.

54. Gianfelice D, Khiat A, Boulanger Y, et al. Feasibility of magnetic resonance imaging-guided focused ultrasound surgery as an adjunct to tamoxifen therapy in high-risk surgical patients with breast carcinoma. J Vasc Interv Radiol 2003;14(10):1275–82.

55. Gianfelice D, Khiat A, Amara M, et al. MR imaging-guided focused ultrasound surgery of breast cancer: correlation of dynamic contrast-enhanced MRI with histopathologic findings. Breast Cancer Res Treat 2003;82(2):93–101.

56. Zippel DB, Papa MZ. The use of MR imaging guided focused ultrasound in breast cancer patients; a preliminary phase one study and review. Breast Cancer 2005;12(1):32–8.

57. Gianfelice D, Khiat A, Amara M, et al. MR imaging-guided focused US ablation of breast cancer: histopathologic assessment of effectiveness– initial experience. Radiology 2003;227(3):849–55.

58. Furusawa H, Namba K, Thomsen S, et al. Magnetic resonance-guided focused ultrasound surgery of breast cancer: reliability and effectiveness. J Am Coll Surg 2006;203(1):54–63.

59. Furusawa H, Yasuda Y. Magnetic resonance image guided focused ultrasound surgery of early breast cancer: efficacy and safety in excisionless study. Cancer Res 2009;69(24):suppl-3.

60. Payne A, Merrill R, Minalga E, et al. Design and characterization of a laterally mounted phased-array transducer breast-specific MRgHIFU device with integrated 11-channel receiver array. Med Phys 2012; 39(3):1552–60.

61. Todd N, Diakite M, Payne A, et al. In vivo evaluation of multi-echo hybrid PRF/T1 approach for temperature monitoring during breast MR-guided focused ultrasound surgery treatments. Magn Reson Med 2014;72(3):793–9.

62. Liberman L, Morris EA, Dershaw DD, et al. MR imaging of the ipsilateral breast in women with percutaneously proven breast cancer. AJR Am J Roentgenol 2003;180(4):901–10.

63. Houssami N, Turner R, Morrow M. Preoperative magnetic resonance imaging in breast cancer: meta-analysis of surgical outcomes. Ann Surg 2013;257(2):249–55.

64. Houssami N, Ciatto S, Macaskill P, et al. Accuracy and surgical impact of magnetic resonance imaging in breast cancer staging: systematic review and meta-analysis in detection of multifocal and multicentric cancer. J Clin Oncol 2008;26(19):3248–58.

65. Holland R, Veling SH, Mravunac M, et al. Histologic multifocality of Tis, T1-2 breast carcinomas. Implications for clinical trials of breast-conserving surgery. Cancer 1985;56(5):979–90.

66. Schelfout K, Van Goethem M, Kersschot E, et al. Contrast-enhanced MR imaging of breast lesions and effect on treatment. Eur J Surg Oncol 2004; 30(5):501–7.

67. Bilimoria KY, Cambic A, Hansen NM, et al. Evaluating the impact of preoperative breast magnetic resonance imaging on the surgical management of newly diagnosed breast cancers. Arch Surg 2007; 142(5):441–5 [discussion: 445–7].

68. Fischer U, Kopka L, Grabbe E. Breast carcinoma: effect of preoperative contrast-enhanced MR imaging on the therapeutic approach. Radiology 1999; 213(3):881–8.

69. Smitt MC, Nowels KW, Zdeblick MJ, et al. The importance of the lumpectomy surgical margin status in long-term results of breast conservation. Cancer 1995;76(2):259–67.

70. Turnbull L, Brown S, Harvey I, et al. Comparative effectiveness of MRI in breast cancer (COMICE) trial: a randomised controlled trial. Lancet 2010; 375(9714):563–71.

71. Peters NH, van Esser S, van den Bosch MA, et al. Preoperative MRI and surgical management in patients with nonpalpable breast cancer: the

MONET - randomised controlled trial. Eur J Cancer 2011;47(6):879–86.

72. Harlow SP, Krag DN, Ames SE, et al. Intraoperative ultrasound localization to guide surgical excision of nonpalpable breast carcinoma. J Am Coll Surg 1999;189(3):241–6.

73. van Riet YE, Jansen FH, van Beek M, et al. Localization of non-palpable breast cancer using a radiolabelled titanium seed. Br J Surg 2010;97(8):1240–5.

74. Cox CE, Whitworth P, Themar-Geck M, et al. Pilot study of a passive non-radioactive electromagnetic wave technology to localize non-palpable breast lesions. 2014. Available at: http://www.ciannamedical.com/wp/wp-content/uploads/2014/12/2014-SABCS-Poster.pdf.

75. Sanchez C, Brem RF, McSwain AP, et al. Factors associated with re-excision in patients with early-stage breast cancer treated with breast conservation therapy. Am Surg 2010;76(3):331–4.

76. Mullenix PS, Cuadrado DG, Steele SR, et al. Secondary operations are frequently required to complete the surgical phase of therapy in the era of breast conservation and sentinel lymph node biopsy. Am J Surg 2004;187(5):643–6.

77. Boughey JC, Peintinger F, Meric-Bernstam F, et al. Impact of preoperative versus postoperative chemotherapy on the extent and number of surgical procedures in patients treated in randomized clinical trials for breast cancer. Ann Surg 2006;244(3):464–70.

78. Fleming FJ, Kavanagh D, Crotty TB, et al. Factors affecting metastases to non-sentinel lymph nodes in breast cancer. J Clin Pathol 2004;57(1):73–6.

79. Bani MR, Lux MP, Heusinger K, et al. Factors correlating with reexcision after breast-conserving therapy. Eur J Surg Oncol 2009;35(1):32–7.

80. O'Sullivan MJ, Li T, Freedman G, et al. The effect of multiple reexcisions on the risk of local recurrence after breast conserving surgery. Ann Surg Oncol 2007;14(11):3133–40.

81. Camp ER, McAuliffe PF, Gilroy JS, et al. Minimizing local recurrence after breast conserving therapy using intraoperative shaved margins to determine pathologic tumor clearance. J Am Coll Surg 2005;201(6):855–61.

82. Kobbermann A, Unzeitig A, Xie XJ, et al. Impact of routine cavity shave margins on breast cancer re-excision rates. Ann Surg Oncol 2011;18(5):1349–55.

83. Sabel MS, Rogers K, Griffith K, et al. Residual disease after re-excision lumpectomy for close margins. J Surg Oncol 2009;99(2):99–103.

84. Cowen D, Houvenaeghel G, Bardou V, et al. Local and distant failures after limited surgery with positive margins and radiotherapy for node-negative breast cancer. Int J Radiat Oncol Biol Phys 2000;47(2):305–12.

85. Clarke M, Collins R, Darby S, et al. Effects of radiotherapy and of differences in the extent of surgery for early breast cancer on local recurrence and 15-year survival: an overview of the randomised trials. Lancet 2005;366(9503):2087–106.

86. Deutsch M, Flickinger JC. Patient characteristics and treatment factors affecting cosmesis following lumpectomy and breast irradiation. Am J Clin Oncol 2003;26(4):350–3.

87. Cochrane RA, Valasiadou P, Wilson AR, et al. Cosmesis and satisfaction after breast-conserving surgery correlates with the percentage of breast volume excised. Br J Surg 2003;90(12):1505–9.

88. Heil J, Breitkreuz K, Golatta M, et al. Do reexcisions impair aesthetic outcome in breast conservation surgery? Exploratory analysis of a prospective cohort study. Ann Surg Oncol 2012;19(2):541–7.

89. Risholm P, Golby AJ, Wells W 3rd. Multimodal image registration for preoperative planning and image-guided neurosurgical procedures. Neurosurg Clin N Am 2011;22(2):197–206, viii.

90. Gould SW, Lamb G, Lomax D, et al. Interventional MR-guided excisional biopsy of breast lesions. J Magn Reson Imaging 1998;8(1):26–30.

91. Hirose M, Kacher DF, Smith DN, et al. Feasibility of MR imaging-guided breast lumpectomy for malignant tumors in a 0.5-T open-configuration MR imaging system. Acad Radiol 2002;9(8):933–41.

92. Jagadeesan J, Golshan M, Narayan V, et al. Gombos, Clinical impact and quantification of prone to supine position in breast MRI 2015.

93. Gombos E, Jagadeesan J, Golshan M, et al. Intraprocedural high field MRI imaging in breast conserving surgery: initial clinical experience. Abstract 129. Proceedings of the 9th International MRI Symposium, Boston, MA, September 22–23, 2012.

Magnetic Resonance Imaging–Guided Cardiac Interventions

Ehud J. Schmidt, PhD

KEYWORDS

• MR imaging • Cardiac • Interventions • Electrophysiology • Therapy • Outcomes • Acute ischemia

KEY POINTS

• Advantages of MR imaging for cardiac interventions include visualizing vessel lumen and wall anatomy, scar tissue, acute ischemia and hemorrhage.
• Therapeutic outcomes may be improved utilizing real-time MR monitoring.
• MR imaging–guided cardiac intervention is finally becoming a clinical reality, after years of technological development and preclinical testing.
• Cardiac electrophysiology (EP) is the first field for which clinical grade device development is complete and in which human clinical trials are currently underway.

INTRODUCTION

Specific issues that result from performing procedures inside the beating heart are as follows: (1) the complex and nonrigid respiratory and cardiac motion of the heart affects both MR imaging and MR imaging–guided navigation and (2) the lack of robustness of MR imaging, in tissues other than the lumen and wall of the major vessels, makes the imaging of small and moving vessels difficult.[1–10] A practical result of the current MR imaging limitations has been the concentration of efforts on regions where diagnostic cardiac MR imaging is more mature, namely, procedures in the greater cardiac vessels such as the ventricles and the atria.

With diagnostic cardiac MR imaging increasingly available in hospitals and clinics throughout the world, the most well-developed MR imaging–guided procedures are those in which the cardiac MR imaging is performed before or after the actual intervention, while the interventional procedure itself is performed in the classical X-ray-guided operating room (OR) or interventional suite. All commercial medical imaging equipment vendors now offer "X-MR suites," which are MR imaging scanners and X-ray interventional suites that share a transport table, facilitating patient transfer between the imaging and interventional modalities. Commercial image processing tools are also available from these vendors and from the major catheter companies, which allows transformation of the images from the MR imaging to the X-ray or OR frame of reference (which can also be the frame of reference of an interventional workstation with integrated electromagnetic positional tracking[11–16]). As a result, in preoperative planning of cardiac EP procedures, in valve repair procedures, and for implantable cardioverter-defibrillator (ICD) placement procedures, use of MR vascular and scar images has become routine. Excellent reviews on these subjects are available.[17–32]

This review focuses on intraoperative use of MR imaging during cardiovascular interventions. This field is clinically in its infancy. Present work is primarily dedicated to removing some of the major hurdles to its use, although several clinical efficacy studies have recently emerged. Prior reviews on this subject exist.[3,33–46]

E.J. Schmidt acknowledges funding from NIH U41-RR019703, NIH R03 EB013873-01A1, and AHA 10SDG261039. E.J. Schmidt receives research funding support from E-TROTZ Inc, St. Jude Medical, and Siemens Healthcare.
Radiology Department, Brigham and Women's Hospital, 221 Longwood Avenue, Room BRB 34C, Boston, MA 02115, USA
E-mail address: ESCHMIDT3@PARTNERS.ORG

Magn Reson Imaging Clin N Am 23 (2015) 563–577
http://dx.doi.org/10.1016/j.mric.2015.05.011
1064-9689/15/$

Although MR imaging–guided procedure development began with coronary intervention, the greatest effort today is on MR imaging–guided therapeutic cardiac EP, primarily using radiofrequency ablation. It is clear that MR imaging provides several imaging contrasts that are useful for the diagnosis of chronic (or temporally stable) cardiac disease. The ability to visualize fat, see scar tissue, detect fibrosis, separate edema and hemorrhage from myocardial tissue, visualize the vascular tree, and assess mechanical function are well-known advantages of MR imaging. In the context of intraoperative MR imaging, however, there is also a need to assess acute or temporally changing conditions. Understanding the appearance of pathologic conditions during the interventional procedure is an evolving field that may weigh heavily on the ultimate utility of MR imaging–guided procedures in the heart. Predicting the ultimate state of myocardium from its intraoperative appearance, where transient effects such as blood by-products, edema, hemorrhage, and reduced perfusion are prevalent, is a challenge that several research groups are currently addressing.

In addition, the need to provide solutions for emergency interventions inside the MR imaging suite is a challenge that must be resolved, because large patient populations are excluded from MR imaging–guided interventions because of the lack of equipment for rapidly detecting and treating cardiac events.

The most dramatic recent progress has been in the field of MR imaging–guided EP. (1) In Europe,[4–6,47] clinical trials are being carried out to assess the effectiveness of MR imaging–guided atrial ablation. (2) Several entrepreneurial companies, such as Imricor Medical Systems, Inc, and MRI Interventions, Inc, are developing MR imaging–compatible clinical grade EP catheters, sheathes, and guidewires in collaboration with major MR imaging vendors, such as Philips Healthcare and Siemens Healthcare. (3) It has been established that there is close agreement between the EP intracardiac voltage mapping as performed with commercial electroanatomic mapping (EAM) systems, such as the NavX-Velocity (St. Jude Medical, Inc, St Paul, MN, USA) or the CarTo3 (Biosense-Webster, Inc, Diamond Bar, CA, USA), and MR imaging–based late gadolinium enhancement (LGE) images in the case of chronic ischemic lesions.[48,49] (4) There are pioneering results on visualizing acute tissue necrosis using T1 or T2* mapping methods, which are critical to the use of MR imaging for monitoring the quality of ablation lesions in the intraoperative acute setting.[50–52]

TOPICS

Coronary Artery Interventions for the Diagnosis or Treatment of Coronary Artery Disease

Coronary artery disease (CAD) is one of the most frequent causes of patient morbidity. The common intervention for CAD is X-ray-fluoroscopy-guided angioplasty in which the culprit (partially or completely) occluded vessels are either opened by balloon expansion followed by stent placement or replaced with a grafted bypassing vessel.

There are several reasons for replacing X-ray as the modality used for procedural guidance. (1) X-rays can visualize only the vessel lumen and not the surrounding soft tissue such as the vessel wall; this reduces the clinician's ability to gauge the extent of injury to surrounding myocardial tissue during the procedure or the amount of restenosis that occurs afterward because of soft tissue regrowth. (2) When the coronary vessel is entirely occluded, chronic total occlusion (CTO), X-rays cannot visualize the occluded region because contrast cannot enter this region, which makes it difficult to guide a device to the proper location for opening the occlusion. Such poor visualization may result in vessel perforation. (3) The X-ray dose that clinicians carrying out coronary procedures are exposed to is quite high, which limits the number of procedures they perform. In addition, the heavy lead aprons clinicians wear to shield from radiation are a significant cause of back pain.

Another role for MR imaging guidance is to monitor the treatment of preexisting cardiac myocardial infarcts. Several innovative therapeutic strategies have been proposed to prevent the remodeling of the myocardium postinfarction and the ensuing progression to heart failure. There are also experimental therapies to induce the (re) growth of myocytes within the infarct such as the induction of specific pharmaceuticals, viruses, and stem cells. For these applications, MR imaging–guided therapy delivery is highly advantageous because of the following reasons. (1) MR imaging visualizes the infarct borders, including the inactive but perfused (stunned) myocardium that surrounds the necrotic area, identifying optimal regions for therapy delivery. (2) MR imaging can monitor the concentration of agents that enters into the injected region during the delivery process. (3) Longitudinal MR imaging can be used to assess the effectiveness of therapy, such as the improvement in myocardial mechanical function.

Coronary vascular access

In animal models, MR imaging–guided navigation through the arterial tree and into the coronary artery was performed early on,[53,54] using dedicated MR imaging–compatible guidewires and sheathes.

The invasive devices were visualized (1) passively, by virtue of their enhanced susceptibility to artifacts,[55] usually resulting in a hypointense appearance of the device on MR imaging; (2) semi-actively, by adding radiofrequency coils onto portions of the device[54,56] so that these regions appear hyperintense on MR imaging, or (3) actively, via microcoils placed on the device's shaft, combined with specific positional tracking sequences to detect the position of these coils.[57] Collectively, such procedures generally required collection of vascular roadmaps using MR angiography,[58] followed by navigation of the devices on these roadmaps by using imaging sequences that provided the position of the devices over time.

Building MR imaging–compatible coronary devices, such as guidewires and sheathes, was a serious challenge because coronary artery diameter is small (<2 mm) and its path tortuous, requiring the construction of small and highly flexible interventional devices. Commercial interventional devices for coronary use require the use of highly specialized materials and fabrication methods. In order to make the devices compatible for MR imaging, it was necessary to replace many of the conventionally used materials (such as stainless steel) with materials with inferior mechanical properties, which sometimes required use of larger dimensions in order to attain equivalent performance. SurgiVision, Inc (now MRI Interventions, Inc) built the first MR imaging–compatible guidewire, based on a simple radiofrequency coil design (the loopless antenna),[56] which was subsequently cleared for clinical use. Other devices were subsequently built by other groups.[57,59,60]

In most cases, the MR imaging–guided coronary procedures required much greater time to perform vascular navigation into the coronaries than equivalent X-ray procedures. More importantly, problems with the robustness of MR coronary imaging, such as high-resolution imaging of the lumen or wall of the coronaries, prevented capitalization on the advantages of MR imaging.

In opening coronary CTOs, extensive animal experimentation was performed,[61] and it was shown that MR imaging guidance has distinct advantages that could be captured with greater ease in occlusions in larger vessels.[62] From the scientific perspective, the coronary MR imaging procedures were very instructive. These procedures forced the development of novel MR imaging–compatible materials[60] and taught the field about the complex motion of the coronary

arteries.[57] At present, there are 2 companies, MaRVis Medical GmbH, Hannover, Germany, and Nano4imaging GmBH, Aachen, Germany, that are engaged in the construction and testing of MR imaging–compatible guidewires, so MR imaging–guided coronary intervention may soon be reexamined. Some of the devices that were developed for coronary intervention are used for less-complex vascular procedures, such as for MR imaging–guided carotid,[63,64] aortic, and peripheral interventions.

Ventricular access and therapy for coronary artery disease

Obtaining vascular access into the lumen of right ventricle or left ventricle (LV) was possible from the early days of MR imaging–guided intervention. As traversing the intra-atrial septum with MR imaging was difficult before the development of an MR imaging-compatible transseptal needle,[65] the left side of the heart was mostly accessed through the arterial vasculature.

Injection of therapeutic agents into the infarcted left ventricular wall was performed primarily by the National Heart, Lung, and Blood Institute[66–71] and Johns Hopkins[72–79] groups. Much of this work used MR imaging–compatible myocardial injection needles[68,80] for this purpose (**Fig. 1**). As initially the stem cells did not survive for a long time after implantation, methods were devised to feed and protect the stem cells in situ.[72,73,76,77,81]

In recent years, most myocardial injections have been performed using a combined X-ray and MR imaging (X-MR) suite, which allows for a faster procedure[81,82] and reduces the mechanical demands on the MR imaging–compatible myocardial injection needles.

Cardiac Electrophysiology Procedure for the Diagnosis and Treatment of Rhythm Disorders

Some of the pioneering work in MR imaging–guided cardiac interventions was directed at the treatment of EP disorders.[1,32] This focus resulted from multiple factors. (1) The incidence of ventricular and atrial rhythm disorders is growing rapidly, as the population ages, with the incidence of atrial fibrillation (AF) and ventricular tachycardia (VT) now approaching 4 million and half a million subjects, respectively, in the United States. (2) The pharmaceutical treatments of these diseases are not very effective and carry considerable side effects. (3) Despite the large increase in the number of ablative procedures for treating VT and AF, the success rate for such procedures, as measured by the lack of recurrence of syndromes, is only approximately 50% and 70%, respectively. Much of the failure is attributed to insufficient

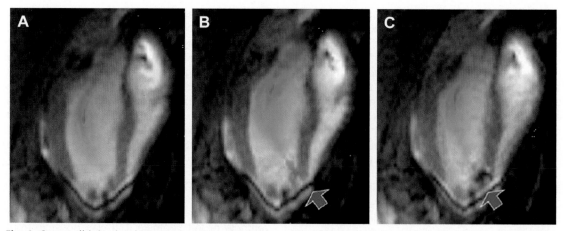

Fig. 1. Stem cell injection into a swine LV under MR imaging guidance. (*A*) Device is inside LV but not touching the wall; (*B*) contact with the apical wall of the LV. Red area denotes tip. (*C*) Injection into the wall. *Blue arrow* denotes area of injection. (*Courtesy of* Dr Robert J. Letterman, NIH-NHLBI Intramural Program, Bethesda, MD.)

ablation of the electrical circuits that cause the arrhythmias due to the creation of ablation lesions that are insufficiently deep or interconnected. (4) EP procedures form a major source of income for cardiology departments. There is great commercial interest in developing solutions, with several catheter companies developing clinical systems for diagnosing and treating rhythm disorders. (6) MR imaging of the ventricles has been a robust clinical technique for several years, and with the development of navigator echo methods, several MR imaging contrasts for use in the atrium are commercially available. When the above-mentioned facts are combined with the unique MR imaging intertissue contrasts, MR imaging guidance for EP procedures is quite attractive.

Use of MR imaging or computed tomographic (CT) imaging for preoperative planning, performed before VT or AF procedures, has become routine in the field. CT or MR angiography is used to map the cardiovascular luminal anatomy. When scar tissue from a prior infarct or previous ablations is present in the LV or left atrium (LA), performing preoperative LGE MR imaging to map the scar tissue provides distinct advantages. This technique can reduce the duration and increase the sensitivity of intracardiac EAM, the diagnostic portion of the EP procedure, by pointing to interventional electrophysiologists as to where, within the LV or the LA, they should go with the mapping catheters to map the pathology. This feature becomes extremely important when the scar tissue is located in regions that are difficult to access or contact with the EP mapping catheters. One example is when the scar tissue is located behind the papillary muscle in the LV[83] (**Fig. 2**). Another

important case is when the scar does not cover the entire width of the chamber wall (a nontransmural lesion),[48,84] where conventional catheter-based EAM requires extensive mapping to provide the scar dimensions. It has recently been shown that some of the LGE image characteristics (intensity, shape) observed in infarcts correlate extremely well with some EAM voltage characteristics (size and shape of voltage), enabling the prediction of the location of reentry circuits within the LV lesions, areas that should be ablated to prevent tachycardia[48] (**Fig. 3**).

Ventricular Diagnostic and Therapeutic Interventions

This section focuses on the use of interventional methods to diagnose and treat, with radio-frequency ablation, inducible VT, the cause of sudden cardiac death. In brief, the diagnostic approach requires finding the regions within the LV (or right ventricle) where the errant electrical circuits can occur during a cardiac event. The common practice is to move along the LV walls with an EP catheter whose location is identified by the EAM system, deliver a voltage to the wall (pace), and use a second EP catheter to measure the tissue electrical response, which is recorded by the EAM system in the form of an intracardiac electrocardiographic trace (EGM) that is then associated with the specific point on the LV wall. If a strong response is obtained when pacing is performed at a certain location, a potential aberrant circuit is identified. At the end of EAM mapping, the regions identified as possible sources of VT are ablated. These areas can be along the borders of, or within, the scar tissue, which was

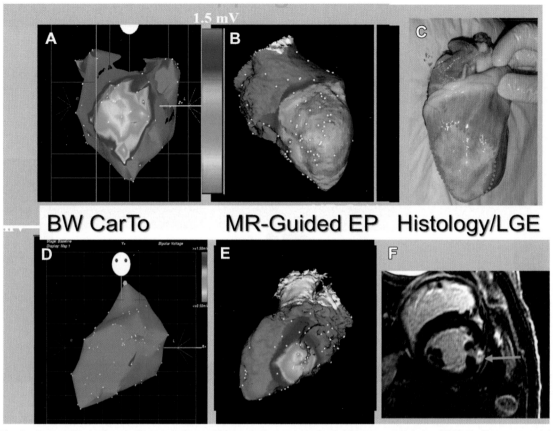

Fig. 2. Comparison of mapping an infarcted swine using a commercial Biosense-Webster (BW) CarTo system with mapping performed in an MR imaging scanner using LGE guidance. (*A–C*) Large infarct. The CarTo map (*A*) is acceptable, but the MR imaging–guided map (*B*) is obtained faster and shows more detail around the infarct, which is similar to gross histologic shape of the infarct (*C*). *Red dotted* line denotes infarct borders. A small infarct behind the papillary wall. The CarTo map (*D*) missed the infarct entirely because it was hard to find with the mapping catheter, whereas the MR imaging–guided map (*E*), with a catheter guided to the infarct by the LGE image (*F*), depicted it nicely. (*Courtesy of* Dr Ehud J. Schmidt, Harvard University, Boston, MA.)

left over after the heart attack that the subject incurred. After each ablation, catheter-induced pacing is performed, and if the previously recorded EGM tissue response is no longer observed, it is assumed that the source of VT has been terminated. However, this is not always the case. Recurrence occurs if some live circuits are not treated or if some circuits are insufficiently ablated, so that the conducting elements (chains of myocytes) reconnect when transient effects resulting from the ablation (edema, hemorrhage) recede.

Intraoperative use of MR imaging improves the localization of the aberrant circuits, and it can also assist in monitoring the radiofrequency ablation process, by determining that the lesions created are sufficient to prevent recurrence of inducible VT.

Although LV interventions are easier to perform from the MR imaging perspective, they primarily treat life-threatening diseases such as sudden

cardiac death. As a result, a LV ablation procedure typically requires a high standard of physiologic monitoring, such as for rapid detection of acute ischemia, via the clear observation of ECG S-T segment elevation, and/or for the rapid detection of ventricular fibrillation. There is also a need for MR imaging–compatible means for rapid resuscitation, principally based on a defibrillation unit that can be rapidly used within the MR imaging suite. An additional issue with performing ventricular interventions is that many of the LV patients already have implanted pacemakers or ICDs. Although increasing numbers of MR imaging sites are performing diagnostic cardiac MR imaging on such patients,[85,86] most of the sites shy away from the increased procedural risk that may be incurred because of malfunctioning of these devices inside the MRI.

As the required monitoring and resuscitation devices are not yet available, LV EP therapeutic

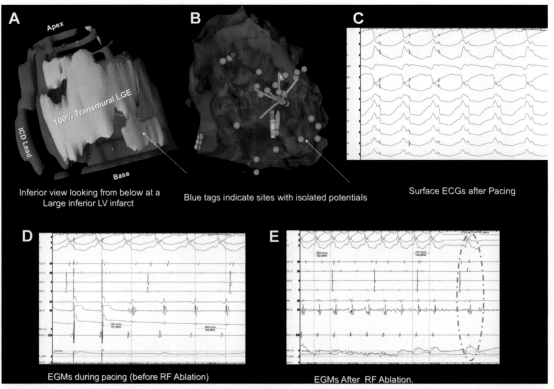

Fig. 3. Human case of ischemic cardiomyopathy treated for possible inducible tachycardia. (*A*) The intensity and geometric shape of LGE lesions were used to construct a map of the LV (note that the apex of the heart is at the top) that shows the regions of scar and their transmurality. The region at the bottom right (*white arrow*) was suspected as the source of inducible tachycardia, based on its LGE appearance. (*B*) The LV was mapped, and indeed, high voltages were seen in this region. When this area was paced (*C*), very-high-rate tachycardia (heart rate of 150 beats per minute) was observed on all the surface ECG leads and on the intracardiac EGMs (*D*). Following radiofrequency (RF) ablation (*E*), the tachycardia was terminated (*dotted red area*) and the patient returned to a lower heart rate. (*Courtesy of* Dr Saman Nazarian, Johns Hopkins University, Baltimore, MD.)

interventions have only been performed in animals. MR imaging–compatible 12-lead ECG and defibrillation systems are currently under development,[87,88] so human MR imaging–guided ventricular ablation procedures may begin soon.

An integrated MR imaging–guided EP laboratory, which included many of the devices and visualization tools required for the performance of interventions inside the MR imaging, was constructed in the mid-2000s as a collaboration between General Electric and St. Jude Medical[83,89] and installed at Massachusetts General Hospital. MR imaging–compatible radiofrequency ablation generators, ablation catheters, and sheathes were developed at that time. Animal interventions were performed, demonstrating the clinical advantages of MR imaging–guided EP ablation. One of the chief novelties of the system was use of MR-tracking-based catheter positional localization, which required that the entire toolset (**Fig. 4**) be equipped with MR-tracking coils. MR tracking provided catheter navigation capabilities of a similar

spatial resolution and temporal rate (**Fig. 5**) as available in the conventional EP laboratory with EAM mapping systems, which rely on electromagnetic tracking. Without MR tracking, navigation inside the MR imaging relied on real-time MR imaging,[3,10,90] which is of a substantially lower spatial and temporal resolution than that possible with commercial EAM systems.

A short time later, the proton resonance shift temperature mapping method was applied during EP ablation in the LV of dog models[91] in order to record the temperatures of the ablated tissues over time (**Fig. 6**). This method has enormous promise because it determines the thermal dose delivered to a given tissue region. Temperature mapping provides tool to discriminate between tissues that have been sufficiently ablated so that they become necrotic and those tissues that have received insufficient thermal dose, which primarily creates transient edema so that the arrhythmia circuits later reconnect, causing recurrence. There are challenges to the application of

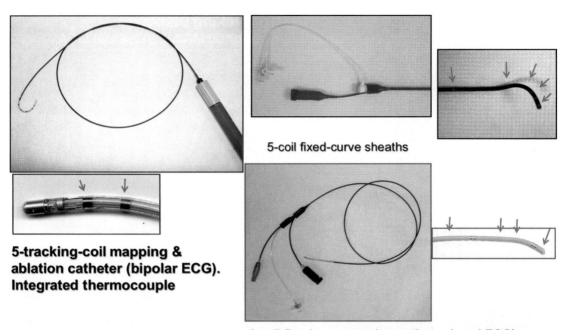

Fig. 4. MR imaging–compatible EP tool set, which can be positionally tracked inside the MR imaging scanner. Toolkit was constructed for the first integrated MR imaging–guided EP suite. Red arrows show microcoils placed on the devices that are tracking them using MR-tracking pulse sequence. This method is used by all the vendors and used in the human trials. (*Courtesy of* Dale Just, St. Jude Medical Inc, St Paul, MN.)

temperature mapping in the human heart, but these may be surmountable.[92]

Atrial Interventions

This section focuses on the use of interventional methods to diagnose and treat, with radiofrequency ablation, paroxysmal and persistent AF. In brief, the diagnostic approach requires finding the regions within the LA where reentry electrical circuits occur. The primary suspect regions are the entries (or ostia) of the 4 pulmonary veins (PVs) into the LA and the top (roof) of the LA.

Common practice is, therefore, to navigate to the PV ostia with an EP catheter, whose location is identified by the EAM system, and map the voltages on the wall. The EP catheters are then moved to other locations until the entire LA wall is mapped. At the end of the EAM mapping phase, the regions that are identified as possible sources of AF are ablated. Circular (circumferential) ablations are performed at all the ostia. To validate that each circumferential ablation is complete and that there are no gaps, one EP catheter is placed inside the respective PV, while the other is placed on the other side of the ablation lesion, that is, just inside the LA. Pacing is performed from the catheter inside the PV, and if no ECG trace is picked up by the second catheter, the ostia is considered isolated.

It is desired that each reentry circuit that contributes to AF be permanently destroyed by the ablation, but this is not always the case. Recurrence can occur if some live circuits are not treated or if some circuits are insufficiently ablated or insufficiently connected (**Fig. 7**) so that the conducting elements (chains of myocytes) reconnect once transient effects resulting from the ablation recede.

Intraoperative MR imaging can assist in monitoring the radiofrequency ablation process by determining that the LA lesions that are created are sufficiently deep and interconnected in order to prevent recurrence of AF.

MR imaging–guided LA interventions were enabled by the development of navigated 3-dimensional LGE imaging (3D LGE)[93,94] that allowed visualizing the scar resulting from radiofrequency ablation in the thin (2–3 mm diameter) atrial wall. Later, it was shown[12] that 3D LGE could be used to visualize gaps in atrial ablation lesions remaining after radiofrequency ablation that resulted in the recurrence of AF in humans (**Fig. 8**). This finding provided an important tool for preoperative use of 3D LGE in the treatment of cases of AF recurrence, constituting approximately 30% of procedures at some sites.[41,95,96]

However, 3D LGE, which measured fibrosis in the chronic scar, proved to be an imperfect tool

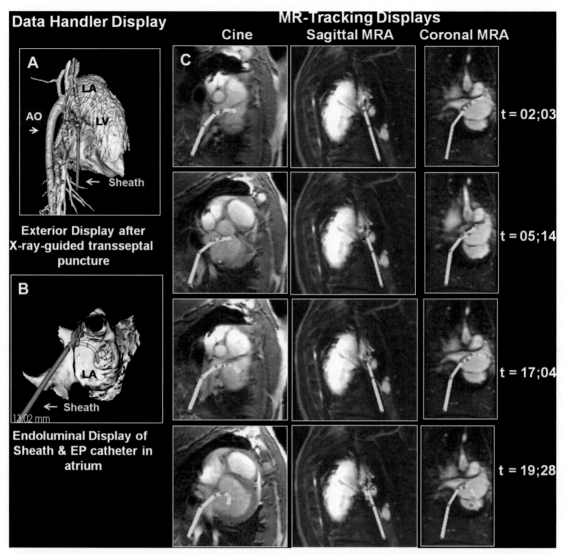

Fig. 5. With a tracked EP toolkit, monitoring the intervention is quite easy because the electrophysiologists visualizing EAM mapping are accustomed to its use. Multiple devices are visualized during manipulation either on a 3-dimensional rendering of anatomy (*A, B*) or on multiple directional or multiple contrast (*C*) viewports. Catheters manipulated are those of **Fig. 4**. AO, Aorta; MRA, MR angiography. (*Courtesy of* Dr Richard P. Mallozzi, The Phantom Laboratory Inc, Salem, NY.)

for assessing the degree of tissue necrosis in the acute phase of injury, such as a few minutes after radiofrequency ablation. During acute injury, the ablated region is surrounded by edema and hemorrhage so that the hyperintense signal seen in 3D LGE tended to overestimate the size of the ablated lesion[47,96–98] compared with the lesion size in the chronic phase, after the edema had receded. There was some evidence that lack of hyperenhancement in the LGE images in the first minutes after ablation was correlated to some extent with the degree of necrosis,[97] but this was not a reliable marker to determine whether the

degree of radiofrequency ablation that had been applied was sufficient.

There are recent publications that suggest that this issue may be resolved[50,52,99,100] (**Fig. 9**). It seems that provision of sufficient thermal dose to myocardial tissue changes the hemoglobin in the cells into a paramagnetic substance. This paramagnetic iron oxide acts as a contrast agent, shortening the T1 of the myocardial tissue. As a result, it may be possible to use quantitative T1 mapping sequences to differentiate between sufficiently and insufficiently ablated atrial (or ventricular) tissue (see **Fig. 9**).

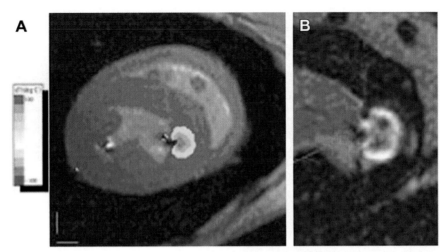

Fig. 6. Temperature mapping of a radiofrequency ablation lesion in a dog model. (*A*) The temperature profile of the lesion that corresponds closely (*B*) to its appearance on LGE images obtained after the ablation is shown. (*Courtesy of* Dr Henry R. Halperin, Johns Hopkins University, Baltimore, MD.)

A human clinical trial of MR imaging–guided atrial flutter ablation, a relatively simple EP procedure in which a single ablation line is drawn, using CE-approved (European Union medical device regulatory authority) equipment developed by Imricor Medical Systems, Inc, together with Philips Healthcare, began in 2012 in Germany. The first phase of the trial, which relied on passive tracking of the EP catheters, was disappointing because it resulted in incomplete MR imaging–based termination of the atrial flutter in most patients.[6] A subsequent study, using active MR-tracked catheters, is now being performed. This study has had better results,[4] with most of the patients reporting complete termination of the flutter. It is expected that future trials will progress to treating AF.

Congenital Procedures (Pediatric Disorders)

There has long been interest in performing interventions in children using MR imaging guidance. This interest is a result of the more damaging effects of X-rays on children, such as the increased incidence of tumors. There was hope that congenital conditions that required interventions in the pulmonary arteries (PAs), such as stenting, could be performed in the MR imaging environment with minimal device development because many of the commercial catheters used were inherently safe for MR imaging. In addition, a major advantage resulted from the ability of phase-contrast MR imaging to noninvasively measure flow rates and pressure gradients,[101,102] replacing the invasive catheters previously required.

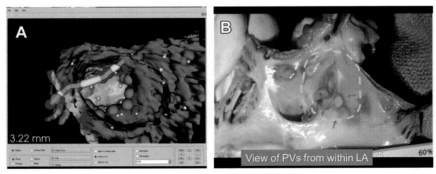

Fig. 7. Incomplete AF ablation in a swine model. (*A*) Three-dimensional rendering of a PV as seen from the LA, showing wall voltages before ablation (*wall colors*). MR-tracked catheter is shown creating lesions (*red balls*), showing areas where lesions were placed. (*B*) Histologic view of the same PV (*yellow dashed line*). Red arrows show the lesions actually created. Note that fewer lesions were actually created and some are not interconnected. (*Courtesy of* Dr Ehud J. Schmidt, Harvard University, Boston, MA.)

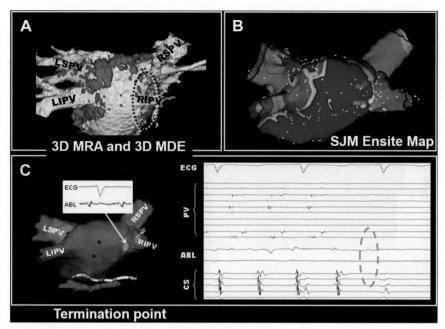

Fig. 8. First human AF recurrence treatment using MR imaging information. (*A*) Three-dimensional navigated LGE (*red overlays*) shows gaps in right inferior PV (*yellow dotted region*). (*B*) EAM mapping using St. Jude Medical (SJM) NavX shows the same region. (*C*) EP catheter brought to the location was used to ablate the region, resulting in the termination of fibrillation (*red dotted region* on EGM trace). This method is widely used today. ABL refers to the EGM trace acquired by the EP ablation catheter. LIPV, left inferior pulmonary veins; LSPV, left superior pulmonary veins; MRA, MR angiography; RIPV, right inferior pulmonary veins; RSPV, right superior pulmonary veins. (*Courtesy of* Dr Vivek Y. Reddy, Mount Sinai School of Medicine, New York, NY.)

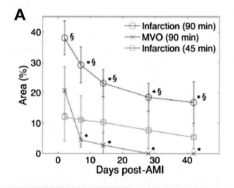

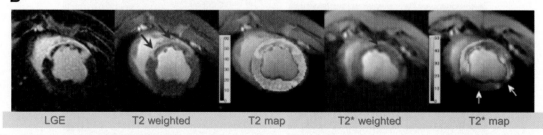

Fig. 9. Changes in a LV infarct over time. Infarct was created by a 45- or 90-minute coronary occlusion. (*A*) Graph showing the reduction in size of the apparent infarct over time. Note that the true necrotic region (labeled microvascular obstruction [MVO]) does not substantially decrease over time. (*B*) Several imaging sequences conducted on a 90-minute occlusion infarct. LGE, T2-weighted image, and T2 map show both the infarct core and the surrounding edema (*thick blue arrows*), whereas T2*-weighted image and T2* map show true infarct core as dark (*thin blue arrows*) region. AMI, acute myocardial infarction. (*Courtesy of* Dr Graham A. Wright, University of Toronto, Toronto, Ontario, Canada.)

Unfortunately, navigation in the PAs is quite difficult without MR imaging–compatible guidewires so that although a few human interventions have been performed,[2,34,103–108] their frequency has tapered off or they have been replaced by X-MR imaging approaches in which X-ray is used for navigation. The recent development of MR imaging–compatible guidewires may rekindle this field.

Valve and Septal Defect Repair

There is an increasing trend for endovascular performance of valve replacement and for the closure of septal defects, namely, ventricular septal defects (VSDs) and atrial septal defects (ASDs). Endovascular procedures may reduce the considerable risks entailed in open heart surgery. Performing such procedures in MR imaging is advantageous, if the MR images provide superior visualization and assist in the implantation process. To perform such procedures with MR imaging, the implanted devices and their deployment aids (guiding catheters, guiding needles, etc.) have to be made compatible for MR imaging, and there is a need to add passive or active markers to the devices, enabling navigation and device deployment under MR imaging guidance.

Experimental devices and navigational aids for VSD and ASD placement[109–113] and for valve replacement[110,114,115] have been tested in animal models.

Miscellaneous Percutaneous and Endovascular Biopsies

Performance of percutaneous (skin access) biopsies under MR imaging guidance is commonplace in several areas of the body. In the heart, there are several instances in which biopsies are also required. The largest volume of procedures requiring cardiac biopsies are diagnosis and staging of cardiac masses and determination of the success of heart transplants. In addition, there are also devices, such as the bioptome, that enable performing cardiac biopsies using endovascular approaches. When such procedures are performed with X-ray guidance, the visualization of the heart area sampled is frequently quite poor, requiring multiple samples to be obtained, which also increases the risk of complications.

MR imaging–compatible percutaneous needles have been developed[116,117] and tested in swine models. H. Maslanka Chirurgische Instrumente GmbH has also developed an MR imaging–compatible bioptome, which includes passive MR imaging markers and is currently undergoing phantom trials.

SUMMARY

MR imaging–guided cardiac intervention is finally becoming a clinical reality, after years of technological development and preclinical testing. Cardiac EP is the first field for which clinical grade device development is complete and in which human clinical trials are currently underway. Important clinical hurdles that remain are understanding acute tissue response to surgical/interventional injury and use of MR imaging markers (T1, T2*, diffusion, etc.) to predict which regions of the acute injury will transform into chronic necrosis.

REFERENCES

1. Lardo AC, McVeigh ER, Jumrussirikul P, et al. Visualization and temporal/spatial characterization of cardiac radiofrequency ablation lesions using magnetic resonance imaging. Circulation 2000; 102:698–705.
2. Razavi R, Hill DL, Keevil SF, et al. Cardiac catheterisation guided by MRI in children and adults with congenital heart disease. Lancet 2003;362:1877–82.
3. Nazarian S, Kolandaivelu A, Zviman MM, et al. Feasibility of real-time magnetic resonance imaging for catheter guidance in electrophysiology studies. Circulation 2008;118:223–9.
4. Harrison JL, Sohns C, Linton NW, et al. Repeat left atrial catheter ablation: cardiac magnetic resonance prediction of endocardial voltage and gaps in ablation lesion sets. Circ Arrhythm Electrophysiol 2015;8:270–8.
5. Nordbeck P, Quick HH, Bauer WR, et al. Initial clinical application of real-time MR imaging-guided ablation of cardiac arrhythmia in patients with atrial flutter. Radiology 2014;273:310–1.
6. Grothoff M, Piorkowski C, Eitel C, et al. MR imaging-guided electrophysiological ablation studies in humans with passive catheter tracking: initial results. Radiology 2014;271:695–702.
7. Eitel C, Hindricks G, Grothoff M, et al. Catheter ablation guided by real-time MRI. Curr Cardiol Rep 2014;16:511.
8. Nordbeck P, Quick HH, Ladd ME, et al. Real-time magnetic resonance guidance of interventional electrophysiology procedures with passive catheter visualization and tracking. Heart Rhythm 2013;10:938–9.
9. Reiter T, Ritter O, Nordbeck P, et al. MRI-guided ablation of wide complex tachycardia in a univentricular heart. World J Cardiol 2012;4:260–3.
10. Nordbeck P, Beer M, Köstler H, et al. Cardiac catheter ablation under real-time magnetic resonance guidance. Eur Heart J 2012;33:1977.

11. Vergara GR, Marrouche NF. Tailored management of atrial fibrillation using a LGE-MRI based model: from the clinic to the electrophysiology laboratory. J Cardiovasc Electrophysiol 2011;22:481–7.

12. Reddy VY, Schmidt EJ, Holmvang G, et al. Arrhythmia recurrence after atrial fibrillation ablation: can magnetic resonance imaging identify gaps in atrial ablation lines? J Cardiovasc Electrophysiol 2008;19:434–7.

13. Malchano ZJ, Neuzil P, Cury RC, et al. Integration of cardiac CT/MR imaging with three-dimensional electroanatomical mapping to guide catheter manipulation in the left atrium: implications for catheter ablation of atrial fibrillation. J Cardiovasc Electrophysiol 2006;17:1221–9.

14. Reddy VY, Malchano ZJ, Holmvang G, et al. Integration of cardiac magnetic resonance imaging with three-dimensional electroanatomic mapping to guide left ventricular catheter manipulation: feasibility in a porcine model of healed myocardial infarction. J Am Coll Cardiol 2004;44:2202–13.

15. Dickfeld T, Calkins H, Zviman M, et al. Stereotactic magnetic resonance guidance for anatomically targeted ablations of the fossa ovalis and the left atrium. J Interv Card Electrophysiol 2004;11: 105–15.

16. Dickfeld T, Calkins H, Zviman M, et al. Anatomic stereotactic catheter ablation on three-dimensional magnetic resonance images in real time. Circulation 2003;108:2407–13.

17. Prakosa A, Malamas P, Zhang S, et al. Methodology for image-based reconstruction of ventricular geometry for patient-specific modeling of cardiac electrophysiology. Prog Biophys Mol Biol 2014; 115:226–34.

18. Faranesh AZ, Lederman RJ. Roadmaps show the way: coregistration to enhance structural heart interventions. Catheter Cardiovasc Interv 2013;82: 443–4.

19. Faranesh AZ, Kellman P, Ratnayaka K, et al. Integration of cardiac and respiratory motion into MRI roadmaps fused with X-ray. Med Phys 2013;40: 032302.

20. Ma YL, Shetty AK, Duckett S, et al. An integrated platform for image-guided cardiac resynchronization therapy. Phys Med Biol 2012;57:2953–68.

21. George AK, Sonmez M, Lederman RJ, et al. Robust automatic rigid registration of MRI and X-ray using external fiducial markers for XFM-guided interventional procedures. Med Phys 2011;38:125–41.

22. Duckett SG, Ginks MR, Knowles BR, et al. Advanced image fusion to overlay coronary sinus anatomy with real-time fluoroscopy to facilitate left ventricular lead implantation in CRT. Pacing Clin Electrophysiol 2011;34:226–34.

23. Duckett SG, Ginks M, Shetty AK, et al. Realtime fusion of cardiac magnetic resonance imaging and computed tomography venography with X-ray fluoroscopy to aid cardiac resynchronisation therapy implantation in patients with persistent left superior vena cava. Europace 2011;13:285–6.

24. Saybasili H, Faranesh AZ, Saikus CE, et al. Interventional MRI using multiple 3d angiography roadmaps with real-time imaging. J Magn Reson Imaging 2010;31:1015–9.

25. Ma Y, Penney GP, Bos D, et al. Hybrid echo and X-ray image guidance for cardiac catheterization procedures by using a robotic arm: a feasibility study. Phys Med Biol 2010;55:N371–82.

26. Ma YL, Penney GP, Rinaldi CA, et al. Echocardiography to magnetic resonance image registration for use in image-guided cardiac catheterization procedures. Phys Med Biol 2009;54: 5039–55.

27. Gutierrez LF, Silva R, Ozturk C, et al. Technology preview: X-ray fused with magnetic resonance during invasive cardiovascular procedures. Catheter Cardiovasc Interv 2007;70:773–82.

28. Dong J, Dickfeld T, Dalal D, et al. Initial experience in the use of integrated electroanatomic mapping with three-dimensional MR/CT images to guide catheter ablation of atrial fibrillation. J Cardiovasc Electrophysiol 2006;17:459–66.

29. Dong J, Calkins H, Solomon S, et al. Integrated electroanatomic mapping with three-dimensional computed tomographic images for real-time guided ablations. Circulation 2006;113:186–94.

30. Rhode KS, Sermesant M, Brogan D, et al. A system for real-time XMR guided cardiovascular intervention. IEEE Trans Med Imaging 2005;24:1428–40.

31. Dick AJ, Raman VK, Raval AN, et al. Invasive human magnetic resonance imaging: feasibility during revascularization in a combined XMR suite. Catheter Cardiovasc Interv 2005;64:265–74.

32. Rhode KS, Hill DL, Edwards PJ, et al. Registration and tracking to integrate X-ray and MR images in an XMR facility. IEEE Trans Med Imaging 2003; 22:1369–78.

33. Valverde I, Hussain T, Razavi R, et al. MR-guided interventions and beyond. Future Cardiol 2012;8: 149–52.

34. Tzifa A, Schaeffter T, Razavi R. MR imaging-guided cardiovascular interventions in young children. Magn Reson Imaging Clin N Am 2012;20:117–28.

35. Mahnkopf C, Halbfass P, Turschner O, et al. Use of cardiac MRI in the field of electrophysiology. Present status and future aspects. Herzschrittmacherther Elektrophysiol 2012;23:275–80.

36. Mahnkopf C, Halbfass P, Holzmann S, et al. interventional electrophysiology in cardiac MRI: what is the current status? Herz 2012;37:146–52.

37. Halperin HR, Kolandaivelu A. MRI-guided electro-physiology intervention. Rambam Maimonides Med J 2010;1:e0015.

38. Saikus CE, Lederman RJ. Interventional cardio-vascular magnetic resonance imaging: a new opportunity for image-guided interventions. JACC Cardiovasc Imaging 2009;2:1321–31.

39. Nazarian S, Bluemke DA, Halperin HR. Applica-tions of cardiac magnetic resonance in electro-physiology. Circ Arrhythm Electrophysiol 2009;2:63–71.

40. Kolandaivelu A, Lardo AC, Halperin HR. Cardio-vascular magnetic resonance guided electro-physiology studies. J Cardiovasc Magn Reson 2009;11:21.

41. Badger TJ, Adjei-Poku YA, Marrouche NF. MRI in cardiac electrophysiology: the emerging role of delayed-enhancement MRI in atrial fibrillation abla-tion. Future Cardiol 2009;5:63–70.

42. Ratnayaka K, Faranesh AZ, Guttman MA, et al. In-terventional cardiovascular magnetic resonance: still tantalizing. J Cardiovasc Magn Reson 2008;10:62.

43. Raman VK, Lederman RJ. Interventional cardiovas-cular magnetic resonance imaging. Trends Cardio-vasc Med 2007;17:196–202.

44. Raman VK, Lederman RJ. Advances in interven-tional cardiovascular MRI. Curr Cardiol Rep 2006;8:70–5.

45. Muthurangu V, Razavi RS. The value of magnetic resonance guided cardiac catheterisation. Heart 2005;91:995–6.

46. Moore P. MRI-guided congenital cardiac catheteri-zation and intervention: the future? Catheter Cardi-ovasc Interv 2005;66:1–8.

47. Parmar BR, Jarrett TR, Burgon NS, et al. Compari-son of left atrial area marked ablated in electroana-tomical maps with scar in MRI. J Cardiovasc Electrophysiol 2014;25:457–63.

48. Sasaki T, Miller CF, Hansford R, et al. Myocardial structural associations with local electrograms: a study of postinfarct ventricular tachycardia patho-physiology and magnetic resonance-based nonin-vasive mapping. Circ Arrhythm Electrophysiol 2012;5:1081–90.

49. Spragg DD, Khurram I, Zimmerman SL, et al. Initial experience with magnetic resonance imaging of atrial scar and co-registration with electroanatomic voltage mapping during atrial fibrillation: success and limitations. Heart Rhythm 2012;9:2003–9.

50. Ghugre NR, Ramanan V, Pop M, et al. Quantitative tracking of edema, hemorrhage, and microvas-cular obstruction in subacute myocardial infarction in a porcine model by MRI. Magn Reson Med 2011;66:1129–41.

51. Zia MI, Ghugre NR, Connelly KA, et al. Character-izing myocardial edema and hemorrhage using quantitative t2 and t2* mapping at multiple time inter-vals post ST-segment elevation myocardial infarc-tion. Circ Cardiovasc Imaging 2012;5:566–72.

52. Yang Y, Graham JJ, Connelly K, et al. MRI manifes-tations of persistent microvascular obstruction and acute left ventricular remodeling in an experimental reperfused myocardial infarction. Quant Imaging Med Surg 2012;2:12–20.

53. Spuentrup E, Ruebben A, Schaeffter T, et al. Mag-netic resonance–guided coronary artery stent placement in a swine model. Circulation 2002;105:874–9.

54. Serfaty JM, Yang X, Foo TK, et al. MRI-guided coro-nary catheterization and PTCA: a feasibility study on a dog model. Magn Reson Med 2003;49:258–63.

55. Buecker A, Spuentrup E, Schmitz-Rode T, et al. Use of a nonmetallic guide wire for magnetic resonance-guided coronary artery catheterization. Invest Radiol 2004;39:656–60.

56. Botnar RM, Bucker A, Kim WY, et al. Initial experi-ences with in vivo intravascular coronary vessel wall imaging. J Magn Reson Imaging 2003;17:615–9.

57. Schmidt EJ, Yoneyama R, Dumoulin CL, et al. 3D coronary motion tracking in swine models with MR tracking catheters. J Magn Reson Imaging 2009;29:86–98.

58. Serfaty JM, Atalar E, Declerck J, et al. Real-time projection MR angiography: feasibility study. Radi-ology 2000;217:290–5.

59. Qiu B, Gao F, Karmarkar P, et al. Intracoronary MR imaging using a 0.014-inch MR imaging-guidewire: toward MRI-guided coronary interventions. J Magn Reson Imaging 2008;28:515–8.

60. Qiu B, Karmarkar P, Brushett C, et al. Develop-ment of a 0.014-inch magnetic resonance imaging guidewire. Magn Reson Med 2005;53:986–90.

61. Raval AN, Karmarkar PV, Guttman MA, et al. Real-time magnetic resonance imaging-guided endo-vascular recanalization of chronic total arterial occlusion in a swine model. Circulation 2006;113:1101–7.

62. Courtney BK, Munce NR, Anderson KJ, et al. Inno-vations in imaging for chronic total occlusions: a glimpse into the future of angiography's blind-spot. Eur Heart J 2008;29:583–93.

63. Feng L, Dumoulin CL, Dashnaw S, et al. Feasibility of stent placement in carotid arteries with real-time MR imaging guidance in pigs. Radiology 2005;234:558–62.

64. Feng L, Dumoulin CL, Dashnaw S, et al. Transfe-moral catheterization of carotid arteries with real-time MR imaging guidance in pigs. Radiology 2005;234:551–7.

65. Arepally A, Karmarkar PV, Weiss C, et al. Magnetic resonance image-guided trans-septal puncture in a swine heart. J Magn Reson Imaging 2005;21: 463–7.

66. de Silva R, Lederman RJ. Delivery and tracking of therapeutic cell preparations for clinical cardiovascular applications. Cytotherapy 2004;6:608–14.

67. Dick AJ, Guttman MA, Raman VK, et al. Magnetic resonance fluoroscopy allows targeted delivery of mesenchymal stem cells to infarct borders in swine. Circulation 2003;108:2899–904.

68. Dick AJ, Lederman RJ. MRI-guided myocardial cell therapy. Int J Cardiovasc Intervent 2005;7: 165–70.

69. Graham JJ, Lederman RJ, Dick AJ. Magnetic resonance imaging and its role in myocardial regenerative therapy. Regen Med 2006;1:347–55.

70. Guttman MA, Dick AJ, Raman VK, et al. Imaging of myocardial infarction for diagnosis and intervention using real-time interactive MRI without ECG-gating or breath-holding. Magn Reson Med 2004; 52:354–61.

71. Lederman RJ, Guttman MA, Peters DC, et al. Catheter-based endomyocardial injection with real-time magnetic resonance imaging. Circulation 2002; 105:1282–4.

72. Arifin DR, Kedziorek DA, Fu Y, et al. Microencapsulated cell tracking. NMR Biomed 2013;26: 850–9.

73. Bulte JW. Science to practice: highly shifted proton MR imaging–a shift toward better cell tracking? Radiology 2014;272:615–7.

74. Cromer Berman SM, Walczak P, Bulte JW. Tracking stem cells using magnetic nanoparticles. Wiley Interdiscip Rev Nanomed Nanobiotechnol 2011;3: 343–55.

75. Kraitchman DL, Gilson WD, Lorenz CH. Stem cell therapy: MRI guidance and monitoring. J Magn Reson Imaging 2008;27:299–310.

76. Kraitchman DL, Kedziorek DA, Bulte JW. MR imaging of transplanted stem cells in myocardial infarction. Methods Mol Biol 2011;680:141–52.

77. Long CM, Bulte JW. In vivo tracking of cellular therapeutics using magnetic resonance imaging. Expert Opin Biol Ther 2009;9:293–306.

78. Rickers C, Kraitchman D, Fischer G, et al. Cardiovascular interventional MR imaging: a new road for therapy and repair in the heart. Magn Reson Imaging Clin N Am 2005;13:465–79.

79. Wu JC, Abraham MR, Kraitchman DL. Current perspectives on imaging cardiac stem cell therapy. J Nucl Med 2010;51(Suppl 1):128S–36S.

80. Karmarkar PV, Kraitchman DL, Izbudak I, et al. MR-trackable intramyocardial injection catheter. Magn Reson Med 2004;51:1163–72.

81. Barnett BP, Arepally A, Stuber M, et al. Synthesis of magnetic resonance-, X-ray- and ultrasound-visible alginate microcapsules for immunoisolation and noninvasive imaging of cellular therapeutics. Nat Protoc 2011;6:1142–51.

82. Fu Y, Azene N, Ehtiati T, et al. Fused X-ray and MR imaging guidance of intrapericardial delivery of microencapsulated human mesenchymal stem cells in immunocompetent swine. Radiology 2014;272: 427–37.

83. Dukkipati SR, Mallozzi R, Schmidt EJ, et al. Electroanatomic mapping of the left ventricle in a porcine model of chronic myocardial infarction with magnetic resonance-based catheter tracking. Circulation 2008;118:853–62.

84. Shokrollahi E, Pop M, Safri M, et al. In-vivo MRI and in-vivo electro-anatomical voltage map characteristics of infarct heterogeneity in a swine model. Conf Proc IEEE Eng Med Biol Soc 2011;2011:2792–5.

85. Nazarian S, Roguin A, Zviman MM, et al. Clinical utility and safety of a protocol for noncardiac and cardiac magnetic resonance imaging of patients with permanent pacemakers and implantable-cardioverter defibrillators at 1.5 tesla. Circulation 2006;114:1277–84.

86. Nazarian S, Halperin HR. How to perform magnetic resonance imaging on patients with implantable cardiac arrhythmia devices. Heart Rhythm 2009; 6:138–43.

87. Tse ZT, Dumoulin CL, Clifford GD, et al. A 1.5t MRI-conditional 12-lead electrocardiogram for MRI and intra-MR intervention. Magn Reson Med 2014;71: 1336–47.

88. Gregory TS, Schmidt EJ, Zhang SH, et al. 3DQRS: a method to obtain reliable QRS complex detection within high field MRI using 12-lead electrocardiogram traces. Magn Reson Med 2014;71: 1374–80.

89. Schmidt EJ, Mallozzi RP, Thiagalingam A, et al. Electroanatomic mapping and radiofrequency ablation of porcine left atria and atrioventricular nodes using magnetic resonance catheter tracking. Circ Arrhythm Electrophysiol 2009;2: 695–704.

90. Nordbeck P, Bauer WR, Fidler F, et al. Feasibility of real-time MRI with a novel carbon catheter for interventional electrophysiology. Circ Arrhythm Electrophysiol 2009;2:258–67.

91. Kolandaivelu A, Zviman MM, Castro V, et al. Noninvasive assessment of tissue heating during cardiac radiofrequency ablation using MRI thermography. Circ Arrhythm Electrophysiol 2010;3:521–9.

92. Volland NA, Kholmovski EG, Parker DL, et al. Initial feasibility testing of limited field of view magnetic resonance thermometry using a local cardiac radiofrequency coil. Magn Reson Med 2013;70: 994–1004.

93. Peters DC, Wylie JV, Hauser TH, et al. Detection of pulmonary vein and left atrial scar after catheter

ablation with three-dimensional navigator-gated delayed enhancement MR imaging: initial experience. Radiology 2007;243:690–5.

94. Wylie JV Jr, Peters DC, Essebag V, et al. Left atrial function and scar after catheter ablation of atrial fibrillation. Heart Rhythm 2008;5:656–62.

95. McGann CJ, Kholmovski EG, Oakes RS, et al. New magnetic resonance imaging-based method for defining the extent of left atrial wall injury after the ablation of atrial fibrillation. J Am Coll Cardiol 2008;52:1263–71.

96. Badger TJ, Daccarett M, Akoum NW, et al. Evaluation of left atrial lesions after initial and repeat atrial fibrillation ablation: lessons learned from delayed-enhancement MRI in repeat ablation procedures. Circ Arrhythm Electrophysiol 2010;3:249–59.

97. Vergara GR, Vijayakumar S, Kholmovski EG, et al. Real-time magnetic resonance imaging-guided radiofrequency atrial ablation and visualization of lesion formation at 3 tesla. Heart Rhythm 2011;8: 295–303.

98. Ranjan R, Kholmovski EG, Blauer J, et al. Identification and acute targeting of gaps in atrial ablation lesion sets using a real-time magnetic resonance imaging system. Circ Arrhythm Electrophysiol 2012;5:1130–5.

99. Ghugre NR, Pop M, Barry J, et al. Quantitative magnetic resonance imaging can distinguish remodeling mechanisms after acute myocardial infarction based on the severity of ischemic insult. Magn Reson Med 2013;70:1095–105.

100. Fitts M, Breton E, Kholmovski EG, et al. Arrhythmia insensitive rapid cardiac t1 mapping pulse sequence. Magn Reson Med 2013;70:1274–82.

101. Steeden JA, Atkinson D, Taylor AM, et al. Split-acquisition real-time cine phase-contrast MR flow measurements. Magn Reson Med 2010;64: 1664–70.

102. Steeden JA, Atkinson D. Rapid flow assessment of congenital heart disease with high-spatiotemporal-resolution gated spiral phase-contrast MR imaging. Radiology 2011;260:79–87.

103. Razavi RS, Hill DL, Muthurangu V, et al. Three-dimensional magnetic resonance imaging of congenital cardiac anomalies. Cardiol Young 2003;13:461–5.

104. Heathfield E, Hussain T, Qureshi S, et al. Cardiovascular magnetic resonance imaging in congenital heart disease as an alternative to diagnostic invasive cardiac catheterization: a single center experience. Congenit Heart Dis 2013;8:322–7.

105. Rickers C, Seethamraju RT, Jerosch-Herold M, et al. Magnetic resonance imaging guided cardiovascular interventions in congenital heart diseases. J Interv Cardiol 2003;16:143–7.

106. Tzifa A, Krombach GA, Krämer N, et al. Magnetic resonance-guided cardiac interventions using magnetic resonance-compatible devices: a preclinical study and first-in-man congenital interventions. Circ Cardiovasc Interv 2010;3:585–92.

107. Tzifa A, Razavi R. Test occlusion of Fontan fenestration: unique contribution of interventional MRI. Heart 2011;97:89.

108. Rogers T, Ratnayaka K, Lederman RJ. MRI catheterization in cardiopulmonary disease. Chest 2014;145:30–6.

109. Rickers C, Jerosch-Herold M, Hu X, et al. Magnetic resonance image-guided transcatheter closure of atrial septal defects. Circulation 2003;107:132–8.

110. McVeigh ER, Guttman MA, Lederman RJ, et al. Real-time interactive MRI-guided cardiac surgery: aortic valve replacement using a direct apical approach. Magn Reson Med 2006;56:958–64.

111. Elagha AA, Kocaturk O, Guttman MA, et al. Real-time MR imaging-guided laser atrial septal puncture in swine. J Vasc Interv Radiol 2008;19: 1347–53.

112. Ratnayaka K, Raman VK, Faranesh AZ, et al. Antegrade percutaneous closure of membranous ventricular septal defect using X-ray fused with magnetic resonance imaging. JACC Cardiovasc Interv 2009;2:224–30.

113. Ratnayaka K, Saikus CE, Faranesh AZ, et al. Closed-chest transthoracic magnetic resonance imaging-guided ventricular septal defect closure in swine. JACC Cardiovasc Interv 2011;4:1326–34.

114. Horvath KA, Guttman M, Li M, et al. Beating heart aortic valve replacement using real-time MRI guidance. Innovations 2007;2:51–5.

115. Voges I, Brasen JH, Entenmann A, et al. Adverse results of a decellularized tissue-engineered pulmonary valve in humans assessed with magnetic resonance imaging. Eur J Cardiothorac Surg 2013;44:e272–9.

116. Borchert B, Lawrenz T, Bartelsmeier M, et al. Utility of endomyocardial biopsy guided by delayed enhancement areas on magnetic resonance imaging in the diagnosis of cardiac sarcoidosis. Clin Res Cardiol 2007;96:759–62.

117. Saikus CE, Ratnayaka K, Barbash IM, et al. MRI-guided vascular access with an active visualization needle. J Magn Reson Imaging 2011;34:1159–66.

Magnetic Resonance–guided Active Catheter Tracking

Wei Wang, PhD

KEYWORDS

- Active tracking • MR-guided device tracking • Microcoil • MR-compatible catheters
- Electrophysiology

KEY POINTS

- MR imaging shows great promise as a tool for guiding interventions because it provides three-dimensional imaging capabilities with excellent soft tissue contrast and functional information without ionizing radiation.
- MR-guided active catheter tracking can provide rapid and robust catheter visualization.
- Combined with MR imaging, it allows simultaneous visualization of the device and the surrounding anatomy.
- Active catheter tracking provides several features that may prove valuable for clinical applications.
- The development of active catheter tracking is an indispensable step toward fully MR-guided clinical interventions.

INTRODUCTION

In recent years, there has been growing interest in using MR imaging to provide guidance for catheter-based interventions. Traditionally, most catheter interventions are performed under x-ray fluoroscopy, which allows good visualization of the device but lacks surrounding anatomic information. Most importantly, ionizing radiation involved in x-ray fluoroscopy is harmful for both the patients and the physicians. MR imaging is a promising alternative to guide intervention because it provides several advantages compared with other imaging modalities, including excellent soft tissue contrast, the ability to provide functional information, and a lack of ionizing radiation. An essential requirement for MR-guided intervention is to track and navigate the interventional devices, such as catheters, needles, and implants, to the target.

For device tracking inside an MR environment, 2 different approaches are commonly used: passive tracking and active tracking. There are approaches proposed that do not belong to these 2 categories and can be classified into a third category of hybrid techniques,[1,2] which is beyond the scope of this article. MR-guided passive tracking is for visualizing a device within MR images based on the negative or positive contrast generated by intrinsic material characteristics. The contrast can be created and enhanced by incorporating ferromagnetic or paramagnetic materials into the device,[3,4] or by using contrast agents.[5] Specific imaging sequences have also been proposed to improve the visualization.[6–9] In contrast, active devices with embedded radiofrequency (RF) coils, antennas, or other sensors can generate conspicuous signals for localization. The major advantage of active tracking compared with passive tracking is that the unambiguous three-dimensional (3D)

Disclosure: The author has nothing to disclose.

Radiology, Brigham and Women's Hospital, Harvard Medical School, 221 Longwood Avenue, Boston, MA 02115, USA

E-mail address: wwang21@partners.org

Magn Reson Imaging Clin N Am 23 (2015) 579–589
http://dx.doi.org/10.1016/j.mric.2015.05.009
1064-9689/15/$ – see front matter © 2015 Elsevier Inc. All rights reserved.

information is generated with high temporal and spatial resolution, which potentially leads to shorter procedure times and improved procedure outcome.

This article reviews state-of-the-art MR-guided active catheter tracking techniques, focusing on the principles and implementation in a clinical setting. Safety issues related to active tracking in MR-guided intervention are discussed, and several preclinical and clinical applications are presented.

METHODS OF MAGNETIC RESONANCE–GUIDED ACTIVE TRACKING
Active Magnetic Resonance Tracking with Microcoils

Active MR tracking can be achieved using an MR tracking pulse sequence with small RF receive coils (microcoils) that are incorporated into interventional instruments[10,11] (**Fig. 1**). The sequence begins with a spatially nonselective RF pulse to excite all the spins within a large volume inside the RF transmit coil (eg, body coil). Then, a magnetic field gradient is applied along 1 spatial direction, making the magnetic field vary monotonically with the position along that direction. Hence, the frequency of the spins at different locations, which is also the frequency of the MR signal received, linearly depends on the spins' location. Different from a conventional MR receive coil, a microcoil has a limited receive sensitivity profile. It can only detect MR signals from the spins in the immediate vicinity of the microcoil. As a consequence, the MR signal received by a microcoil is shown as a sharp peak in the frequency spectrum (see

Fig. 1C). The location of the signal peak in the frequency domain indicates the microcoil's spatial location along the axis of the applied gradient. If this process is performed with the magnetic gradient applied along 3 orthogonal directions, the 3D coordinates of the coil can be obtained. By integrating different coils connected to individual receive channels, this approach is capable of tracking multiple coils simultaneously for visualizing the trajectory of a catheter rather than only its tip position.

For robust tracking with microcoils, several strategies can be applied. First, any variation to the static magnetic field (B_0) distorts the linear relationship between the MR tracking signal frequency and the microcoil's location. This resonance frequency offset may be caused by the transmitter and receiver frequency offset, or B_0 inhomogeneities created by the device. In active tracking, the microcoils are usually at or near the interface between the tissue and the device where the magnetic susceptibility difference between the two greatly distorts the local magnetic field. This situation leads to either loss of the received tracking signal or imprecise calculation of the device location. Several multiplexing acquisition schemes have been proposed to eliminate the resonance offset errors.[11] In these schemes, 4 excitations are usually required with certain modulation of the gradients' appearance and polarity along x, y, and z axes. Another important strategy is phase field dithering, which is especially useful in low signal-to-noise ratio conditions.[12] It uses dephasing gradients in a rotating fashion on the orthogonal plane to the frequency-encoding gradient.

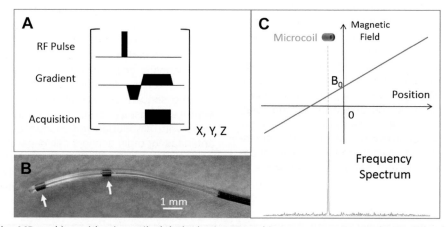

Fig. 1. Active MR tracking with microcoils. (*A*) The basic MR tracking sequence. A nonselective RF pulse is applied followed by frequency-encoding gradient along 1 axis during data acquisition. The 3D position of a microcoil can be acquired by playing the tracking sequence 3 times with the gradients applied along X, Y and Z axes respectively. (*B*) A catheter equipped with 2 tracking solenoid microcoils (*arrows*). (*C*) MR signal received by the microcoil is shown as a sharp peak in the frequency domain. The frequency at which the peak is located is proportional to the microcoil's position along the applied gradient direction.

This strategy dramatically improves the tracking quality by reducing the undesirable coupling with the body coils or other conducting devices.

Active Magnetic Resonance Tracking with Antennas

To enable the whole-shaft visibility of the catheter, active visualization methods using antennas connected to an MR receiver were proposed. Different from passive tracking, the active visualization (profiling) of the device is based on the conspicuous signal received by tracking antennas on separate channels other than conventional imaging channels. There are 2 main types of antennas: magnetically coupled loop antennas (coils)[13–15] and electrically coupled loopless (rod) antennas.[16,17]

A loop antenna is a loop coil wound thinly and extended along a certain length of the interventional instrument (eg, catheters). Because of limited receive sensitivity of the coil, conventional MR imaging with the loop antenna can outline the instrument. Different coil geometries can be used so long as the coil's sensitivity can be highly localized.

A loopless antenna is essentially a wire that can be easily integrated into more flexible and thinner interventional instruments. Similar to a loop antenna, it also serves as a receive-only antenna that can detect signals from its surroundings, and the resultant MR image delineates the instrument. The difference is that such an antenna has extremely high sensitivity in a cylindrical volume with a significantly greater size than that of the catheter. This property hinders sharp delineation of the instrument, but it can reveal the anatomy surrounding the instrument.

Active Tracking with Measurement of Gradients

Another active tracking technique that does not rely on visualization with MR imaging uses the spatially varying gradients of the MR system. Robin Medical, Inc (Baltimore, MD) developed a miniature tracking sensor that has 3 orthogonal pickup coils to measure the voltages induced by the changing magnetic fields (gradients) inside the MR scanner. By comparing the measured signals with the gradient field map of the scanner, which is acquired in advance, the current location and orientation of the sensor (6 degrees of freedom) can immediately be determined. Specifically, for catheter-based applications, such sensors were integrated into the tip of MR imaging–compatible catheters (**Fig. 2**). Another

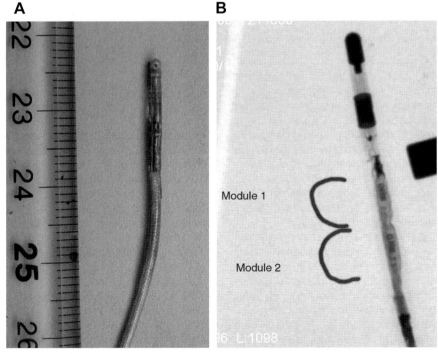

Fig. 2. CatheScout developed by Robin Medical, Inc (Baltimore, MD). (*A*) Two CatheScout tracking modules with a transmission wire. Each module includes 3 orthogonal coils and can generate 6 degrees of freedom information. (*B*) A radiograph image of an MR-compatible ablation catheter with 2 CatheScout tracking modules embedded near the tip of the catheter. (*Courtesy of* Erez Nevo, PhD, Robin Medical, Inc Baltimore, MD; Atsushi Yamada, PhD, Tohru Tani, PhD, Shigehiro Morikawa, PhD, and Shigeyuki Naka, PhD, Shiga University of Medical Science, Japan.)

mechanism for measuring the gradient fields is to use an optical sensor using the Faraday effect, which can also generate position and orientation information in the MR scanner.[18]

VISUALIZATION OF MAGNETIC RESONANCE–GUIDED ACTIVE TRACKING
Visualization on MR Images

In MR-guided active tracking with microcoils, the calculated coil positions use the same MR scanner coordinate system as MR imaging because the same frequency-encoding principle of MR tracking also applies to MR imaging. As a consequence, virtual markers representing microcoil positions from MR tracking can be directly overlaid on the preacquired MR images for visualization without time-consuming registration (Fig. 3A, B).

In MR-guided active tracking with antennas, the catheter-related signal is intrinsically visualized as part of the MR image. In addition, for better identification, the signals from the active device channels can be depicted in color and displayed with the conventional gray-scale images acquired by the body coil (see Fig. 3C, D). The visualization of the whole device requires the full length of the device contained within the imaging slice. Therefore, a thick imaging slice is usually prescribed and the slice may need to be manually repositioned when the catheter is moving.

Combining Active Tracking with Real-time Imaging

For the active tracking methods with numeric output of locational information (eg, tracking with microcoil and tracking with sensors measuring magnetic field), tracking sequence can be interleaved with a fast MR imaging sequence so that the 3D spatial coordinates of the device can be used by a subsequent imaging sequence to automatically shift the imaging plane with movement of the device. This property allows two-dimensional images of the surrounding anatomy to be updated in real time at the location of the device.

For active tracking with antennas, the real-time imaging plane needs to be adjusted interactively in real time to contain the device in the image plane, which sometimes causes delays and inaccuracies, so this approach is not ideal for real-time tracking. One solution to this problem is to perform device-only projection imaging that allows the entire device to be seen even if the portion is outside the conventional imaging slice.[19,20] A further improvement is an iterative predication correction algorithm that can reconstruct the 3D trajectory of the catheter based on the projection images in a fraction of a second.[21]

Visualization Interface of Active Catheter Tracking

The development of graphical interfaces is one of the key components of applying active catheter tracking in a clinical setting. It should allow clear and real-time visualization of both the catheters and the surrounding anatomic and functional information revealed by imaging with an easy-to-operate interactive user interface.

All the major MR scanner vendors have developed interactive graphical interfaces that support active catheter tracking. Siemens introduced the Interactive Front End (Siemens Corporate Research, Baltimore, MD), which can provide flexible control over the scan plane orientation and imaging parameters.[22] The signals from the catheter coil channels can be color coded and visualized as part of the real-time MR images. For active catheter tracking with microcoils, graphical representations of catheters are displayed based on the curve fitted to the tracked coil positions and superimposed on the incoming real-time MR images (Fig. 4). Similarly, Philips Healthcare developed the iSuite real-time interactive interface, which integrated active catheter visualization and real-time imaging options (Fig. 5). Besides these vendor-specific applications, in-house solutions for visualization of active catheter tracking were developed under open-source software; for example, Visual Understanding of Real-Time Image Guided Operations (VURTIGO),[23] which focuses on electrophysiology applications, and 3D Slicer,[24,25] which is a more generic platform for image-guided device tracking.

SAFETY

The primary concern when performing any intervention is ensuring the safety of the patient. All the potential safety problems of MR-guided intervention techniques need to be addressed before clinical usage. The most basic requirement is that all of the devices used in the MR environment should be nonmagnetic so that their normal functionality is not affected inside the magnetic field. However, the focus here is the safety issues associated with active catheter tracking, rather than MR safety.

The major safety risk of active catheter tracking is the possibility of localized increases in the RF specific absorption rate (SAR) near the catheter. This problem applies generally for MR-guided interventions involving metallic devices (eg, needles, guidewires). Although metallic devices have no ferromagnetic components and are safe to use in an MR environment, they are electrically conductive. The RF pulses applied in the MR scanner can induce electric currents in and around these

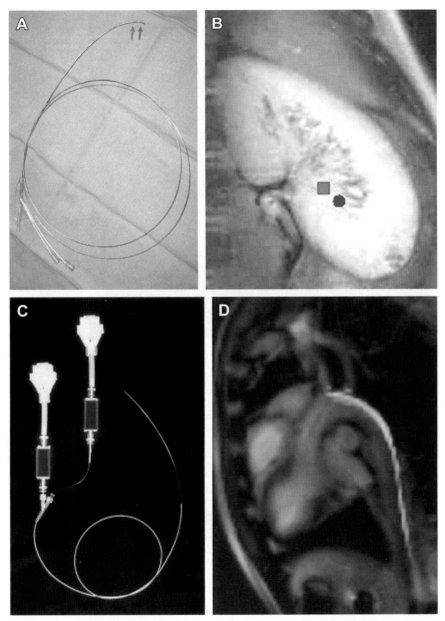

Fig. 3. (A) Two microcoils (*arrows*) affixed to a guidewire inside a catheter. (B) The microcoils' positions (the *red square* and *blue dot* corresponding with the 2 microcoils shown in A) acquired by active tracking are superimposed on a preacquired MR image during renal catheterization. (C) A 6-French catheter and guidewire with integrated loopless antennas for active tracking. Two individual RF-shielded boxes at the proximal end contain the antenna tuning, matching, and decoupling electronics, and can be connected to separate receive channels of the MR scanner. (D) Tracking of an active catheter shown in (C) inside the aortic arch with a fast real-time imaging sequence (balanced steady state free precession). A hot-metal color table was used to coat the signal from the tracking antenna's channel for visualization. This technique allows a simultaneous visualization and tracking of the intravascular catheter and the anatomy despite cardiac and respiratory motion. ([A, B] *Courtesy of* E.J. Schmidt, PhD, Brigham and Women's Hospital, Boston, MA, and C.L. Dumoulin, PhD, Cincinnati Children's Hospital Medical Center, Cincinnati, OH. [C, D] *Adapted from* Quick HH, Kuehl H, Kaiser G, et al. Interventional MRA using actively visualized catheters, TrueFISP, and real-time image fusion. Magn Reson Med 2003;49(1):130, 133; with permission.)

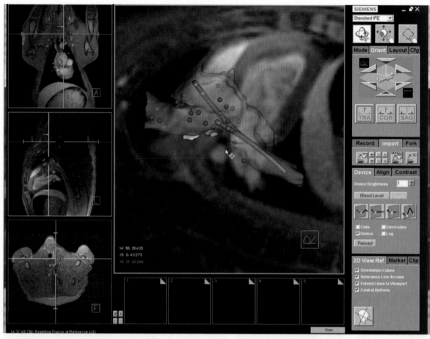

Fig. 4. The Siemens Interactive Front End interface acquired during a cardiac RF ablation procedure. Two active tracked catheters are displayed as colored geometric models by curve fitting of the detected microcoils' positions, and are overlaid on a set of incoming real-time MR images, together with a 3D model built from preacquired MR angiography (MRA) images. User-placed ablation markers are shown as magenta spheres. (*Courtesy of* L. Pan, PhD, Siemens Healthcare, Baltimore, MD.)

conductors, resulting in so-called RF heating. In particular, when using microcoils or RF antennas for active catheter tracking, long cables need to be incorporated along the full length of the catheter to transport electrical signals from active tracking coils to the MR receiver system. Under certain conditions, these long conductive transmission lines can cause significant heating because of the high electric fields induced by the RF pulses.[26–28]

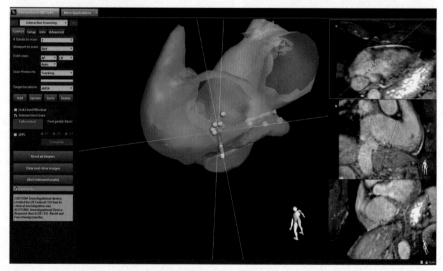

Fig. 5. The iSuite real-time interactive interface (Philips Healthcare, Best, Netherlands) acquired during an atrial flutter ablation study. Actively tracked ablation catheter (*red cylinder*) and reference catheter in coronary sinus (*green cylinder*) are displayed in real time in the autosegmented/autoregistered 3D model of right atrium (*blue*) and left atrium (*orange*) (*central window*) and in MR images in the 3 small windows on the right. The red spheres are the ablation sites. (*Courtesy of* S. Weiss, PhD, Philips GmbH Innovative Technologies, Hamburg, Germany.)

One approach that can significantly reduce the heating near the tip of the cable/coil combination is to avoid a resonant length of the cable and place coaxial chokes on the cables to disrupt the standing wave pattern on the outer conducting surface of the cable.[29] However, the chokes resonate at Larmor frequency, so the local heating generated by the high electric fields is not eliminated but is confined to the choke region. A different method for modifying the transmission line is to use miniature transformers to segment the line, which can suppress common-mode current associated with RF heating by shifting the lowest common-mode resonance of the device far beyond the Larmor frequency.[30,31] Another strategy for safe active catheter tracking is to use nonconductive transmission lines, such as optical fibers, that are inherently RF safe. A miniaturized optical link needs to be integrated into the catheter to convert the electric signal into an optical signal.[32,33]

APPLICATIONS
Cardiac Electrophysiology

Catheter ablation, a treatment of choice for cardiac arrhythmias, is generally performed under functional guidance using electrophysiologic mapping in conjunction with x-ray fluoroscopy or ultrasonography. However, because of the suboptimal success rate, the risk of significant complication, and the prolonged radiation exposure, MR-guided electrophysiology (EP) has moved toward the goal of improving ablation efficacy and safety. Compared with other imaging modalities, MR imaging offers complex 3D cardiovascular anatomic information with improved soft tissue resolution, allows visualization of myocardial scar and ablation lesions, permits catheter visualization relative to soft tissue structure, and reduces radiation exposure. MR-guided active catheter tracking techniques along with passive tracking techniques have been developed as important advances toward fully MR-guided EP procedures. In the first study to report the feasibility of real-time MR imaging–guided EP procedures, an active catheter with a loop antenna extending along the entire shaft was successfully positioned at the right ventricular target sites of a canine model.[34] Later, active tracking using microcoils were shown in swine to navigate catheters to the left atrium and atrioventricular node, followed by electroanatomic mapping and RF ablation.[35,36] The tracked catheter and coil locations were superimposed on time-resolved high-resolution MR image roadmaps to provide real-time guidance during in vivo manipulation (**Fig. 6**).

Recently, an MR-guided actively tracked electroanatomic mapping and ablation system was used in a human for ablation of typical right atrial flutter.[37] Deflectable MR-EP RF Vision catheters (Imricor, Burnsville, MN) were guided into the coronary sinus and right atrium using active MR tracking alone. The catheters were shown as a virtual catheter icon displayed in real time in a previously generated 3D model created from MR images. RF ablation of a cavotricuspid isthmus was also performed under active MR guidance.

Other Intravascular Interventions

In addition to cardiac applications, active catheter tracking techniques have been successfully applied to several different MR-guided endovascular interventions. These interventions generally require precise and fast localization of catheters in the complex and moving anatomy in which MR-guided active tracking may offer some benefits. Studies using active MR catheter tracking have been reported for angioplasty,[38] stenting of aortic aneurysms,[39] renal arteries,[40,41] carotid arteries,[42] renal embolization,[43,44] and creation of a transcatheter shunt.[45] Because of the lack of clinically approved instruments to date, these are all limited to animal studies.

Cell Therapy Delivery

The hybrid cell therapy delivery procedure combining transvascular and percutaneous approaches could benefit from MR guidance because therapeutics can be precisely targeted to the desired location with MR guidance and the results can be evaluated by MR imaging. Their feasibility was first shown in swine for targeted left ventricular mural injection under MR guidance.[46] A commercially available guiding catheter (Stiletto, Boston Scientific, Natick, MA) was converted to an active receive coil that was easily localized in the interactive real-time MR images for targeted left ventricular mural injection. Based on this work, the injection catheter was further modified to incorporate 2 receive coils to precisely deliver regenerative cellular treatments to the infarcted myocardium.[47] In addition to the active antenna along the guiding catheter allowing the visualization of the entire shaft, the new design added a microcoil at the tip of the injection needle to enhance the precision of positioning. Modifying commercially available injection catheters, which are usually designed specifically for x-ray fluoroscopy, has limitations in becoming fully optimized for MR-guided procedures. Dedicated devices need to be designed and built for MR-guided procedures. A steerable intramyocardial injection catheter was developed with a deflectable distal section by using the components of the catheter to form a loopless antenna

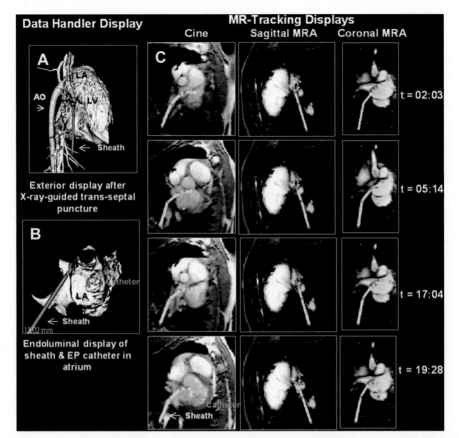

Fig. 6. Navigation to and within the atrium. (*A*) Data Handler 3D surface display, showing MR-tracked EP catheter and torqueable sheath passing through the transseptal hole. (*B*) Endoluminal Data Handler display, taken at the time of (*A*), showing the anterior portion of the left atrium (LA) with the EP catheter inside. (*C*) Three of the MR tracking in-room displays used by the clinicians showing (*left column*) axial (S/I) cine wall motion, (*middle column*) sagittal (L/R) MRA, and (*right column*) coronal (A/P) MRA, during atrial mapping. The real-time displays can be appreciated from the image in the left column, second row, where the catheter is close to the coronary trifurcation; ablation here could have serious repercussions. (*From* Schmidt EJ, Mallozzi RP, Thiagalingam A, et al. Electroanatomic mapping and radiofrequency ablation of porcine left atria and atrioventricular nodes using magnetic resonance catheter tracking. Circ Arrhythm Electrophysiol 2009;2(6):699, with permission.)

for active tracking. This prototype was used under MR guidance to deliver labeled stem cells to the infarcted myocardium.[48] Another active tracking method using loop antennas was also adapted to steerable catheter therapeutic interventional MR imaging procedures.[49]

Interstitial Tumor Therapy

Interstitial therapy delivered directly to the tumor can be achieved with radiation, chemicals, or thermal coagulation. MR imaging has been increasingly used to guide and monitor therapy deliveries because of its excellent anatomic and functional imaging capabilities. Recently, an active MR tracking system was developed to facilitate accurate and time-efficient catheter placement in interstitial brachytherapy for radiation delivery to

treat gynecologic cancer[24] (**Fig. 7**). The active catheter tracking was achieved by attaching flexible printed-circuit microcoils to the inner metallic stylet that fits into the catheter. The tracking system, including an active device, an advanced MR tracking sequence, and a visualization interface, has been successfully applied in clinical cases.

For thermal therapy, MR imaging has frequently been used to monitor the therapy progress because multiple MR imaging techniques are suitable for thermometry. Active MR tracking can be added to guide the therapy delivery catheter and improve the monitoring. The catheter positional information provided by active catheter tracking could be used to prescribe thermometry slice position.[50] For improved MR thermometry, continuous tracking can also provide motion information on the therapy probe to compensate motion.[51]

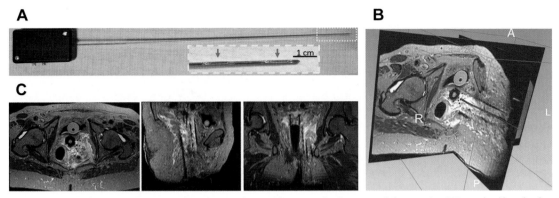

Fig. 7. MR-guided active catheter tracking in a patient with gynecologic cancer. (*A*) An active MR-tracked brachytherapy catheter that consists of a plastic hollow catheter and inner metallic stylet. The dashed window shows an enlarged view of the inner stylet with 2 printed-circuit tracking coils (*arrows*) attached at the distal end. 3D rendering (*B*) and axial, sagittal, and coronal views (*C*) of 1 catheter trajectory (*Red dots* are tracked positions to which the line is fitted) were reconstructed by actively tracking the stylet's tip position during the stylet withdrawal from the catheter and fitting to a smooth curve. A, Anterior; P, Posterior; R, Right; L, Left.

SUMMARY

Within the last 2 decades, great efforts have been made in developing robust active catheter tracking techniques for MR-guided interventions. Active tracking can provide accurate and rapid localization of catheters in an MR environment. It requires fewer personnel during intervention procedures than image-based passive tracking approaches and may result in more efficient intervention procedures. To date, numerous MR-guided active catheter tracking techniques have been applied in many preclinical applications and they may soon be applicable in clinical routines. To facilitate MR imaging becoming mainstream for image-guided intervention, further research on active device tracking is needed, together with other MR imaging techniques, to fully exploit the unique strengths of MR and to thoroughly address the practical and safety issues in clinical settings.

REFERENCES

1. Burl M, Coutts GA, Young IR. Tuned fiducial markers to identify body locations with minimal perturbation of tissue magnetization. Magn Reson Med 1996; 36(3):491–3.

2. Quick HH, Zenge MO, Kuehl H, et al. Interventional magnetic resonance angiography with no strings attached: wireless active catheter visualization. Magn Reson Med 2005;53(2):446–55.

3. Rubin DL, Ratner AV, Young SW. Magnetic susceptibility effects and their application in the development of new ferromagnetic catheters for magnetic resonance imaging. Invest Radiol 1990;25(12): 1325–32.

4. Bakker CJ, Hoogeveen RM, Weber J, et al. Visualization of dedicated catheters using fast scanning techniques with potential for MR-guided vascular interventions. Magn Reson Med 1996; 36(6):816–20.

5. Omary RA, Unal O, Koscielski DS, et al. Real-Time MR Imaging-guided passive catheter tracking with use of gadolinium-filled catheters. J Vasc Interv Radiol 2000;11(8):1079–85.

6. Seevinck PR, de Leeuw H, Bos C, et al. Highly localized positive contrast of small paramagnetic objects using 3D center-out radial sampling with off-resonance reception. Magn Reson Med 2011;65(1):146–56.

7. Seppenwoolde JH, Viergever MA, Bakker CJ. Passive tracking exploiting local signal conservation: the white marker phenomenon. Magn Reson Med 2003;50(4):784–90.

8. Mani V, Briley-Saebo KC, Itskovich VV, et al. Gradient echo acquisition for superparamagnetic particles with positive contrast (GRASP): sequence characterization in membrane and glass superparamagnetic iron oxide phantoms at 1.5 T and 3T. Magn Reson Med 2006;55(1):126–35.

9. Dahnke H, Liu W, Herzka D, et al. Susceptibility gradient mapping (SGM): a new postprocessing method for positive contrast generation applied to superparamagnetic iron oxide particle (SPIO)-labeled cells. Magn Reson Med 2008; 60(3):595–603.

10. Ackerman J, Offutt M, Buxton R, et al. Rapid 3D tracking of small RF coils. Paper presented at: proceedings of the 5th annual meeting of SMRM. Montreal (Canada), August 19-22, 1986.

11. Dumoulin CL, Souza SP, Darrow RD. Real-time position monitoring of invasive devices using magnetic resonance. Magn Reson Med 1993;29(3):411–5.

12. Dumoulin CL, Mallozzi RP, Darrow RD, et al. Phase-field dithering for active catheter tracking. Magn Reson Med 2010;63(5):1398–403.

13. Ladd ME, Zimmermann GG, Quick HH, et al. Active MR visualization of a vascular guidewire in vivo. J Magn Reson Imaging 1998;8(1):220–5.

14. Burl M, Coutts GA, Herlihy DJ, et al. Twisted-pair RF coil suitable for locating the track of a catheter. Magn Reson Med 1999;41(3):636–8.

15. Ladd ME, Erhart P, Debatin JF, et al. Guidewire antennas for MR fluoroscopy. Magn Reson Med 1997;37(6):891–7.

16. McKinnon G, Debatin J, Leung D, et al. Towards active guidewire visualization in interventional magnetic resonance imaging. MAGMA 1996;4(1):13–8.

17. Ocali O, Atalar E. Intravascular magnetic resonance imaging using a loopless catheter antenna. Magn Reson Med 1997;37(1):112–8.

18. Bock M, Umathum R, Sikora J, et al. Faraday effect position sensor for interventional magnetic resonance imaging. Phys Med Biol 2006;51(4):999–1009.

19. Guttman MA, Ozturk C, Raval AN, et al. Interventional cardiovascular procedures guided by real-time MR imaging: an interactive interface using multiple slices, adaptive projection modes and live 3D renderings. J Magn Reson Imaging 2007;26(6):1429–35.

20. Peters DC, Lederman RJ, Dick AJ, et al. Undersampled projection reconstruction for active catheter imaging with adaptable temporal resolution and catheter-only views. Magn Reson Med 2003;49(2):216–22.

21. George AK, Derbyshire JA, Saybasili H, et al. Visualization of active devices and automatic slice repositioning ("SnapTo") for MRI-guided interventions. Magn Reson Med 2010;63(4):1070–9.

22. Lorenz S, Kirchberg K, Zuehlsdorff S, et al. Interactive frontend (IFE): a platform for graphical MR scanner control and scan automation. Paper presented at: Proceedings of the ISMRM 13th Scientific Meeting. Miami Beach (USA), May 7-13, 1995.

23. Radau P, Pintilie S, Flor R, et al. VURTIGO: visualization platform for real-time, MRI-guided cardiac electroanatomic mapping. In: Camara O, Konukoglu E, Pop M, et al, editors. Statistical atlases and computational models of the heart. Imaging and modelling challenges, vol. 7085. Berlin; Heidelberg (Germany): Springer; 2012. p. 244–53.

24. Wang W, Dumoulin CL, Viswanathan AN, et al. Real-time active MR-tracking of metallic stylets in MR-guided radiation therapy. Magn Reson Med 2014;73(5):1803–11.

25. Fedorov A, Beichel R, Kalpathy-Cramer J, et al. 3D Slicer as an image computing platform for the Quantitative Imaging Network. Magn Reson Imaging 2012;30(9):1323–41.

26. Maier S, Wildermuth S, Darrow R, et al. Safety of MR tracking catheters. Paper presented at:

proceedings of the ISMRM 3rd Scientific Meeting. Nice (France), August 19-25, 1995.

27. Wildermuth S, Debatin JF, Leung DA, et al. MR imaging-guided intravascular procedures: initial demonstration in a pig model. Radiology 1997; 202(2):578–83.

28. Ladd M, Quick H, Boesiger P, et al. RF heating of actively visualized catheters and guidewires. Paper presented at: Proceedings of the 6th annual meeting of ISMRM. Sydney (Australia), April 18-24, 1998.

29. Ladd ME, Quick HH. Reduction of resonant RF heating in intravascular catheters using coaxial chokes. Magn Reson Med 2000;43(4):615–9.

30. Weiss S, Vernickel P, Schaeffter T, et al. Transmission line for improved RF safety of interventional devices. Magn Reson Med 2005;54(1):182–9.

31. Weiss S, Wirtz D, David B, et al. In vivo evaluation and proof of radiofrequency safety of a novel diagnostic MR-electrophysiology catheter. Magn Reson Med 2011;65(3):770–7.

32. Fandrey S, Weiss S, Müller J. Development of an active intravascular MR device with an optical transmission system. IEEE Trans Med Imaging 2008; 27(12):1723–7.

33. Fandrey S, Weiss S, Muller J. A novel active MR probe using a miniaturized optical link for a 1.5-T MRI scanner. Magn Reson Med 2012;67(1):148–55.

34. Nazarian S, Kolandaivelu A, Zviman MM, et al. Feasibility of real-time magnetic resonance imaging for catheter guidance in electrophysiology studies. Circulation 2008;118(3):223–9.

35. Dukkipati SR, Mallozzi R, Schmidt EJ, et al. Electroanatomic mapping of the left ventricle in a porcine model of chronic myocardial infarction with magnetic resonance-based catheter tracking. Circulation 2008;118(8):853–62.

36. Schmidt EJ, Mallozzi RP, Thiagalingam A, et al. Electroanatomic mapping and radiofrequency ablation of porcine left atria and atrioventricular nodes using magnetic resonance catheter tracking. Circ Arrhythm Electrophysiol 2009;2(6):695–704.

37. Chubb H, Harrison J, Williams SE, et al. First in man: real-time magnetic resonance-guided ablation of typical right atrial flutter using active catheter tracking. Europace 2014;16(suppl 3):iii25.

38. Yang X, Atalar E. Intravascular MR imaging-guided balloon angioplasty with an MR imaging guide wire: feasibility study in rabbits. Radiology 2000; 217(2):501–6.

39. Raman VK, Karmarkar PV, Guttman MA, et al. Real-time magnetic resonance-guided endovascular repair of experimental abdominal aortic aneurysm in swine. J Am Coll Cardiol 2005;45(12):2069–77.

40. Elgort DR, Hillenbrand CM, Zhang S, et al. Image-guided and -monitored renal artery stenting using only MRI. J Magn Reson Imaging 2006;23(5):619–27.

41. Omary RA, Gehl JA, Schirf BE, et al. MR imaging-versus conventional X-ray fluoroscopy-guided renal angioplasty in swine: prospective randomized comparison. Radiology 2006;238(2):489–96.

42. Feng L, Dumoulin CL, Dashnaw S, et al. Transfemoral catheterization of carotid arteries with real-time MR imaging guidance in pigs. Radiology 2005;234(2):551–7.

43. Fink C, Bock M, Umathum R, et al. Renal embolization: feasibility of magnetic resonance-guidance using active catheter tracking and intraarterial magnetic resonance angiography. Invest Radiol 2004;39(2):111–9.

44. Homagk AK, Umathum R, Bock M, et al. Initial in vivo experience with a novel type of MR-safe pushable coils for MR-guided embolizations. Invest Radiol 2013;48(6):485–91.

45. Weiss C, Karmarkar P, Arepally A, et al. Real time MR guided meso-caval puncture: towards the development of a percutaneous MR guided mesocaval shunt. Radiology 1999;10(5):529–35.

46. Lederman RJ, Guttman MA, Peters DC, et al. Catheter-based endomyocardial injection with real-time magnetic resonance imaging. Circulation 2002; 105(11):1282–4.

47. Dick AJ, Guttman MA, Raman VK, et al. Magnetic resonance fluoroscopy allows targeted delivery of mesenchymal stem cells to infarct borders in Swine. Circulation 2003;108(23):2899–904.

48. Karmarkar PV, Kraitchman DL, Izbudak I, et al. MR-trackable intramyocardial injection catheter. Magn Reson Med 2004;51(6):1163–72.

49. Bell JA, Saikus CE, Ratnayaka K, et al. A deflectable guiding catheter for real-time MRI-guided interventions. J Magn Reson Imaging 2012;35(4):908–15.

50. Prakash P, Salgaonkar VA, Scott SJ, et al. MR guided thermal therapy of pancreatic tumors with endoluminal, intraluminal and interstitial catheter-based ultrasound devices: preliminary theoretical and experimental investigations. Proc SPIE Int Soc Opt Eng 2013;8584:85840V.

51. Wang P, Unal O. Motion-compensated real-time MR thermometry augmented by tracking coils. J Magn Reson Imaging 2014;41(3):851–7.

Magnetic Resonance–Guided Passive Catheter Tracking for Endovascular Therapy

Fabio Settecase, MD, MSc[a],*, Alastair J. Martin, PhD[b],
Prasheel Lillaney, PhD[c], Aaron Losey, MD[c],
Steven W. Hetts, MD[d]

KEYWORDS

- Endovascular intervention • MR imaging • Passive tracking • Device tracking • MR angiography
- Real-time MR imaging

KEY POINTS

- Steady-state free precession (SSFP) sequences have become the preferred sequences for endovascular interventional MR imaging.
- Passive tracking using negative contrast uses marker materials in device construction that cause localized magnetic field inhomogeneities resulting in dephasing of adjacent proton spins and a local signal void or susceptibility artifact on MR imaging without the use of active radiofrequency (RF) components.
- Passive tracking can also be achieved with positive contrast using paramagnetic materials that cause focal T1 shortening (bright spot), such as gadolinium, within the lumen or on the surface of a catheter. Additional passive tracking methods include nonproton multispectral, and direct current techniques.
- The main advantage of passive catheter tracking over active tracking is simplicity and absence of radiofrequency (RF) heating, as no additional MR imaging scanner software, wires or electronics are required for most passive tracking techniques.
- Because device coordinates are not registered with passive tracking methods and imaging plane is not automatically updated, automatic visualization and correct imaging plane selection is difficult.

 Videos on the XMR suite at UCSF Medical Center and magnetic resonance imaging–guided electrophysiological ablation accompanies this article at http://www.mri.theclinics.com/

Disclosures: Dr S.W. Hetts: Chief Medical Officer: ChemoFilter; Scientific advisory: Medina Medical; Consulting: Stryker, Silk Road Medical, Penumbra; Data Safety and Monitoring Committee: DAWN trial; Core Imaging Lab: MAPS trial, FRED trial; Grant support: NIBIB 1R01EB012031, NCI 1R01CA194533, ASNR Foundation. Dr F. Settecase, Dr A.J. Martin, Dr P. Lillaney, and Dr A. Losey have nothing to disclose.
The authors were funded by NIH R01 grant EB012031-01A1.
^a Department of Radiology and Biomedical Imaging, University of California San Francisco, 505 Parnassus Avenue, L351, San Francisco, CA 94143-0628, USA; ^b Department of Radiology and Biomedical Imaging, University of California San Francisco, 505 Parnassus Avenue, L-310, San Francisco, CA 94143-0628, USA; ^c Department of Radiology and Biomedical Imaging, University of California San Francisco, 185 Berry Street, Suite 350, San Francisco, CA 94107, USA; ^d Department of Radiology and Biomedical Imaging, University of California San Francisco, 505 Parnassus Avenue, L-349, San Francisco, CA 94143-0628, USA
* Corresponding author.
E-mail address: fabio.settecase@ucsf.edu

Magn Reson Imaging Clin N Am 23 (2015) 591–605
http://dx.doi.org/10.1016/j.mric.2015.05.003
1064-9689/15/$ – see front matter © 2015 Elsevier Inc. All rights reserved.

INTRODUCTION

The use of MR imaging for guidance of endovascular interventions has emerged as a feasible alternative or adjunctive imaging modality to digital subtraction angiography (DSA). MR imaging guidance offers several potential advantages. The absence of ionizing radiation during MR imaging is particularly attractive, as there may be substantial radiation exposures to both the patient and the interventionalist during DSA.[1,2] In addition, although DSA is limited to luminal information, MR imaging can also provide high-contrast visualization of the vessel wall and adjacent soft tissues with moderately high spatial resolution, allowing for the identification of vulnerable atherosclerotic plaques, the ability to monitor the effect of endovascular therapy on adjacent tissues, and to recognize possible complications, such as vascular perforation, hemorrhage, and infarction, all in real time. MR imaging also offers unrestricted multiplanar imaging capabilities and the opportunity to obtain physiologic and functional information such as flow velocity, 4D flow imaging and computational fluid dynamics, temperature, diffusion, and perfusion.

Concurrent advances in the design of real-time MR fluoroscopy and MR angiography pulse sequences and the development of MR safe and compatible endovascular devices have facilitated progress from in vitro and animal feasibility studies of MR guidance for endovascular interventions to their translation into clinical care. This review highlights state-of-the-art imaging techniques and hardware used for passive tracking of devices in endovascular interventional MR imaging.

THE VASCULAR INTERVENTIONAL MR IMAGING SUITE

The use of MR imaging guidance for endovascular intervention requires balancing multiple trade-offs involving image quality, spatial and temporal resolution, patient accessibility, field of view, and cost. Higher-field-strength cylindrical bore scanners are capable of better image quality; however, they require small diameter bores compared with open MR imaging scanners and therefore limit patient accessibility. At present, open bore MR imaging scanners do not provide adequate field strength, gradient strength, or field uniformity for endovascular intervention.[3] Clamshell and double-doughnut–shaped bores were initially introduced to improve patient accessibility during intraoperative MR imaging. Fortunately, arterial access at the groin for most endovascular procedures permits longer distances (40–80 cm)

between the interventionist standing at the opening of the magnet bore and the target tissue of interest in the head, neck, chest, or abdomen, making commonly available cylindrical (or closed) bore clinical MR scanners suitable. Cylindrical bore magnets with shorter bore lengths (125 cm instead of 160 cm) and/or with larger bore diameters (70 cm instead of 60 cm) have been developed, allowing easier patient access and are commercially available. Most research sites now have hybrid systems consisting of a short-bore cylindrical MR imaging and DSA unit connected by a single floating table, also known as XMR systems (**Fig. 1**, Video 1). This system allows for use of either imaging modality for different parts of a procedure and permits the use of DSA backup in case of difficulties during MR guidance.

REAL-TIME MR IMAGING AND MR ANGIOGRAPHY TECHNIQUES FOR ENDOVASCULAR INTERVENTIONAL MR IMAGING

Image acquisition during MR-guided endovascular procedures must be rapid enough to allow the interventionist to visualize changes within the patient as devices are externally manipulated in real time. Several pulse sequence approaches to achieve higher-temporal-resolution MR imaging for MR-guided interventions, also known as real-time MR imaging or MR fluoroscopy, have been explored. Higher temporal resolution usually comes at the expense of spatial resolution. Nevertheless, MR fluoroscopy sequences used today allow sufficient spatial and temporal resolution to track endovascular devices. Because each pulse sequence offers unique contrast characteristics, the ideal sequence depends on the properties of the device being tracked and the passive tracking method being used for device tracking (see passive tracking section), the contrast properties of the tissue of interest, and the need for intravascular contrast. Commonly used MR fluoroscopy sequences are summarized in **Table 1**.

SSFP sequences have become the preferred sequences for endovascular interventional MR imaging. SSFP provides excellent bright blood contrast and visualization of devices using passive tracking because of the high temporal resolution (short repetition time [TR]), high signal-to-noise ratio (SNR), and greater sensitivity to magnetic field inhomogeneities[4–13] (**Fig. 2**).

T2-weighted turbo spin echo, rapid acquisition with relaxation enhancement (RARE, HASTE) sequences, may also be used for verification of device location because of the flexibility in image contrast and fast acquisition of the pulse

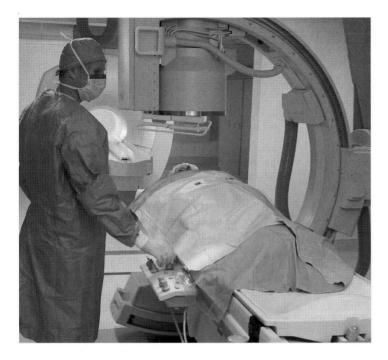

Fig. 1. Philips hybrid interventional XMR system at the University of California, San Francisco Medical Center, combining a clinical 1.5-T MR imaging scanner (background) and fully functional DSA unit (foreground), connected by a floating dockable table.

sequence. Additional methods to decrease image acquisition time include the use of parallel imaging,[14] key-hole imaging,[15] alternative k-space sampling such as spiral or radial trajectories, asymmetric truncated k-space sampling strategies,[16] and recently the exploitation of k-space data sparsity using compressed sensing.[17] Coupled with high-performance multiprocessor computers, real-time MR guidance is now capable of up to 10 frames per second, which is comparable to the temporal resolution of x-ray fluoroscopic guidance for most clinical endovascular interventions (4–15 frames per second).

MR angiograms with intra-arterial gadolinium contrast may also be used for MR guidance of endovascular procedures[18] (**Fig. 3**). Similar to DSA, contrast-enhanced MR angiography can be overlaid onto subsequent image acquisitions for

Table 1		
Characteristics of commonly used MR fluoroscopy sequences		
Contrast Weighting	**Sequence**	**Comments**
T1/T2	Balanced SSFP (aka FIESTA, TrueFISP, or balanced FFE)	• Fast • No gadolinium required • At low flip angles, SSFP (or FLAPS) can be used for positive contrast passive tracking of susceptibility markers • Susceptible to B_0 disturbances and blood flow artifacts in setting of slow or turbulent flow
T1+T2*	GRASS, FISP, FFE	• Fast, but less SNR efficient than SSFP
T2	TOSSI (RARE, HASTE) TSE	• Flexibility in image contrast • Fast acquisition
T1	FSPGR FLASH T1-FFE	• May be used with IA gadolinium for road-map guidance

Abbreviations: FFE, fast field echo; FIESTA, fast imaging employing steady-state acquisition; FISP, fast imaging with steady-state precession; FLASH, fast low-angle shot; FSPGR, fast spoiled gradient echo; FSPGR, fast spoiled gradient recalled echo; GRASS, gradient-recalled acquisition in the steady state; HASTE, half-fourier acquisition single-shot turbo spin-echo; IA, intra-arterial; RARE, rapid acquisition with relaxation enhancement; SSFP, steady-state free precession; TOSSI, T1-insensitive steady-state imaging; TSE, turbo spin echo.

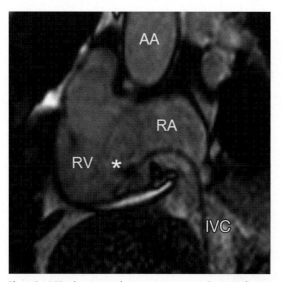

Fig. 2. MR images demonstrate passive catheter tracking within a human heart using a steady-state free precession sequence. The catheter tip is located above the cavotricuspid isthmus. *, passive marker near the catheter tip; AA, ascending aorta; IVC, inferior vena cava; RA, right atrium; RV, right ventricle. (*From* Grothoff M, Piorkowski C, Eitel C, et al. MR imaging-guided electrophysiological ablation studies in humans with passive catheter tracking: initial results. Radiology 2014;271(3):698; with permission.)

vascular road-map guidance.[19–21] Although intra-arterial injection of gadolinium chelate is an off-label use, no adverse events have been reported so far. The US Food and Drug Administration total dose limit for gadolinium chelate is 0.3 mmol/L/kg body weight. A low-dose gadolinium injection protocol requires[18,22] taking into account the blood flow rate in the artery of interest and avoids excess concentrations of gadolinium (resulting in T2/T2* spin-dephasing effects) or inadequate gadolinium concentrations (resulting in lack of T1 shortening).[20,22] Because contrast delivery is local rather than systemic, much lower doses are needed, and thus, repeat intra-arterial contrast administration is practical. Gadolinium contrast dose limit issues may be at least partially ameliorated by using new gadolinium-based contrast agents that remain in the blood pool for longer periods and provide prolonged vascular enhancement (eg, Gadomer-17, Vasovist).[23,24]

Different MR imaging pulse sequences may be interleaved and swapped as the procedure demands as the ideal pulse sequence for device visualization or tracking often differs from that needed for vascular road mapping, 2- and 3-dimensional visualization of tissue near the device, or therapeutic monitoring. Endovascular interventional MR imaging requires real-time changes in scan plane and pulse sequence parameters, and MR imaging vendors and third-party providers have started to develop interactive display and MR imaging control software that allow adaptation of parameters (eg, slice orientation, slab thickness, field of view (FOV), or contrast) (**Fig. 4**).

TRACKING OF ENDOVASCULAR DEVICES

Accurate, fast, and reliable visualization and localization of endovascular devices are essential requirements for safe and successful endovascular procedures. In DSA, catheters, guidewires, stents, clips, and pacemaker leads are visible because of the increased x-ray absorption of high-atomic-number metal components and markers relative to blood and tissues. The strong magnetic field in the MR imaging environment, however, restricts the use of ferromagnetic metals commonly used in the manufacture of guidewires and stents and in the braiding incorporated within catheter walls for improved torquability and pushability. In addition, the plastic polymers commonly used in catheter construction are difficult to visualize on MR imaging. The increasing availability and clinical utility of MR imaging scanners have created a significant demand for MR-compatible implants and devices such as titanium aneurysm clips and MR-compatible pacemakers. MR-compatible devices for endovascular interventional procedures, in contrast, are lacking because of a lower demand, high costs, paucity of MR imaging scanners dedicated to image-guided procedures, relative familiarity with alternate modalities for image guidance of procedures, and lack of training in MR-guided intervention. Nevertheless, several investigators have developed methods for endovascular device localization and visualization, or tracking, in the interventional MR imaging environment. These methods of device tracking are divided into 2 main categories: active and passive.

PASSIVE TRACKING METHODS

With passive tracking, endovascular devices can be tracked on MR imaging by incorporating markers or materials in their construction that enhance, reduce, or distort the T1- and/or T2-weighted MR signal relative to blood or tissues, either focally using a marker at the tip or along the length of the device. Passive tracking methods are summarized in **Table 2**.

NEGATIVE CONTRAST

Passive tracking using negative contrast uses marker materials in device construction that cause localized magnetic field inhomogeneities resulting

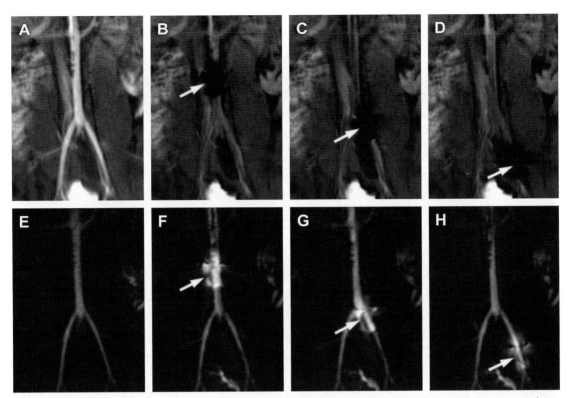

Fig. 3. The road-mapping approach is demonstrated in the distal aorta of a swine. The source images are shown on the top row, and the road-mapping mode images are on the bottom row. An intra-arterial injection of Gd is initially used to highlight arterial anatomy (*A*) and establish the road map (*E*). The magnetically assisted remote control catheter is then activated, producing a substantial signal void on the source images (*arrows* in *B–D*) and a signal enhancement pattern on the road-map images that is superimposed on the arterial anatomy (*arrows* in *F–H*). The road-map images can be used to track the device without losing visibility of the local arterial anatomy. (*From* Martin AJ, Lillaney P, Saeed M, et al. Digital subtraction MR angiography roadmapping for magnetic steerable catheter tracking. J Magn Reson Imaging 2015;41(4):1161; with permission.)

in dephasing of adjacent proton spins and a local signal void or susceptibility artifact on MR imaging without the use of active RF components[9,25–32] (see **Fig. 2**, **Table 2**).

The marker materials may be ferromagnetic (eg, stainless steel type AISI 410, nickel), ferrimagnetic (eg, copper zinc ferrite), or strongly paramagnetic (eg, dysprosium oxide). The focal susceptibility artifact associated with this kind of marker is most easily visualized on T2*-weighted MR imaging sequences. To increase the contrast between a passively tracked MR-compatible catheter or guidewire and background tissues, subtraction of a baseline tracking image can be used for background tissue suppression and can be overlaid onto a previously acquired MR angiogram for road-mapping.[33–35] An adaptive subtraction technique that automatically selects the most suitable reference image from a dynamic series for subtraction resulting in reduction in degradation of imaging by patient motion has also been described.[35]

During negative contrast passive device tracking, reliable device visualization depends on the contrast to noise ratio (CNR) and the visibility of the susceptibility artifact in the subtraction image. The CNR in the tracking images depends on the susceptibility artifact induced by the marker and the SNR of the tracking image.[31] The SNR can be controlled by sequence design, the size and amount of susceptibility artifact by the magnetic moment (m) of the marker material, and the echo time.[36] For diamagnetic and paramagnetic materials, m is proportional to the main magnetic field of the MR scanner. For ferromagnetic and ferrimagnetic materials, a nonlinear relationship exists, meaning the size of susceptibility artifact is similar through a range of field strengths.[31] As a result, with ferromagnetic and ferrimagnetic markers, to achieve the same size of artifact, less material is required than with paramagnetic markers.[31] If the entire catheter is doped with the negative contrast material, the artifact visibility depends on field strength and device orientation

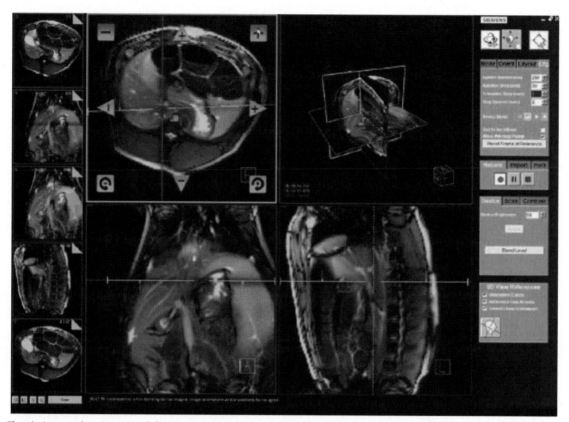

Fig. 4. Interactive Front End (Siemens, Munich, Germany) user interface for MR imaging–guided navigation. (*From* Saikus CE, Lederman RJ. Interventional cardiovascular magnetic resonance imaging: a new opportunity for image-guided interventions. JACC Cardiovasc Imaging 2009;2(11):1327; with permission.)

to B_0 (main magnetic field).[25,26,37] The artifact is less dependent on device orientation and field strength, however, if using focal rings as markers.[37]

Similar to diagnostic MR imaging, susceptibility artifact size also depends on the imaging sequence used. Gradient recalled echo sequences, for example, result in larger susceptibility artifacts and consequently poorer information on surrounding tissues, whereas spin-echo sequences produce smaller areas of signal cancellation.[38] The relative importance of loss of the anatomic information around the artifact on MR imaging varies with different procedures.

The signal void created by negative contrast markers can also be converted to a bright spot, or white marker (**Fig. 5**). The white marker phenomenon can be elicited by dephasing the background signal with application of a slice gradient, whereas the signal near the marker is conserved because a dipole field induced by the marker compensates the dephasing gradient.[39] The MR imaging appearance of the white marker is determined by the marker magnetic susceptibility, echo time, slice thickness, and gradient strength.[39] A white marker phenomenon for negative contrast markers can

also be achieved using off-resonance techniques such as low flip angle SSFP sequences (or FLAPS).[32,40] The intensity and the spatial extent of the off-resonance contrast strongly depend on TR, flip angle, field strength, and T2/T1 of the medium. Although off-resonance techniques may result in increased accuracy of the location of the marker, this technique does not eliminate the potential for loss of signal from adjacent anatomic structures due to the local magnetic field inhomogeneities caused by the markers.

A distinct feature of most passive tracking techniques is that the tracking mechanism cannot be switched on or off because the markers are built into the catheter. However, it was shown that a passive marker using negative contrast, in this case, a titanium cylinder built into a catheter tip, could be mechanically switched on or off by sliding a graphite cylinder with a layer thickness calculated to cancel out the susceptibility artifact of the titanium marker.[41] However, this setup did not allow for use of the inner lumen of a catheter, and the outer diameter of the device measured a large 9F.

Negative contrast passive tracking has also been shown using CO_2, either injected into a

Table 2
Passive tracking techniques

Passive Tracking Mechanism	Technology	Advantages	Disadvantages
Negative contrast	Markers with susceptibility artifact (material creating signal void)	• Simple • Safe • Lower cost • Negative contrast can be converted to positive (white marker phenomenon)	• Susceptible to motion and flow artifacts when using subtraction • Loss of the anatomic information around the artifact • White marker phenomenon requires prior knowledge of field distortion gradients
Positive contrast	Markers with T1 shortening (eg, gadolinium)	• Preserves anatomic information around marker	• Positive contrast coating materials unstable • Inability to use lumen of gadolinium-filled catheters/need for larger multilumen catheters
Nonproton multispectral	Catheters filled with ^{19}F or ^{13}C	High CNR and/or SNR	• Additional hardware needed for non-^{1}H magnetic resonance • Additional software for postprocessing • ^{1}H-MR imaging road-map overlay is obligatory • Decreased spatial and temporal resolution • Requires use of larger multilumen catheters
Direct current	Current applied to wire and/or coils create a local field distortion/signal void (negative contrast)	• Simple • Cost-effective • Negative contrast can be converted to positive contrast using subtraction (current on/off) • Coil can also be used for catheter steering and endovascular imaging	• Coil/wires add to outer diameter of catheter • Requires additional hardware • With subtraction technique, time per image doubles • Potential RF and resistive heating of wires/coils • Not commercially available

Abbreviation: CNR, contrast to noise ratio.

catheter after gadolinium contrast-enhanced T1-weighted MR angiography[24] or using balloon catheters inflated with CO_2.[10]

POSITIVE CONTRAST

Passive tracking can also be achieved with positive contrast, using paramagnetic materials that cause focal T1 shortening (bright spot), such as gadolinium, within the lumen[9,30] or on the surface of a catheter[42,43] (**Fig. 6**, see **Table 2**). This image is best visualized on a T1-weighted pulse sequence. The main drawbacks of passive tracking with positive contrast are the inability to use the lumen of contrast-filled single-lumen catheters and need for larger-diameter multilumen catheters. Furthermore, positive contrast materials used for catheter coating are unstable. The

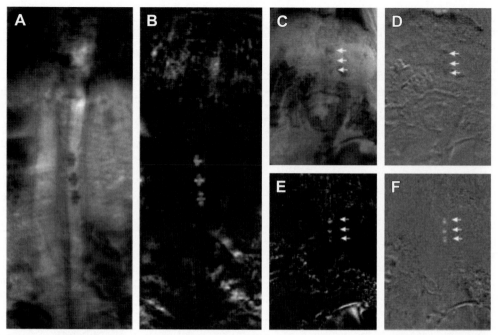

Fig. 5. Passive catheter tracking using white marker phenomenon. (*A, B*) In vivo imaging of 3 paramagnetic markers, mounted on a 5F catheter, located in the abdominal aorta of a living pig, as visualized with (*A*) conventional gradient echo sequence (slice 30 mm, echo time[TE]/TR = 4.6/60 milliseconds, duration 22 seconds) and (*B*) dephased positive contrast gradient echo imaging (white marker sequence with 1.9 cycles of phase across the slice) for similar acquisition parameters. (*C–F*) Demonstration of performance of in vivo application of white marker tracking for a case with significant obscuring of the markers (*arrows*) during in vivo tracking. For (*C*) unsubtracted and (*D*) subtracted conventional tracking, the markers are hardly seen, whereas the white marker tracking allows easy detection of the markers for both (*E*) unsubtracted and (*F*) subtracted positive contrast tracking. (*From* Seppenwoolde JH, Viergever MA, Bakker CJ. Passive tracking exploiting local signal conservation: the white marker phenomenon. Magn Reson Med 2003;50(4):789; with permission.)

T2* effect of gadolinium can also be exploited for positive contrast passive tracking. If the excitation frequency and bandwidth are properly chosen, specific concentrations of gadolinium contrast agent within a catheter can be excited without exciting fat or water spins.[44] The authors term this technique off-resonance contrast angiography. In addition, complete background

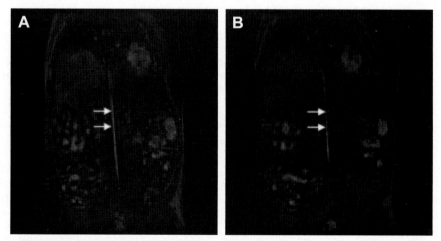

Fig. 6. Positive contrast tracking. Coronal T1 SPGR maximum intensity projection images of a 6F catheter filled with 4% Gd-diethylene triamine pentaacetic acid (*arrows* in *A*) and a 4F catheter coated using Design III (*arrows* in *B*) in a canine aorta. (*From* Unal O, Li J, Cheng W, et al. MR-visible coatings for endovascular device visualization. J Magn Reson Imaging 2006;23(5):767; with permission.)

suppression can be obtained without image subtraction. This method is highly sensitive to catheter orientation within the B_0 field, however, which currently limits practical usefulness.

NONPROTON MULTISPECTRAL CONTRAST

Recently, passive tracking was demonstrated with catheters filled with contrast materials visible with nonproton magnetic resonance such as ^{19}F and hyperpolarized ^{13}C.[45,46] Although these methods are capable of high CNR and SNR, the spatial resolution of this device-tracking technique is lower, additional scanner hardware and software are required, and ^1H- MR imaging road-map overlay is obligatory. In addition, because of the inability to use the lumen of the ^{19}F or hyperpolarized ^{13}C contrast-filled catheters, larger-diameter multilumen catheters are necessary when using this technique as well.

DIRECT CURRENT

Another passive tracking method using negative contrast uses the local field distortions and resulting susceptibility artifact caused by application of small direct currents (DCs) (10–150 mA) running through wire coils wound at a catheter tip (**Fig. 7**).[47–49] Device visualization using this method can be turned on or off using a DC switch controlled by the interventionist and the visualization artifact can be adjusted by varying the amount of current applied. This method can also be combined with road-mapping with intravascular contrast[20] (see **Fig. 3**). With currents higher than those needed for catheter tip visualization, such coils may be used to steer a catheter tip into difficult turns.[48,49] Despite the use of long wires running along the length of the catheter and resultant potential for RF heating, in vivo testing has found endothelial damage from RF heating effects using this method to be negligible.[50] With heat-dissipating saline flowing at 2 mL/s within a guide catheter in a larger vessel, no endothelial damage from ohmic heating of the wire or coil from current application for tip deflection was found at current levels less than 300 mA.[51] The wire coils could also be used as RF receive coils, permitting concurrent active tracking or endovascular imaging.[48]

Passive tracking techniques can also be combined with active tracking techniques and used simultaneously in the same procedure to track different devices. Omary and colleagues[52] actively tracked a 0.030-inch guidewire with a loopless antenna and passively tracked a 5F catheter filled with dilute 4% gadopentate dimeglumine (positive contrast), allowing catheterization and stenting of swine renal arteries under MR guidance.

ADVANTAGES AND DISADVANTAGES RELATIVE TO ACTIVE TRACKING

Active tracking techniques are beyond the scope of this article and discussed in detail elsewhere in this issue.[53] Advantages and disadvantages of passive tracking relative to active tracking are summarized in **Table 3**. The main advantage of passive catheter tracking over active tracking is simplicity, as no additional MR imaging scanner software or electronics are required for most passive tracking techniques. In addition, the absence of a wire connection from the device to the scanner for negative and positive contrast passive tracking eliminates the risk of RF heating posed by long conductive wires needed for active tracking during MR image acquisition.[54–56] The decreased complexity of passive tracking also allows for better miniaturization of devices.

Although a needle can be completely visualized on a single image acquired along the needle shaft, the course of an endovascular catheter within vessels is seldom in a straight line. Visualizing the catheter shaft, which in some cases can become redundant or looped during clinical catheterization procedures, may require prescription of multiple scan planes and placement of tracking markers proximal to the catheter tip. In DSA, the course of an endovascular catheter can be easily obtained using a single projection or orthogonal biplane projections even within a tortuous vessel. Because previously acquired MR angiographic images can be used as an anatomic road-map onto which catheter tracking can be overlayed, catheter guidance shares similarity to conventional DSA road-map guidance. However, visualizing the course of a catheter is more difficult using MR imaging, as the distal catheter may course out of the imaging planes, often unbeknownst to the interventionist during the procedure.

Since device coordinates are not registered with passive tracking methods and imaging plane is not automatically updated, automatic visualization and correct imaging plane selection is not possible with passive techniques; this is the principal disadvantage of passive tracking methods as the process of manually updating the imaging plane may be more time consuming.[57]

In a feasibility study of MR-guided cardiac electrophysiologic ablation in humans, scan plane reorientation, when a passively tracked catheter fell out of plane, was usually achieved within 1 to 3 attempts. In some cases, however, it took up to 15 attempts, with up to 40 seconds until the catheter tip was relocated.[58] Thicker imaging slices are often used to keep the passive marker within the imaging volume; however, increased slice

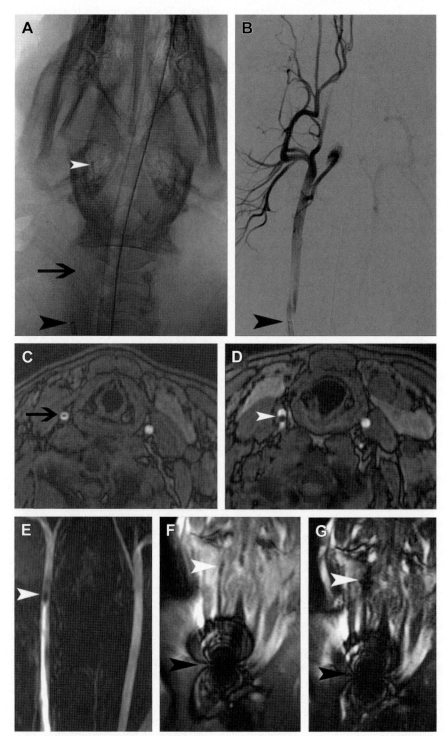

Fig. 7. Passive tracking using direct current coils. In vivo radiography, DSA, axial MR angiography, coronal MR angiography maximum intensity projection (MIP), and coronal SSFP. Unsubtracted radiograph (*A*) demonstrates magnetically assisted remote control catheter tip coils (*white arrowhead*), microcatheter shaft with lead wires (*black arrow*), and guiding catheter (*black arrowhead*) in the right common carotid artery. Only the guiding catheter tip marker (*black arrowhead*) is readily evident on the equivalent DSA image (*B*). Susceptibility from the catheter shaft lead wires (*black arrow*) and catheter tip (*white arrowhead*) is seen on axial MR angiography (*C* and *D*), coronal MR angiography MIP (*E*), and coronal SSFP (*F*). With a 300-mA current applied (*G*), the catheter tip coils are more apparent (*white arrowhead*). Guide catheter tip artifacts resulting from a metallic marker band are prominent on the SSFP sequence (*F* and *G*). (*From* Hetts SW, Saeed M, Martin AJ, et al. Endovascular catheter for magnetic navigation under MR imaging guidance: evaluation of safety in vivo at 1.5T. AJNR Am J Neuroradiol 2013;34(11):2087; with permission.)

Table 3
Passive tracking techniques: advantages and disadvantages compared with active tracking

Advantages	Disadvantages
Simple—no additional hardware or software[a]	Time consuming
Inexpensive	No automatic visualization or plane orientation
Does not require long wires or connection to current source[a]	correction if device tip exits the imaging plane unless using PRIDE sequence
Safe (no RF or ohmic heating risk)[a]	Tracking mechanism cannot be switched on or off[a]
Can be used at different field strengths	Thick slices required to keep device in imaging plane
Easier miniaturization of devices[a]	may result in superimposition of anatomic structures

[a] Exception: direct current passive tracking.

thickness may decrease visibility of the passive marker and increase superimposition of anatomy. Furthermore, passive tracking methods may be hampered by the need for subtraction because of weak negative contrast of the passive markers to their background, especially if thick imaging slices are used. This subtraction leads to an undesired increased sensitivity to motion and flow artifacts.[39] The ability to automatically update the image plane with changes in position of a device using negative contrast susceptibility markers was recently shown, however, by interleaving an SSFP sequence with a projection-reconstruction imaging with echo-dephasing (PRIDE) sequence.[59] The latter sequence detects the focal area of susceptibility artifact due to the marker on an image along all 3 physical axes. After successful localization of the paramagnetic marker with PRIDE (with an absolute error of 4.5 mm), the location of the marker can be used to provide automated SSFP slice positioning using a dedicated real-time feedback link with update times comparable to existing active tracking methods[59] (**Fig. 8**).

CLINICAL APPLICATIONS OF ENDOVASCULAR DEVICE PASSIVE TRACKING

Despite a dearth of commercially available MR-compatible endovascular devices, the feasibility of commonly performed endovascular procedures using MR guidance has been demonstrated in numerous animal studies and early human clinical studies of a variety of vascular and cardiac procedures. Successful transjugular intrahepatic stent placement,[60] coronary stent deployment,[61] closure of atrial septal defects[62] and patent foramen ovale,[63] aortic valve implantation,[64] aortic coarctation repair,[65] aortic dissection repair,[66] renal angioplasty[52] and stenting,[67] iliac artery stenting,[6] placement and retrieval of inferior vena cava filters,[68,69] hepatic artery catheterization,[70] recanalization of complete carotid occlusion,[71] carotid stenting,[72] aortic stent grafting,[73,74] and

hepatic arterial delivery of islet cells[75] have been successfully performed under MR guidance in animals. However, the lack of clinically approved endovascular devices for use in the MR imaging setting has limited the number of human studies.

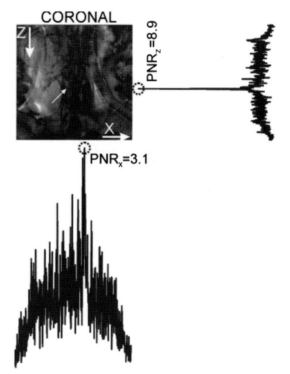

Fig. 8. Use of PRIDE for localization of a passively tracked negative contrast device in vivo: real-time balanced SSFP coronal image displaying the placement of the guidewire tip (*white arrow*) identified by susceptibility artifact. The PRIDE projections along the X and Z directions having peaks (*encircled*) within the close vicinity of the marker position are clearly seen. (*From* Patil S, Bieri O, Jhooti P, et al. Automatic slice positioning (ASP) for passive real-time tracking of interventional devices using projection-reconstruction imaging with echo-dephasing (PRIDE). Magn Reson Med 2009;62(4):941; with permission.)

Endovascular procedures successfully performed with MR guidance in humans include iliac,[76] femoral, and popliteal artery angioplasty[77]; cardiac catheterization[78,79]; cardiac electrophysiological ablation[58] (Video 2); and visualization of intramyocardial injection of gadolinium-diethylene triamine pentaacetic acid.[77]

However, the use of MR guidance for endovascular interventions has not yet been found to be superior, nor of additional benefit, compared with x-ray fluoroscopy/DSA guidance alone. MR guidance currently lacks sufficient spatial or temporal resolution for guiding meaningful clinical endovascular procedures,[80] and the additional costs and procedure time continue to favor DSA. Further development and testing of MR-compatible catheters, guidewires, stents, and other endovascular devices is needed, along with improvements in reliability of device visualization and tracking. Maintenance of a scan plane orientation that keeps the device tip in the field of view at all times remains challenging, especially with passive tracking techniques, but is obligatory for performing any endovascular intervention safely, quickly, and reliably. Future reports of improvements in clinical outcomes and the emergence of new therapies using MR-guided endovascular therapies not possible under x-ray, DSA, or ultrasound guidance have the highest potential for driving further technical evolution of the field.

SUPPLEMENTARY DATA

Supplementary data related to this article can be found online at http://dx.doi.org/10.1016/j.mric.2015.05.003.

REFERENCES

1. Lickfett L, Mahesh M, Vasamreddy C, et al. Radiation exposure during catheter ablation of atrial fibrillation. Circulation 2004;110(19):3003–10.
2. Gkanatsios NA, Huda W, Peters KR. Adult patient doses in interventional neuroradiology. Med Phys 2002;29(5):717–23.
3. Wacker FK, Hillenbrand C, Elgort DR, et al. MR imaging-guided percutaneous angioplasty and stent placement in a swine model comparison of open- and closed-bore scanners. Acad Radiol 2005;12(9):1085–8.
4. Bakker CJ, Hoogeveen RM, Hurtak WF, et al. MR-guided endovascular interventions: susceptibility-based catheter and near-real-time imaging technique. Radiology 1997;202(1):273–6.
5. Smits HF, Bos C, van der Weide R, et al. Interventional MR: vascular applications. Eur Radiol 1999; 9(8):1488–95.
6. Buecker A, Neuerburg JM, Adam GB, et al. Real-time MR fluoroscopy for MR-guided iliac artery stent placement. J Magn Reson Imaging 2000; 12(4):616–22.
7. Yang X, Bolster BD Jr, Kraitchman DL, et al. Intravascular MR-monitored balloon angioplasty: an in vivo feasibility study. J Vasc Interv Radiol 1998; 9(6):953–9.
8. Green JD, Omary RA, Finn JP, et al. Passive catheter tracking using MRI: comparison of conventional and magnetization-prepared FLASH. J Magn Reson Imaging 2002;16(1):104–9.
9. Omary RA, Unal O, Koscielski DS, et al. Real-time MR imaging-guided passive catheter tracking with use of gadolinium-filled catheters. J Vasc Interv Radiol 2000;11(8):1079–85.
10. Miquel ME, Hegde S, Muthurangu V, et al. Visualization and tracking of an inflatable balloon catheter using SSFP in a flow phantom and in the heart and great vessels of patients. Magn Reson Med 2004; 51(5):988–95.
11. Martin AJ, Weber OM, Saeed M, et al. Steady-state imaging for visualization of endovascular interventions. Magn Reson Med 2003;50(2):434–8.
12. Quick HH, Kuehl H, Kaiser G, et al. Interventional MRA using actively visualized catheters, TrueFISP, and real-time image fusion. Magn Reson Med 2003;49(1):129–37.
13. Schmitt P, Jakob PM, Kotas M, et al. T-one insensitive steady state imaging: a framework for purely T2-weighted TrueFISP. Magn Reson Med 2012; 68(2):409–20.
14. Griswold MA, Jakob PM, Heidemann RM, et al. Generalized autocalibrating partially parallel acquisitions (GRAPPA). Magn Reson Med 2002;47(6): 1202–10.
15. van Vaals JJ, Brummer ME, Dixon WT, et al. "Keyhole" method for accelerating imaging of contrast agent uptake. J Magn Reson Imaging 1993;3(4):671–5.
16. Peng H, Draper JN, Frayne R. Rapid passive MR catheter visualization for endovascular therapy using nonsymmetric truncated k-space sampling strategies. Magn Reson Imaging 2008;26(3):293–303.
17. Macdonald ME, Stafford RB, Yerly J, et al. Accelerated passive MR catheter tracking into the carotid artery of canines. Magn Reson Imaging 2013; 31(1):120–9.
18. Potthast S, Schulte AC, Bongartz GM, et al. Low-dose intra-arterial contrast-enhanced MR aortography in patients based on a theoretically derived injection protocol. Eur Radiol 2005;15(11):2347–53.
19. Bos C, Smits HF, Bakker CJ, et al. Selective contrast-enhanced MR angiography. Magn Reson Med 2000; 44(4):575–82.
20. Martin AJ, Lillaney P, Saeed M, et al. Digital subtraction MR angiography roadmapping for magnetic

steerable catheter tracking. J Magn Reson Imaging 2015;41(4):1157–62.

21. Green JD, Omary RA, Finn JP, et al. Two- and three-dimensional MR coronary angiography with intra-arterial injections of contrast agent in dogs: a feasibility study. Radiology 2003;226(1):272–7.

22. Huegli RW, Aschwanden M, Scheffler K, et al. Fluoroscopic contrast-enhanced MR angiography with a magnetization-prepared steady-state free precession technique in peripheral arterial occlusive disease. AJR Am J Roentgenology 2006;187(1):242–7.

23. Goyen M, Shamsi K, Schoenberg SO. Vasovist-enhanced MR angiography. Eur Radiol 2006; 16(Suppl 2):B9–14.

24. Maes RM, Lewin JS, Duerk JL, et al. Combined use of the intravascular blood-pool agent, gadomer, and carbon dioxide: a novel type of double-contrast magnetic resonance angiography (MRA). J Magn Reson Imaging 2005;21(5):645–9.

25. Rubin DL, Ratner AV, Young SW. Magnetic susceptibility effects and their application in the development of new ferromagnetic catheters for magnetic resonance imaging. Invest Radiol 1990;25(12): 1325–32.

26. Kochli VD, McKinnon GC, Hofmann E, et al. Vascular interventions guided by ultrafast MR imaging: evaluation of different materials. Magn Reson Med 1994; 31(3):309–14.

27. Bakker CJ, Hoogeveen RM, Weber J, et al. Visualization of dedicated catheters using fast scanning techniques with potential for MR-guided vascular interventions. Magn Reson Med 1996;36(6):816–20.

28. Leung DA, Debatin JF, Wildermuth S, et al. Intravascular MR tracking catheter: preliminary experimental evaluation. AJR Am J Roentgenol 1995;164(5): 1265–70.

29. Wacker FK, Reither K, Branding G, et al. Magnetic resonance-guided vascular catheterization: feasibility using a passive tracking technique at 0.2 Telsa in a pig model. J Magn Reson Imaging 1999;10(5): 841–4.

30. Unal O, Korosec FR, Frayne R, et al. A rapid 2D time-resolved variable-rate k-space sampling MR technique for passive catheter tracking during endovascular procedures. Magn Reson Med 1998; 40(3):356–62.

31. Peeters JM, Seppenwoolde JH, Bartels LW, et al. Development and testing of passive tracking markers for different field strengths and tracking speeds. Phys Med Biol 2006;51(6):N127–37.

32. Mekle R, Hofmann E, Scheffler K, et al. A polymer-based MR-compatible guidewire: a study to explore new prospects for interventional peripheral magnetic resonance angiography (ipMRA). J Magn Reson Imaging 2006;23(2):145–55.

33. Omary RA, Frayne R, Unal O, et al. MR-guided angioplasty of renal artery stenosis in a pig model: a feasibility study. J Vasc Interv Radiol 2000;11(3): 373–81.

34. Serfaty JM, Yang X, Aksit P, et al. Toward MRI-guided coronary catheterization: visualization of guiding catheters, guidewires, and anatomy in real time. J Magn Reson Imaging 2000;12(4):590–4.

35. Bakker CJ, Seppenwoolde JH, Bartels LW, et al. Adaptive subtraction as an aid in MR-guided placement of catheters and guidewires. J Magn Reson Imaging 2004;20(3):470–4.

36. Bos C, Viergever MA, Bakker CJ. On the artifact of a subvoxel susceptibility deviation in spoiled gradient-echo imaging. Magn Reson Med 2003;50(2):400–4.

37. Ladd ME, Quick HH, Debatin JF. Interventional MRA and intravascular imaging. J Magn Reson Imaging 2000;12(4):534–46.

38. Henk CB, Brodner W, Grampp S, et al. The postoperative spine. Top Magn Reson Imaging 1999;10(4): 247–64.

39. Seppenwoolde JH, Viergever MA, Bakker CJ. Passive tracking exploiting local signal conservation: the white marker phenomenon. Magn Reson Med 2003;50(4):784–90.

40. Dharmakumar R, Koktzoglou I, Tang R, et al. Off-resonance positive contrast imaging of a passive endomyocardial catheter in swine. Phys Med Biol 2008;53(13):N249–57.

41. Dominguez-Viqueira W, Karimi H, Lam WW, et al. A controllable susceptibility marker for passive device tracking. Magn Reson Med 2014;72(1):269–75.

42. Frayne R, WC, Yanng Z, et al. MR evaluation of signal emitting coatings. Paper presented at Seventh Annual Meeting of the International Society for Magnetic Resonance in Medicine. Philadelphia (PA), May 22–28, 1999.

43. Unal O, Li J, Cheng W, et al. MR-visible coatings for endovascular device visualization. J Magn Reson Imaging 2006;23(5):763–9.

44. Edelman RR, Storey P, Dunkle E, et al. Gadolinium-enhanced off-resonance contrast angiography. Magn Reson Med 2007;57(3):475–84.

45. Kozerke S, Hegde S, Schaeffter T, et al. Catheter tracking and visualization using 19F nuclear magnetic resonance. Magn Reson Med 2004;52(3): 693–7.

46. Magnusson P, Johansson E, Mansson S, et al. Passive catheter tracking during interventional MRI using hyperpolarized 13C. Magn Reson Med 2007; 57(6):1140–7.

47. Glowinski A, Adam G, Bucker A, et al. Catheter visualization using locally induced, actively controlled field inhomogeneities. Magn Reson Med 1997; 38(2):253–8.

48. Roberts TP, Hassenzahl WV, Hetts SW, et al. Remote control of catheter tip deflection: an opportunity for interventional MRI. Magn Reson Med 2002;48(6): 1091–5.

49. Settecase F, Sussman MS, Wilson MW, et al. Magnetically assisted remote control (MARC) steering of endovascular catheters for interventional MRI: a model for deflection and design implications. Med Phys 2007;34(8):3135–42.

50. Settecase F, Hetts SW, Martin AJ, et al. RF heating of MRI-assisted catheter steering coils for interventional MRI. Acad Radiol 2011;18(3):277–85.

51. Hetts SW, Saeed M, Martin AJ, et al. Endovascular catheter for magnetic navigation under MR imaging guidance: evaluation of safety in vivo at 1.5T. AJNR Am J Neuroradiology 2013;34(11):2083–91.

52. Omary RA, Gehl JA, Schirf BE, et al. MR imaging-versus conventional X-ray fluoroscopy-guided renal angioplasty in swine: prospective randomized comparison. Radiology 2006;238(2):489–96.

53. Wang W. MR guided active catheter tracking. 2015, in press.

54. Konings MK, Bartels LW, Smits HF, et al. Heating around intravascular guidewires by resonating RF waves. J Magn Reson Imaging 2000;12(1):79–85.

55. Nitz WR, Oppelt A, Renz W, et al. On the heating of linear conductive structures as guidewires and catheters in interventional MRI. J Magn Reson Imaging 2001;13(1):105–14.

56. Shellock FG. Radiofrequency energy-induced heating during MR procedures: a review. J Magn Reson Imaging 2000;12(1):30–6.

57. Frericks BB, Elgort DR, Hillenbrand C, et al. Magnetic resonance imaging-guided renal artery stent placement in a swine model: comparison of two tracking techniques. Acta Radiologica 2009;50(1):21–7.

58. Grothoff M, Piorkowski C, Eitel C, et al. MR imaging-guided electrophysiological ablation studies in humans with passive catheter tracking: initial results. Radiology 2014;271(3):695–702.

59. Patil S, Bieri O, Jhooti P, et al. Automatic slice positioning (ASP) for passive real-time tracking of interventional devices using projection-reconstruction imaging with echo-dephasing (PRIDE). Magn Reson Med 2009;62(4):935–42.

60. Kee ST, Rhee JS, Butts K, et al. 1999 Gary J. Becker Young Investigator Award. MR-guided transjugular portosystemic shunt placement in a swine model. J Vasc Interv Radiol 1999;10(5):529–35.

61. Spuentrup E, Ruebben A, Schaeffter T, et al. Magnetic resonance–guided coronary artery stent placement in a swine model. Circulation 2002;105(7):874–9.

62. Rickers C, Jerosch-Herold M, Hu X, et al. Magnetic resonance image-guided transcatheter closure of atrial septal defects. Circulation 2003;107(1):132–8.

63. Buecker A, Spuentrup E, Grabitz R, et al. Magnetic resonance-guided placement of atrial septal closure device in animal model of patent foramen ovale. Circulation 2002;106(4):511–5.

64. Kuehne T, Yilmaz S, Meinus C, et al. Magnetic resonance imaging-guided transcatheter implantation of a prosthetic valve in aortic valve position: feasibility study in swine. J Am Coll Cardiol 2004;44(11):2247–9.

65. Raval AN, Telep JD, Guttman MA, et al. Real-time magnetic resonance imaging-guided stenting of aortic coarctation with commercially available catheter devices in swine. Circulation 2005;112(5):699–706.

66. Raman VK, Karmarkar PV, Guttman MA, et al. Real-time magnetic resonance-guided endovascular repair of experimental abdominal aortic aneurysm in swine. J Am Coll Cardiol 2005;45(12):2069–77.

67. Elgort DR, Hillenbrand CM, Zhang S, et al. Image-guided and -monitored renal artery stenting using only MRI. J Magn Reson Imaging 2006;23(5):619–27.

68. Shih MC, Rogers WJ, Bonatti H, et al. Real-time MR-guided retrieval of inferior vena cava filters: an in vitro and animal model study. J Vasc Interv Radiol 2011;22(6):843–50.

69. Shih MC, Rogers WJ, Hagspiel KD. Real-time magnetic resonance-guided placement of retrievable inferior vena cava filters: comparison with fluoroscopic guidance with use of in vitro and animal models. J Vasc Interv Radiol 2006;17(2 Pt 1):327–33.

70. Seppenwoolde JH, Bartels LW, van der Weide R, et al. Fully MR-guided hepatic artery catheterization for selective drug delivery: a feasibility study in pigs. J Magn Reson Imaging 2006;23(2):123–9.

71. Raval AN, Karmarkar PV, Guttman MA, et al. Real-time magnetic resonance imaging-guided endovascular recanalization of chronic total arterial occlusion in a swine model. Circulation 2006;113(8):1101–7.

72. Feng L, Dumoulin CL, Dashnaw S, et al. Feasibility of stent placement in carotid arteries with real-time MR imaging guidance in pigs. Radiology 2005;234(2):558–62.

73. Mahnken AH, Chalabi K, Jalali F, et al. Magnetic resonance-guided placement of aortic stents grafts: feasibility with real-time magnetic resonance fluoroscopy. J Vasc Interv Radiol 2004;15(2 Pt 1):189–95.

74. Eggebrecht H, Kuhl H, Kaiser GM, et al. Feasibility of real-time magnetic resonance-guided stent-graft placement in a swine model of descending aortic dissection. Eur Heart J 2006;27(5):613–20.

75. Barnett BP, Arepally A, Karmarkar PV, et al. Magnetic resonance-guided, real-time targeted delivery and imaging of magnetocapsules immunoprotecting pancreatic islet cells. Nat Med 2007;13(8):986–91.

76. Manke C, Nitz WR, Djavidani B, et al. MR imaging-guided stent placement in iliac arterial stenoses: a feasibility study. Radiology 2001;219(2):527–34.

77. Paetzel C, Zorger N, Bachthaler M, et al. Magnetic resonance-guided percutaneous angioplasty of femoral and popliteal artery stenoses using real-time imaging and intra-arterial contrast-enhanced magnetic resonance angiography. Invest Radiol 2005;40(5):257–62.

78. Razavi R, Hill DL, Keevil SF, et al. Cardiac catheterisation guided by MRI in children and adults with congenital heart disease. Lancet 2003;362(9399): 1877–82.

79. Ratnayaka K, Faranesh AZ, Hansen MS, et al. Real-time MRI-guided right heart catheterization in adults using passive catheters. Eur Heart J 2013;34(5): 380–9.

80. Saikus CE, Lederman RJ. Interventional cardiovascular magnetic resonance imaging: a new opportunity for image-guided interventions. JACC Cardiovasc Imaging 2009;2(11):1321–31.

Magnetic Resonance–Guided Thermal Therapy for Localized and Recurrent Prostate Cancer

David A. Woodrum, MD, PhD[a],*,
Akira Kawashima, MD, PhD[a], Krzysztof R. Gorny, PhD[a],
Lance A. Mynderse, MD[b]

KEYWORDS

- MR imaging • Native prostate cancer • Recurrent prostate cancer • Laser ablation • Cryoablation
- Focused ultrasound ablation

KEY POINTS

- Whole-gland and focal MR imaging–guided thermal ablative treatments for native and recurrent prostate cancer include cryoablation, laser, and focused ultrasonography ablation.
- Integrated clinical and imaging workup for the native and recurrent prostate cancer should include optimal multiparametric MR imaging of the prostate, careful mapping/targeted biopsy, and judicial selection of patients with appropriate cross-sectional imaging of the body to assess regional and distant disease.
- Multicenter, prospective clinical trials are critically needed to assess thermal ablative treatment efficacy for native and recurrent prostate cancer.

THE STATE OF THERAPIES FOR PROSTATE CANCER

The American Cancer Society estimates that 220,800 new cases of prostate cancer will be diagnosed in the United States in 2015. Prostate cancer is the most commonly diagnosed cancer in men. With an estimated 27,540 deaths in 2015, prostate cancer is the second-leading cause of cancer death in men.[1] Many men with prostate cancer are often managed with radiotherapy, surgery, or androgen deprivation.[2] No matter how expertly performed, these therapies carry significant risk and morbidity to the patient's health-related quality

of life, with potential impact on sexual, urinary, and bowel function.[3] Active screening programs for prostate cancer have identified increasing numbers of low-risk prostate cancer and have encouraged regimens of active surveillance to delay treatment until cancer progression.[4] Although active debate continues on the suitability of focal or regional therapy for these patients with low-risk prostate cancer, many unresolved issues remain, complicating this management approach, including prostate cancer multifocality, limitations of current biopsy strategies, suboptimal staging by accepted imaging modalities, and less than robust prediction models for indolent prostate

Disclosure: Dr D.A. Woodrum has an NIH grant, Regulation of molecular thermal ablative resistance in hepatocellular carcinoma funded by National Cancer Institute. (R01 CA 177686) but no grant funds or time were used on this project. Drs A. Kawashima, K.R. Gorny, and L.A. Mynderse have nothing to disclose.
[a] Department of Radiology, Mayo Clinic, 200 First Street Southwest, Rochester, MN 55905, USA; [b] Department of Urology, Mayo Clinic, 200 First Street Southwest, Rochester, MN 55905, USA
* Corresponding author.
E-mail address: woodrum.david@mayo.edu

Magn Reson Imaging Clin N Am 23 (2015) 607–619
http://dx.doi.org/10.1016/j.mric.2015.05.014
1064-9689/15/$ – see front matter © 2015 Elsevier Inc. All rights reserved.

cancers. Despite these restrictions, focal therapy continues to confront the current paradigm of therapy for low-risk disease.[5] Furthermore, prostate cancer recurrence rates after established forms of therapy range from 20% to 60%.[6] Advanced, locally recurrent, or metastatic disease has also become more amenable to treatment with new classes of medications and robotic surgical approaches. With such disease volume, the opportunities for treating advancement in early, recurrent, and metastatic disease are almost boundless. In this article, the use of MR imaging to direct focal therapy for native and recurrent prostate cancer is described.

IMPORTANCE OF MR IMAGING FOR PROSTATE CANCER IMAGING

Prostate cancer has traditionally been diagnosed by systematic but random sampling of the entire organ. The recent introduction of multiparametric MR imaging (mpMR imaging) now allows for imaging-based identification of prostate cancer, which may improve diagnostic accuracy for higher-risk tumors.[7] Recently, a consensus panel agreed to PI-RADS v2 (Prostate Imaging-Reporting and Data System), which is designed to improve detection, localization, characterization, and risk stratification in patients with suspected cancer in treatment-naive prostate glands.[8] Targeted biopsy of suspected cancer lesions detected by MR imaging is associated with increased detection of high-risk prostate cancer and decreased detection of low-risk prostate cancer, particularly with the aid of MR imaging/ultrasonography (US) fusion platforms.[9] The use of mpMR imaging has expanded beyond staging to detection, characterization, and monitoring for active surveillance for cases of suspected recurrence. The use of MR imaging for recurrent prostate cancer continues to evolve and has potential to evaluate both local recurrence and distant bony and nodal metastases.[10] In 2013, a consensus panel chaired by Professor Michael Marberger endorsed using mpMR imaging to identify patients for focal therapy.[11] Multiparametric MR imaging is capable of localizing small tumors for focal therapy and is the technique of choice for follow-up of focal ablation. Although mpMR imaging plays an established, critical role in native and recurrent prostate cancer imaging, functional, metabolic imaging for prostate cancer is in its formative years. [11C]Choline PET/computed tomography (CT) has an advantage in showing both local recurrent and distant metastatic prostate cancers. [11C]Choline PET/CT had a sensitivity of 73%, a specificity of 88%, a positive predictive value of 92%, a negative predictive value

of 61%, and an accuracy of 78% for the detection of clinically suspected recurrent prostate cancer in postsurgical patients.[12] In a study of postprostatectomy patients with increasing prostate-specific antigen (PSA) levels, mpMR imaging was superior for the detection of local recurrence, [11C]choline PET/CT superior for pelvic nodal metastasis, and both are equally excellent for pelvic bone metastasis. [11C]Choline PET/CT and mpMR imaging are complementary for restaging prostatectomy patients with suspected recurrent disease.[10] However, [11C]choline PET/CT is not widely available.

With the limitations of US and PET/CT imaging, MR imaging remains preeminent for detection and staging of recurrent prostate tumors. MR imaging provides superior soft tissue contrast resolution, high spatial resolution, multiplanar imaging capabilities, and a large field of view.

If the focal treatment is intended for potential curative treatment, it is important to ensure that there is not distant disease with whole-body CT/MR imaging, bone scan, and [11C]choline PET/CT. None of these imaging modalities is perfect, and appropriate selection of image staging is unique to each patient.

Native Prostate Cancer

In selecting the appropriate patient for focal therapy for the native prostate gland, it is critical to determine that the patient has localized low-risk disease. With low-risk disease, there is level 1 evidence that implies a lack of benefit from radical therapy.[13–15] Patients are often targeted for cancer workup because of increasing PSA levels or nodule on digital rectal examination. Patients are further evaluated with a mapping biopsy or mpMR imaging with targeted biopsy. Patients are classified to have low or intermediate prostate cancer with a focal positive lesion on mpMR imaging, Gleason score 4 + 3 or lower, and PSA level less than 20 ng/mL. For consideration for focal therapy, the target lesion should be confined to 1 lobe of the prostate.[16] Furthermore, the target should be visible with the imaging modality that will be used to guide the focal ablation treatment.

Focal Therapy Treatments for Native Prostate Cancer

Although radical prostatectomy and radiation therapy remain the preferred definitive therapy for choice for men with newly diagnosed prostate cancer and with a life expectancy greater than 10 years,[17,18] there is increasing interest in less radical focal methodologies for treatment, especially in the watchful waiting population. For this population of patients with low-risk and intermediate-risk prostate cancer, active surveillance may be undesirable, yet the complications and comorbidities associated with standard therapies are still not palatable. This patient-driven interest is pushing the development of minimally invasive focal therapies for prostate carcinoma in low-risk patients.[19] As a result, several minimally invasive thermal ablation methods under direct MR guidance, most prominently cryotherapy,[20] laser ablation,[21] and high-intensity focused US (HIFU),[22] have been developed and are being evaluated.

Magnetic resonance–guided cryoablation

MR-guided percutaneous cryoablation offers the combination of superb soft tissue resolution typical of MR imaging coupled with the ablative capacity of cryosurgery. Early experience combining cryoablation with MR imaging has shown a high degree of accuracy in defining normal and frozen tissue on all MR imaging sequences.[23,24] In addition, MR imaging allows visualization of the iceball in multiple planes, which becomes critically important in the pelvis, where there is limited safety for nontarget iceball growth. These features allow for more precise cryoprobe

placement and iceball monitoring during treatment within the confined space of the pelvis. The final advantage is that this procedure is not appreciably limited by previous surgery or radiation to the treated area.[25,26]

There are limited data using MR-guided cryoablation within the native prostate. Two published canine studies reported feasibility and overall safety.[27,28] These studies did bring out 1 limitation of cryoablation, which is that the visualized edge of the ice (°C) does not represent the ablation margin. The ablation margin is best shown with contrast enhancement after the procedure and is at the −2°C isotherm, which is just inside the edge of the iceball. There are 2 published reports of MR-guided cryoablation in native prostate glands, each with small numbers (**Fig. 1**).[25,26] Gangi and colleagues[26] performed MR imaging–guided prostate cryoablation in 11 patients using 1.5-T MR imaging. They had some minor complications of hematuria, dysuria, and urine retention. In addition, they had 1 major complication of rectal fistula, with spontaneous closure after 3 months. The other study[25] examined 18 patients with 2 slightly different methodologies. The group treated with a more aggressive freezing regimen had better

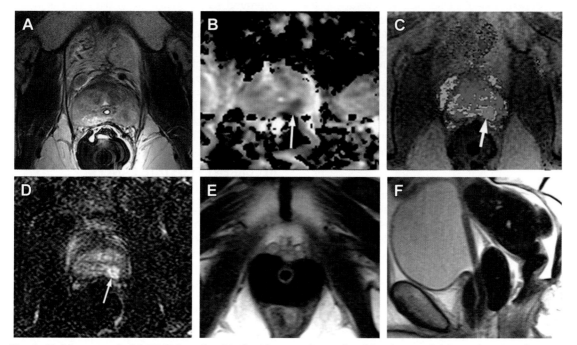

Fig. 1. Multiparametric 3.0-T MR imaging (*A–F*) with an endorectal coil in place. Axial fast relaxation, fast spin echo (FRFSE) images show a focal area of decreased T2 signal in the left posterior prostate (*A*), axial diffusion-weighted imaging shows a corresponding area of restricted diffusion (*arrows, B*), axial dynamic contrast-enhanced LAVA-FLEX images showing abnormal tumor enhancement (*arrows*) in the prostatic bed (*C, D*). Cryoprobe needles are evenly placed throughout the gland to facilitate whole-gland ablation. Axial (*C*) and sagittal (*D*) FRFSE images obtained during treatment showing the final extent of the iceball encompassing the prostate with a urethral warmer present in sparing the urethral mucosa from the iceball (*E, F*).

results over time.[25] These studies confirm that MR-guided cryoablation is technically feasible with relative safety; however, more short-term and long-term data are needed to assess overall efficacy.

Magnetic resonance–guided laser ablation

Laser-induced interstitial thermal therapy (LITT) uses a locally placed laser fiber to deliver targeted thermal ablation. LITT is inherently MR compatible, making it an obvious choice of ablation technologies to couple with MR imaging. MR-based temperature monitoring allows real-time feedback during LITT treatment, because both deposition of light energy and MR signal acquisition can be performed simultaneously without degradation in the MR image.[29] Performance of the ablation within the MR imaging allows use of posttreatment imaging to verify treatment delivery. Because MR images clearly show the prostate anatomy and the surrounding critical structures, MR imaging is critical for monitoring ablation growth to prevent encroachment onto adjacent critical structures.

Examination of the literature shows that LITT began being used in the brain to treat epileptogenic foci and neoplasms and expanded to liver lesions, in which its use is widely accepted.[29–31] However, use of percutaneous laser ablation therapy in the prostate is relatively new. Two studies[32,33] reported feasibility in canine prostate as well. These studies were beneficial because they showed technical feasibility but also correlation of the MR temperature map with contrast-enhanced T1-weighted images. A subsequent study in cadavers reported technical feasibility in the human prostate within a 3-T MR imaging scanner.[34] Lee and colleagues[21] published early results on 23 patients treated with focal laser ablation, showing promising results. Raz and colleagues[35] described using laser ablation for treatment of 2 patients with prostate cancer at 1.5 T, with discharge 3 hours after the procedure. These studies show the potential usefulness of laser ablation in the prostate. However, more data are needed to determine short-term and long-term effects.

Magnetic resonance–guided focused US ablation

Treatment of the prostate with focused US ablation is not new, although an MR imaging–guided version of the procedure has not been approved by the US Food and Drug Administration (FDA) in the United States. It has been performed with transrectal US imaging guidance with success in Europe for many years.[22,36] However, a major limitation of US imaging guidance is the difficulty in visualizing the focus of cancer, especially if the focus is small. Therefore, the treatment strategy used with US-guided HIFU is to ablate the entire prostate, or a relatively large region if the site of biopsy-proven cancer was found using a mapping biopsy or mpMR imaging. This procedure often results in inadequate tumor control or overablation of unnecessary normal/neural tissue, with potential subsequent morbidity. An early study by Gelet and colleagues[37] used US-guided focused US ablation in the prostate of 82 patients who were treated and followed up for 24 months. These patients also received subsequent radiation treatment. Of the patients, 68% were cancer free at the time of follow-up. Because of relatively high complication rates, the treatment device underwent multiple iterations and improvements. A subsequent study by Gelet and colleagues[38] reported incontinence and impotency rates of approximately 14% and 61%, respectively, at 19 months after treatment. In both studies, major limitations were identified as total procedure time as a result of need to cover the entire prostate and inability to monitor temperatures or ablation zone expansion. MR thermal monitoring and localization of lesions/zones within the prostate should allow optimization of an ablation treatment zone, whereas ablation temperature monitoring should allow an improved safety margin regarding vital adjacent tissues. There are 2 MR imaging integrated systems using transrectal or transurethral transmission routes for treatment of prostate lesions with focused US technology. The systems are fully integrated with the MR imaging console with temperature feedback control to adjust power, frequency, and rotation rate. Both systems are being used in patient trials assessing safety and efficacy for evidence for FDA approval.

RECURRENT PROSTATE CANCER
Standard Therapies for Treatment of Recurrent Prostate Cancer

Traditional curative therapy for prostate cancer has been either surgical resection or radiotherapy. Patients are roughly divided with half choosing surgery and half choosing radiotherapy. Recurrences after surgical resection can range from 25% to 40%, which is usually manifested by increasing serum level of PSA.[39–41] Approximately 30,000 men develop biochemical recurrence (BCR) with increasing PSA levels after radical prostatectomy each year in the United States.[40] One study examining where recurrences occur found that 81% had a local prostate bed recurrence that could be shown with MR imaging using an endorectal coil.[42] For those undergoing radiotherapy, BCR can range widely, from 33% to

63%, over 10 years, and contributes another 45,000 men per year with recurrent cancer from radiotherapy in the United States.[43,44] Although 5-year disease-free survival from prostate cancer, including good outcomes from primary therapies, approaches 100% in the United States, these figures clearly show that many men develop recurrent cancer each year. Salvage treatments for recurrent prostate cancer include salvage radical prostatectomy (sRP), salvage radiotherapy, salvage US-guided HIFU, salvage US-guided cryoablation, and newly described salvage MR imaging–guided laser and cryoablation.

Limitations of Current Salvage Therapies for Recurrent Prostate Cancer

Surgery
sRP after radiotherapy is more difficult because of local fibrosis and tissue plane obliteration secondary to the radiation, with limited centers of excellence offering this surgery. Because of the difficulties posed after primary radiation treatment failure, the complication rates for sRP have been higher than primary surgery, with incontinence rates of 58% and major complication rates of 33%.[45]

Radiation
Salvage radiotherapy can be used for BCR after surgery or primary radiotherapy failures. In a large study at the Mayo Clinic, 49 patients with primary external beam radiotherapy failure were treated with salvage low-dose rate brachytherapy. They showed a 3-year biochemical disease-free survival (bDFS) of 48% and a 5-year bDFS of 34%. Complications for salvage brachytherapy were either genitourinary or gastrointestinal. Grade 3 to 4 genitourinary toxicity was 17% as a late complication, and grade 3 to 4 gastrointestinal toxicity was approximately 5.6%.[45,47]

High-intensity focused ultrasonography
Salvage US-guided HIFU has been used for salvage therapy. Three different studies have been published, with relatively short follow-up periods of 7.4 to 18.1 months. These studies reported a highly variable bDFS of 25% to 71%, which was confounded by variable definitions of PSA failure and variable use of hormonal therapy before treatment. The most commonly reported complications are incontinence (10%–49.5%), urethral stricture with retention (17%–17.6%), erectile dysfunction (66.2%–100%), and rectourethral fistula (3%–16%).[45,48–50]

Salvage ultrasound-guided cryotherapy
US-guided cryotherapy was used for salvage therapy in several limited studies. The most recent large study from the Cryo On-Line Data (COLD) registry[51] reported a 5-year bDFS of 58.9% by the American Society for Radiation Oncology definition of BCR and 54.5% by the Phoenix definition of BCR. For patients treated with salvage US-guided cryotherapy after primary radiotherapy failure, the most recent reported complication rates are perineal pain (4%–14%), mild-moderate incontinence (6%–13%), severe incontinence (2%–4%), and urethrorectal fistula (1%–2%). With the use of a urethral warming catheter, the rate of sloughing and urethral stricture has been reduced to near zero. Erectile dysfunction is still high, with rates of 69% to 86%.[45]

Selection of Patients with Recurrent Prostate Cancer for Magnetic Resonance–Guided Focal Therapy

The first issue is to determine whether the increasing PSA levels represent local recurrence, systemic recurrence, or both.[41] The second issue in managing patients with BCR of prostate cancer is assessing the risk of cancer treatment versus the risk of further intervention. Overall, rapid increase in PSA levels, short disease-free interval, and high-grade disease are all poor prognostic indicators, with a higher probability of systemic recurrence, whereas slow increase in PSA levels, long disease-free interval, and low-grade disease are better prognostic indicators, with a higher probability of local recurrence.[41,52]

Suggested criteria for MR-guided focal ablative treatment in recurrent prostate cancer are (1) biopsy-proven local recurrent tumor that can be visualized by MR imaging, (2) absence of distant metastasis confirmed with chest, abdomen, pelvis CT, or MR imaging plus bone scintigraphy, or [^{11}C] choline PET/CT scan.[53] Although these selection criteria are not perfect, they are helpful in avoiding treatment of what is believed to be a local recurrence that is really systemic.

Magnetic resonance–guided cryoablation
MR-guided cryoablation for recurrent prostate cancer has also been shown feasible and successful in several small limited studies. Woodrum and colleagues[25] published a study of 18 patients treated with MR-guided cryoablation for locally recurrent prostate cancer. These investigators broke the cohort into 2 groups of 9 patients each, with alternation of the cryoablation technique between the groups. They reported that tight (5 mm) spacing, 3 freeze–thaw cycles, and sometimes decreasing the urethral warmer temperature produced better short-term recurrence-free intervals. In addition, Gangi and colleagues[26] reported successful MR-guided cryoablation treatment of

several patients with recurrent prostate cancer. Using MR guidance, cryoablation treatment can be tailored to the desired region (**Fig. 2**) or focal area (**Fig. 3**).

Magnetic resonance–guided laser interstitial therapy

Using LITT for recurrent prostate cancer is a relatively recent development. A feasibility study and a case study reported using 3-T MR imaging with Visualase 980 nm diode laser system (Medtronic, Minneapolis, MN) to treat a prostate cancer.[54] A small case series was presented by the same group, reporting the feasibility of treating recurrent prostate cancer with laser ablation (**Fig. 4**).[54] One complicating factor with MR-guided laser ablation in patients with previous surgical resection is the presence of surgical clips, which cause susceptibility artifacts and disrupt the MR-based temperature mapping. Therefore, recurrences with the surgical clips present would be a relative contraindication for this method of treatment.

Magnetic resonance guidance technologies

Interventional MR techniques have used needle guidance devices that have integrated varying amounts of software interface from robotic guidance systems to live imaging during free-hand placement. Several robotic systems have been developed to guide needle placement into the prostate.[55–57] Other systems from Invivo (Invivo Corp, Gainesville, FL) and Sentenelle (Hologic, Toronto, CA) have integrated computer-assisted design diagnostic imaging with needle guidance systems. These systems benefit from the power of separate diagnostic imaging performed preprocedurally and can be fused with intraprocedural imaging to guide needle/probe placement. Many of the MR vendors offer live imaging packages for aiding needle placement with live imaging using an in-room monitor.

MR imaging thermometry

One of the major advantages associated with MR guidance of thermal ablations is the MR imaging thermometry and subsequent dose estimations that are performed in near real time and allow for adjustments of treatment parameters and tumor targeting. The thermometry to monitor local temperatures most commonly is accomplished using the known linear dependence of proton resonance

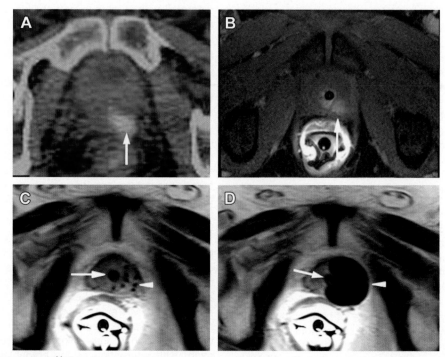

Fig. 2. Axial CT PET/[^{11}C]choline image shows increased activity in the left posterior prostate consistent with recurrent prostate cancer (*arrow, A*). (*B, C,* and *D*) were obtained on an MR imaging Siemens Espree 1.5 T with corresponding axial dynamic contrast-enhanced VIBE (volumetric interpolated breath-hold examination) images demonstrating abnormal tumor enhancement (*arrow*) in the left posterior prostate (*B*). Axial image confirming needle position of 8 cryoneedles (*arrowhead*) within the left half of the prostate and urethral warmer in place (*arrow*) (*C*). Axial image showing the ice ball size (*arrowhead*) with visible indentation secondary to the urethral warmer (*arrow*) (*D*).

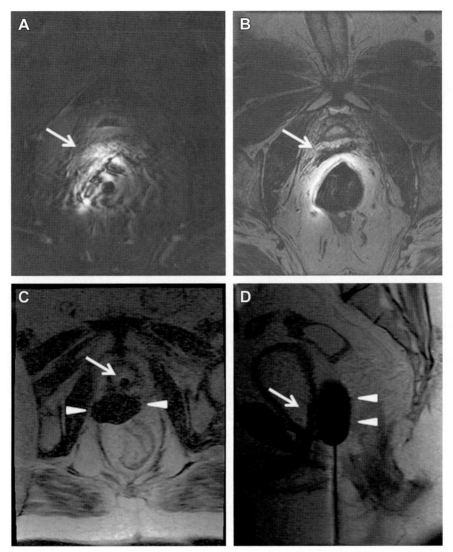

Fig. 3. Multiparametric 3.0-T MR imaging (*A* and *B*) with endorectal coil in place. Axial dynamic contrast-enhanced LAVA-FLEX images showing abnormal tumor enhancement (*arrow*) in the right and left seminal vesicle remnants after previous prostatectomy (*A*). Axial FRFSE images show a focal thickening of the seminal vesicle remnants (*B, arrow*). Axial (*C*) and sagittal (*D*) TSE images obtained during treatment showing the final extent of the iceball (*arrowheads*) encompassing the seminal vesicle prostate cancer recurrence (biopsy proven) with a urethral warmer (*arrow*) present and saline displacement of the rectum.

frequency (PRF) as a function of temperature. During delivery of ablative energy (generated by US transducer or laser applicator), a series of two-dimensional phase-sensitive T1-weighted fast spoiled gradient-recalled echo MR images are acquired on the MR imaging scanner.[58–60] Based on temperature changes, a thermal dose can be calculated to predict a tissue lethal dose.[61]

URETHRAL PROTECTION CATHETER

The Galil Medical Urethral Warming Set (Galil Medical, Minneapolis, MN) is a disposable component used to protect and warm urethral tissue when performing cryogenic destruction of prostatic tissue. The Urethral Warming System is designed to circulate a warm saline solution through a warming double-lumen catheter to maintain urethral tissue near body temperatures while the surrounding prostate tissue is being frozen (**Fig. 5**). During cryoablation therapies of prostate cancer, the urethral warming catheter constitutes an external heat source, which may counter the effects of cryoablations at the lesion site. Although the isotherms around cryoneedles have been investigated,[62] little is still known about the

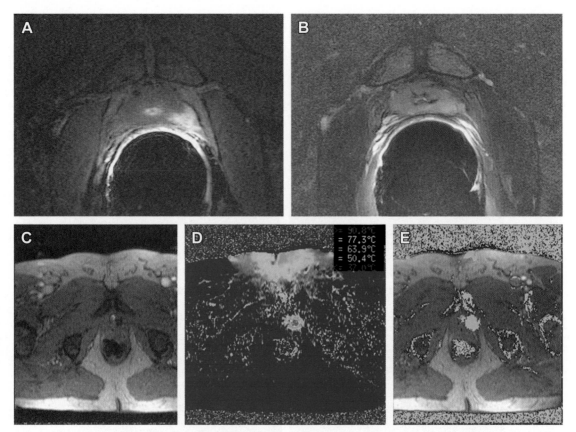

Fig. 4. MR images of the 15W Visualase laser ablation with double applicator (*A–E*) activation. Axial dynamic contrast-enhanced MR image (*A*) and T2-weighted FRFSE image (*B*) showing hyperenhancement and increased T2 signal consistent with biopsy-proven recurrent prostate cancer in the left posterior gland (*A*). Intraablation MR imaging monitoring with corresponding T1-weighted VIBE imaging (*C*), temperature-sensitive phase imaging (*B*) showing color-coded temperature changes, and calculated damage map (*E*). The calculated damage map takes into account the temperature and time variables estimating ablation damage using the Arrhenius model of thermal tissue damage, projected back onto the magnitude images as solid orange (*E*).

interactions between these isotherms and the urethral warmer. Recent numerical simulations[63] and phantom experiments,[64] using single-needle and multineedle configurations in the presence of the warmer, suggest that although the warmer provides sufficient tissue protection, it comes at a detrimental cost to both temperatures inside the cryoablation ice and dimensions of the critical isotherms.[64] Further investigations are needed and could prove to be critical to preoperative planning and treatment.

POSTPROCEDURAL IMAGING AFTER MAGNETIC RESONANCE–DIRECTED TREATMENTS

To appropriately assess the ablative zone after ablative treatment, imaging immediately after ablation includes T1-weighted/T2-weighted images in axial, sagittal, and coronal planes.

Diffusion-weighted images in the axial plane can also be acquired. Dynamic contrast-enhanced (DCE) MR images are critical, with images acquired in the axial plane and also potentially in the sagittal and coronal planes. The contrast-enhanced images provide the best immediate ablation zone examination (**Fig. 6**). However, it is important to be aware that with cryoablation, there can be residual vessel enhancement immediately after ablation and, for several months thereafter, a normal occurrence that does not indicate a failed ablation.[65]

FOLLOW-UP IMAGING

After MR-guided thermal ablation, the best way to monitor the patient is a combination of MR imaging and serum PSA levels. For the salvage patients, PSA levels are expected to be undetectable within several weeks of the salvage procedure. However,

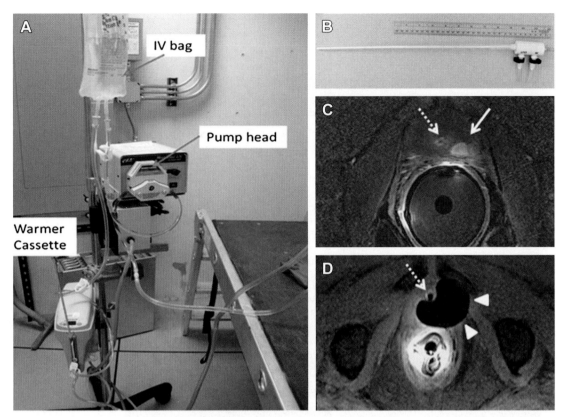

Fig. 5. Urethral warmer schematic showing the components located outside the MR suite (*A*). Setup consists of a sterile saline intravenous (IV) bag, warmer cassette, and peristaltic pump. The warmer temperature can be varied between 38°C and 43°C. The peristaltic pump speed can also be varied. Sterile double-lumen catheter allows circulation of fluid in and out of the urethral catheter through tubing that enters the MR suite through a wave guide in the wall (*B*). This system allows protection of the urethra while treating in close proximity. Axial dynamic contrast-enhanced VIBE images showing abnormal tumor enhancement (*solid arrow*) in the prostate and urethral warmer in place (*dashed arrow*) (*C*). Axial image showing the iceball (*arrowhead*) with visible indentation secondary to the urethral warmer (*dashed arrow*) and close proximity to the rectal wall (*D*).

for the focal gland ablation within the native gland, the PSA levels should decrease and then plateau at a new baseline. MR imaging with repeat biopsies as needed becomes important after ablation for monitoring the involution of the ablation zone. An increase in previously undetectable or stable postoperative PSA levels during posttreatment follow-up raises concerns about recurrent or new prostate cancer. Careful assessment of PSA velocities at 3 and 6 months may trigger concern for systemic disease.

CHALLENGES TO MAGNETIC RESONANCE GUIDANCE
Limitations of MR Imaging Thermometry

PRF temperature mapping uses the phenomenon of linear change of resonance frequency of water protons with temperature. PRF temperature mapping is a powerful tool in MR imaging;

however, there are certain limitations to the technique, mainly because these types of thermometry measure phase changes between an initial baseline image and all subsequent images acquired in real time. Ideally, all these images should be in perfect alignment, with no motion among them. As a consequence, motion is a large problem when the baseline image alignment is disrupted, causing phase registration artifacts. Reference-less temperature mapping has been proposed as a method of alleviating this.[66,67] Another issue is metallic artifact, causing signal dropout, with resulting artifact. In the native prostate, this is less of an issue, but in the postsurgical prostate bed, the surgical clip artifact becomes a problem for phase change–based temperature imaging. Another issue with temperature mapping is the problem with the tissue/fat interface. The PRF temperature mapping method is not much less sensitive

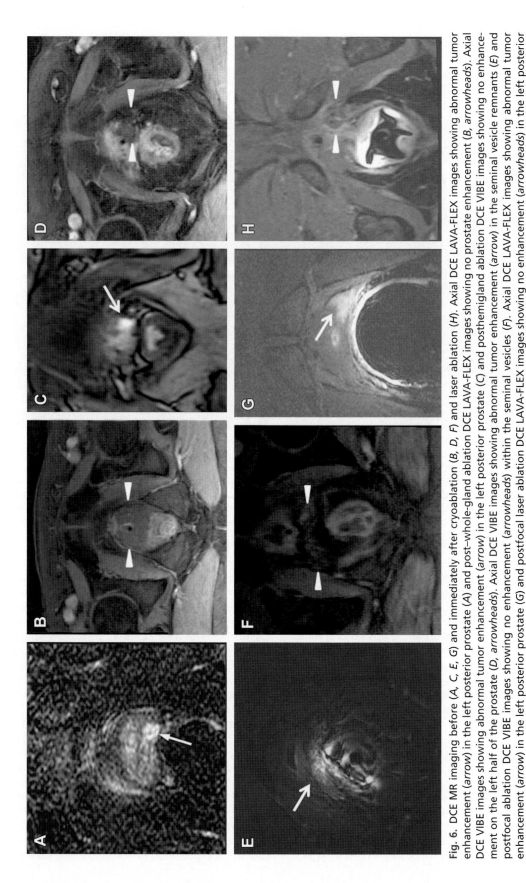

Fig. 6. DCE MR imaging before (*A, C, E, G*) and immediately after cryoablation (*B, D, F*) and laser ablation (*H*). Axial DCE LAVA-FLEX images showing abnormal tumor enhancement (*arrow*) in the left posterior prostate (*A*) and post–whole-gland ablation DCE LAVA-FLEX images showing no prostate enhancement (*B, arrowheads*). Axial DCE VIBE images showing abnormal tumor enhancement (*arrow*) in the left posterior prostate (*C*) and posthemigland ablation DCE VIBE images showing no enhancement on the left half of the prostate (*D, arrowheads*). Axial DCE VIBE images showing abnormal tumor enhancement (*arrow*) in the seminal vesicle remnants (*E*) and postfocal ablation DCE VIBE images showing no enhancement (*arrowheads*) within the seminal vesicles (*F*). Axial DCE LAVA-FLEX images showing abnormal tumor enhancement (*arrow*) in the left posterior prostate (*G*) and postfocal laser ablation DCE LAVA-FLEX images showing no enhancement (*arrowheads*) in the left posterior prostate where lesion was located (*H*).

in fat than in glandular tissue because of differing water content.

Limitations to MR Imaging Visualization of Iceball Temperature Isotherms

A major limitation of MR-guided cryoablation is that the iceball isotherms are not readily visualized. The leading edge of the iceball is readily visualized, but this corresponds to 0°C and may not be lethal. Therefore, it is necessary to carry the edge of the iceball beyond the tumor margin by at least 5 mm. However, this strategy assumes that the iceball lethal isotherms of –4°C are less than 5 mm from the leading edge of the iceball.[68] When other factors such as major vessels or urethral warmers are added to the treatment scenario, then, this assumption may or may not be true.[69] In addition, there are no reliable MR-compatible temperature-monitoring devices. Confounding the need for good margin coverage is the problem that the space in the prostate bed becomes very small with close proximity to the rectum, bladder, and external striated urethral sphincter, with little margin for error.

SUMMARY

As the most commonly diagnosed cancer in men, prostate cancer diagnosis and treatment of newly diagnosed or recurrent disease will demand considerable resources and efforts for years to come. MR imaging plays a seminal role in the management of this disease, although MR-guided focal ablation of native or recurrent prostate cancer is feasible and is rapidly becoming a viable alternative to standard treatment options. All the focal therapy treatments suffer from a small number of patients and need to be compared with established therapies. In addition, it is important that good prospective clinical trials for each treatment modality be performed to assess the advantage of each treatment modality and to determine long-term efficacy.

REFERENCES

1. Siegel RL, Miller KD, Jemal A. Cancer statistics, 2015. CA Cancer J Clin 2015;65(1):5–29.
2. Cooperberg MR, Broering JM, Carroll PR. Time trends and local variation in primary treatment of localized prostate cancer. J Clin Oncol 2010;28(7):1117–23.
3. Potosky AL, Davis WW, Hoffman RM, et al. Five-year outcomes after prostatectomy or radiotherapy for prostate cancer: the prostate cancer outcomes study [see comment]. J Natl Cancer Inst 2004;96(18):1358–67.
4. Jemal A, Siegel R, Ward E, et al. Cancer statistics, 2006. CA Cancer J Clin 2006;56(2):106–30.
5. Onik G, Vaughan D, Lotenfoe R, et al. "Male lumpectomy": focal therapy for prostate cancer using cryoablation. Urology 2007;70(6 Suppl):16–21.
6. Cooperberg MR, D'Amico AV, Karakiewicz PI, et al. Management of biochemical recurrence after primary treatment of prostate cancer: a systematic review of the literature. Eur Urol 2013;64(6):905–15.
7. Turkbey B, Mani H, Shah V, et al. Multiparametric 3T prostate magnetic resonance imaging to detect cancer: histopathological correlation using prostatectomy specimens processed in customized magnetic resonance imaging based molds. J Urol 2011;186(5):1818–24.
8. American College of Radiology. MR prostate imaging reporting and data system version 2.0. Available at: http://wwwacrorg/Quality-Safety/Resources/PIRADS/. 2015. Accessed March 21, 2015.
9. Siddiqui MM, Rais-Bahrami S, Turkbey B, et al. Comparison of MR/ultrasound fusion-guided biopsy with ultrasound-guided biopsy for the diagnosis of prostate cancer. JAMA 2015;313(4):390–7.
10. Kitajima K, Murphy RC, Nathan MA, et al. Detection of recurrent prostate cancer after radical prostatectomy: comparison of 11C-choline PET/CT with pelvic multiparametric MR imaging with endorectal coil. J Nucl Med 2014;55(2):223–32.
11. Futterer JJ, Gupta RT, Katz A, et al. The role of magnetic resonance imaging (MRI) in focal therapy for prostate cancer: recommendations from a consensus panel. BJU Int 2014;113(2):218–27.
12. Reske SN, Blumstein NM, Glatting G. [11C]choline PET/CT imaging in occult local relapse of prostate cancer after radical prostatectomy. Eur J Nucl Med Mol Imaging 2008;35(1):9–17.
13. Silberstein JL, Vickers AJ, Power NE, et al. Reverse stage shift at a tertiary care center: escalating risk in men undergoing radical prostatectomy. Cancer 2011;117(21):4855–60.
14. Wilt TJ, Brawer MK, Jones KM, et al. Radical prostatectomy versus observation for localized prostate cancer. N Engl J Med 2012;367(3):203–13.
15. Budaus L, Spethmann J, Isbarn H, et al. Inverse stage migration in patients undergoing radical prostatectomy: results of 8916 European patients treated within the last decade. BJU Int 2011;108(8):1256–61.
16. van den Bos W, Pinto PA, de la Rosette JJ. Imaging modalities in focal therapy: patient selection, treatment guidance, and follow-up. Curr Opin Urol 2014;24(3):218–24.
17. Hakimi AA, Feder M, Ghavamian R. Minimally invasive approaches to prostate cancer: a review of the current literature. Urol J 2007;4(3):130–7.
18. Menon M, Tewari A, Peabody JO, et al. Vattikuti Institute prostatectomy, a technique of robotic radical prostatectomy for management of localized

carcinoma of the prostate: experience of over 1100 cases. Urol Clin North Am 2004;31(4):701–17.

19. Polascik TJ. How to select the right patients for focal therapy of prostate cancer? Curr Opin Urol 2014; 24(3):203–8.

20. Katz AE. Prostate cryotherapy: current status. Curr Opin Urol 2009;19(2):177–81.

21. Lee T, Mendhiratta N, Sperling D, et al. Focal laser ablation for localized prostate cancer: principles, clinical trials, and our initial experience. Rev Urol 2014;16(2):55–66.

22. Blana A, Rogenhofer S, Ganzer R, et al. Eight years' experience with high-intensity focused ultrasonography for treatment of localized prostate cancer. Urology 2008;72(6):1329–33 [discussion: 1333–4].

23. Tacke J, Adam G, Haage P, et al. MR-guided percutaneous cryotherapy of the liver: in vivo evaluation with histologic correlation in an animal model. J Magn Reson Imaging 2001;13(1):50–6.

24. Tuncali K, Morrison PR, Tatli S, et al. MRI-guided percutaneous cryoablation of renal tumors: use of external manual displacement of adjacent bowel loops. Eur J Radiol 2006;59(2):198–202.

25. Woodrum DA, Kawashima A, Karnes RJ, et al. Magnetic resonance imaging-guided cryoablation of recurrent prostate cancer after radical prostatectomy: initial single institution experience. Urology 2013;82(4):870–5.

26. Gangi A, Tsoumakidou G, Abdelli O, et al. Percutaneous MR-guided cryoablation of prostate cancer: initial experience. Eur Radiol 2012;22(8):1829–35.

27. Josan S, Bouley DM, van den Bosch M, et al. MRI-guided cryoablation: in vivo assessment of focal canine prostate cryolesions. J Magn Reson Imaging 2009;30(1):169–76.

28. van den Bosch MA, Josan S, Bouley DM, et al. MR imaging-guided percutaneous cryoablation of the prostate in an animal model: in vivo imaging of cryoablation-induced tissue necrosis with immediate histopathologic correlation. J Vasc Interv Radiol 2009;20(2):252–8.

29. McNichols RJ, Gowda A, Kangasniemi M, et al. MR thermometry-based feedback control of laser interstitial thermal therapy at 980 nm. Lasers Surg Med 2004;34(1):48–55.

30. McNichols RJ, Kangasniemi M, Gowda A, et al. Technical developments for cerebral thermal treatment: water-cooled diffusing laser fibre tips and temperature-sensitive MRI using intersecting image planes. Int J Hyperthermia 2004;20(1):45–56.

31. Vogl TJ, Straub R, Zangos S, et al. MR-guided laser-induced thermotherapy (LITT) of liver tumours: experimental and clinical data. Int J Hyperthermia 2004;20(7):713–24.

32. McNichols RJ, Gowda A, Gelnett MD, et al. Percutaneous MRI-guided laser thermal therapy in canine

prostate. Paper presented at Photonic Therapeutics and Diagnostics. San Diego (CA), August 2–6, 2005.

33. Stafford RJ, Shetty A, Elliott AM, et al. Magnetic resonance guided, focal laser induced interstitial thermal therapy in a canine prostate model. J Urol 2010;184(4):1514–20.

34. Woodrum DA, Gorny KR, Mynderse LA, et al. Feasibility of 3.0T magnetic resonance imaging-guided laser ablation of a cadaveric prostate. Urology 2010;75(6):1514.e1–6.

35. Raz O, Haider MA, Davidson SR, et al. Real-time magnetic resonance imaging-guided focal laser therapy in patients with low-risk prostate cancer. Eur Urol 2010;58(1):173–7.

36. Thuroff S, Chaussy C, Vallancien G, et al. High-intensity focused ultrasound and localized prostate cancer: efficacy results from the European multicentric study. J Endourol 2003;17(8):673–7.

37. Gelet A, Chapelon JY, Bouvier R, et al. Transrectal high-intensity focused ultrasound: minimally invasive therapy of localized prostate cancer. J Endourol 2000;14(6):519–28.

38. Gelet A, Chapelon JY, Bouvier R, et al. Transrectal high intensity focused ultrasound for the treatment of localized prostate cancer: factors influencing the outcome. Eur Urol 2001;40(2):124–9.

39. Brandeis J, Pashos CL, Henning JM, et al. A nationwide charge comparison of the principal treatments for early stage prostate carcinoma. Cancer 2000;89(8):1792–9.

40. Moul JW. Prostate specific antigen only progression of prostate cancer. J Urol 2000;163(6):1632–42.

41. Stephenson AJ, Slawin KM. The value of radiotherapy in treating recurrent prostate cancer after radical prostatectomy. Nat Clin Pract Urol 2004; 1(2):90–6.

42. Sella T, Schwartz LH, Swindle PW, et al. Suspected local recurrence after radical prostatectomy: endorectal coil MR imaging. Radiology 2004;231(2): 379–85.

43. Agarwal PK, Sadetsky N, Konety BR, et al. Treatment failure after primary and salvage therapy for prostate cancer: likelihood, patterns of care, and outcomes. Cancer 2008;112(2):307–14.

44. Kuban DA, Thames HD, Levy LB, et al. Long-term multi-institutional analysis of stage T1-T2 prostate cancer treated with radiotherapy in the PSA era. Int J Radiat Oncol Biol Phys 2003;57(4):915–28.

45. Kimura M, Mouraviev V, Tsivian M, et al. Current salvage methods for recurrent prostate cancer after failure of primary radiotherapy. BJU Int 2010;105(2): 191–201.

46. Grado GL, Collins JM, Kriegshauser JS, et al. Salvage brachytherapy for localized prostate cancer after radiotherapy failure. Urology 1999;53(1):2–10.

47. Koutrouvelis P, Hendricks F, Lailas N, et al. Salvage reimplantation in patient with local recurrent prostate

carcinoma after brachytherapy with three dimensional computed tomography-guided permanent pararectal implant. Technol Cancer Res Treat 2003; 2(4):339–44.

48. Zacharakis E, Ahmed HU, Ishaq A, et al. The feasibility and safety of high-intensity focused ultrasound as salvage therapy for recurrent prostate cancer following external beam radiotherapy. BJU Int 2008;102(7):786–92.

49. Murat F-J, Poissonnier L, Rabilloud M, et al. Mid-term results demonstrate salvage high-intensity focused ultrasound (HIFU) as an effective and acceptably morbid salvage treatment option for locally radiorecurrent prostate cancer. Eur Urol 2009;55(3):640–7.

50. Gelet A, Chapelon JY, Poissonnier L, et al. Local recurrence of prostate cancer after external beam radiotherapy: early experience of salvage therapy using high-intensity focused ultrasonography. Urology 2004;63(4):625–9.

51. Pisters LL, Rewcastle JC, Donnelly BJ, et al. Salvage prostate cryoablation: initial results from the Cryo On-Line Data Registry. J Urol 2008;180(2):559–63 [discussion: 563–4].

52. Partin AW, Pearson JD, Landis PK, et al. Evaluation of serum prostate-specific antigen velocity after radical prostatectomy to distinguish local recurrence from distant metastases. Urology 1994;43(5):649–59.

53. Uchida T, Shoji S, Nakano M, et al. High-intensity focused ultrasound as salvage therapy for patients with recurrent prostate cancer after external beam radiation, brachytherapy or proton therapy. BJU Int 2011;107(3):378–82.

54. Woodrum DA, Mynderse LA, Gorny KR, et al. 3.0T MR-guided laser ablation of a prostate cancer recurrence in the postsurgical prostate bed. J Vasc Interv Radiol 2011;22(7):929–34.

55. Elhawary H, Zivanovic A, Rea M, et al. The feasibility of MR-image guided prostate biopsy using piezoceramic motors inside or near to the magnet isocentre. Med Image Comput Comput Assist Interv 2006;9(Pt 1):519–26.

56. Lagerburg V, Moerland MA, van Vulpen M, et al. A new robotic needle insertion method to minimise attendant prostate motion. Radiother Oncol 2006; 80(1):73–7.

57. van den Bosch MR, Moman MR, van Vulpen M, et al. MRI-guided robotic system for transperineal prostate interventions: proof of principle. Phys Med Biol 2010;55(5):N133–40.

58. Vitkin IA, Moriarty JA, Peters RD, et al. Magnetic resonance imaging of temperature changes during interstitial microwave heating: a phantom study. Med Phys 1997;24(2):269–77.

59. Hynynen K, Freund WR, Cline HE, et al. A clinical, noninvasive, MR imaging-monitored ultrasound surgery method. Radiographics 1996;16(1):185–95.

60. Ishihara Y, Calderon A, Watanabe H, et al. A precise and fast temperature mapping using water proton chemical shift. Magn Reson Med 1995;34(6):814–23.

61. Sapareto SA, Dewey WC. Thermal dose determination in cancer therapy. Int J Radiat Oncol Biol Phys 1984;10(6):787–800.

62. Young JL, Kolla SB, Pick DL, et al. In vitro, ex vivo and in vivo isotherms for renal cryotherapy. J Urol 2010;183(2):752–8.

63. Baissalov R, Sandison GA, Donnelly BJ, et al. A semi-empirical treatment planning model for optimization of multiprobe cryosurgery. Phys Med Biol 2000;45(5):1085–98.

64. Favazza CP, Gorny KR, King DM, et al. An investigation of the effects from a urethral warming system on temperature distributions during cryoablation treatment of the prostate: A phantom study. Cryobiology 2014;69(1):128–33.

65. Porter CA, Woodrum DA, Callstrom MR, et al. MRI after technically successful renal cryoablation: early contrast enhancement as a common finding. AJR Am J Roentgenol 2010;194(3):790–3.

66. Rieke V, Kinsey AM, Ross AB, et al. Referenceless MR thermometry for monitoring thermal ablation in the prostate. IEEE Trans Med Imaging 2007;26(6): 813–21.

67. Rieke V, Vigen KK, Sommer G, et al. Referenceless PRF shift thermometry. Magn Reson Med 2004; 51(6):1223–31.

68. Gage AA, Baust J. Mechanisms of tissue injury in cryosurgery. Cryobiology 1998;37(3):171–86.

69. Favazza CP, Gorny KR, King DM, et al. An investigation of the effects from a urethral warming system on temperature distributions during cryoablation treatment of the prostate: a phantom study. Cryobiology 2014;69(1):128–33.

Magnetic Resonance-Guided Prostate Biopsy

S. Saeid Dianat, MD[a], H. Ballentine Carter, MD[b], Katarzyna J. Macura, MD, PhD[c],*

KEYWORDS

- Prostate cancer • Prostate biopsy • MR imaging • Magnetic resonance-guided biopsy
- Targeted biopsy

KEY POINTS

- Magnetic resonance (MR)-targeted prostate biopsy is beneficial in most scenarios of prostate cancer diagnosis and management.
- Targeted biopsies can detect more clinically significant disease requiring curative treatment, and avoid detection of insignificant disease that is commonly diagnosed on random systematic biopsy.
- Fewer biopsy cores are needed when targeted prostate biopsy is used and can reduce complication rate.
- MR-targeted biopsy limitations are a potential for missing small volume prostate cancer on multiparametric MR imaging, equipment complexity and availability, and operator training requirement.

INTRODUCTION

The optimal strategy for prostate cancer (PCa) diagnosis is to avoid overdiagnosis, defined as diagnosis of clinically insignificant disease, and undersampling of the gland, which leads to missing clinically significant disease (CSD). Targeted prostate biopsy is a potential solution for decreasing the rate of both overdiagnosis and undersampling PCa.[1]

Recent applications of multiparametric prostate MR imaging (MP-MR imaging) have been documented as aiding more accurate risk stratification of PCa and treatment selection.[2] MR-invisible PCa has been shown to be associated with lower risk of adverse biopsy pathology.[3]

The management of patients with an increased prostate-specific antigen (PSA) level and negative standard transrectal ultrasound (TRUS)-guided prostate biopsy results is a challenging clinical setting in which MP-MR imaging may detect cancer lesions missed on standard TRUS-guided biopsy. The anterior prostate is the primary site of missed tumors and these can be detected on MP-MR imaging. It has been suggested that MP-MR imaging could be used as a triage test for the management of patients with increasing PSA levels and negative prior biopsy.[4]

In this article, we focus on different techniques for targeting prostate lesions identified on MP-MR imaging and review different clinical settings in which MR imaging–targeted prostate biopsies are performed.

UTILITY OF MULTIPARAMETRIC MR IMAGING

With the MP-MR imaging approach to imaging of the prostate, the use of functional MR imaging sequences such as diffusion-weighted imaging and dynamic-contrast enhanced imaging in addition

The authors have nothing to disclose.
[a] Department of Radiology, University of Minnesota, 420 Delaware Street, SE Minneapolis, MN 55455, USA;
[b] The James Buchanan Brady Urological Institute, The Johns Hopkins University, 600 North Wolfe Street, Marburg 100, Baltimore, MD 21287, USA; [c] The Russell H. Morgan Department of Radiology and Radiological Science, The James Buchanan Brady Urological Institute, The Johns Hopkins University, 601 North Caroline Street, JHOC 3140C, Baltimore, MD 21287, USA
* Corresponding author.
E-mail address: kmacura@jhmi.edu

Magn Reson Imaging Clin N Am 23 (2015) 621–631
http://dx.doi.org/10.1016/j.mric.2015.05.005

to anatomic assessment offers an important advantage in the diagnosis and localization of PCa. It has been reported that MP-MR imaging may decrease the number of unnecessary repeat biopsies in approximately 31% of men with initial negative extended transperineal biopsy. The sensitivity and specificity of MP-MR imaging in the overall diagnosis of PCa versus diagnosis of CSD was reported as 82.2% versus 100% and 77.8% versus 78.9%, respectively.[5]

Bratan and colleagues[6] showed that 3T MP-MR imaging could detect 93% of high-grade PCa (Gleason score of >7) with any volume, and 95.8% of those greater than 0.5 mL in reference to radical prostatectomy pathology findings. The sensitivity to diagnose PCa with unfavorable grade (Gleason score of ≥7) was 88.1%. The sensitivity for diagnosing low-grade (Gleason score of 6) and large volume disease (>0.5 mL) was 69.6%.

Risk stratification is the other potential application of MP-MR imaging. In a study by Marcus and colleagues,[7] the highest yield of MP-MR imaging for risk stratification with impact on disease management was demonstrated in intermediate risk disease in which MR imaging led to upstaging in 25.6% of cases. MR level of suspicion for PCa was shown to be correlated significantly with D'Amico risk stratification.[8]

Although MP-MR imaging is an adjunct tool for PCa diagnosis and management, its role is being evaluated in different patient workup algorithms. MR-detected suspicious lesions of the prostate can be targeted for tissue sampling using a variety of image-guided biopsy techniques in many PCa management scenarios.

TARGETED BIOPSY TECHNIQUES

Targeting suspicious lesions in the prostate can be achieved directly within the MR imaging scanner, "in-bore" MR-guided biopsy (MR-GB), or outside the MR imaging using fusion techniques that allow utilization of preprocedure MP-MR imaging and application of TRUS for imaging guidance during the procedure. Two image fusion techniques can be used: (1) a "cognitive" fusion by an operator performing the US-guided procedure who is familiar with MR imaging results and TRUS, and (2) software-based coregistration of MR images to TRUS images (MR-TRUS fusion) enabling the real-time TRUS-guided biopsy.

Known challenges to MR-guided "in-bore" biopsies include limited access within the scanner for manual instrument handling. A solution to this problem is the use of MR-compatible robots designed to operate in the space and environmental restrictions inside the MR scanner. Application of MR imaging compatible robotic devices involves sophisticated engineering solutions because, in addition to restrictions in materials that can be used to build these tools, robots require actuators and sensors that can only use a certain type of energies, and dedicated software applications are needed for image to robot registration. A number of MR-compatible robots, ranging from simple manipulator to fully automated systems, have been developed over the years.[9–11] The robotic approach to prostate biopsy offers a possibility of more precise targeting that may be crucial to the success of prostate interventions.

There are several platforms currently available for MR-TRUS fusion biopsies. The advantages on these fusion techniques include performance in the standard clinical setting familiar to the patient and the operator, and shorter procedure times. The disadvantages may be the lower targeting accuracy for small lesions and complicated fusion software handling.

In-Bore Magnetic Resonance-Guided Biopsy

In the "in-bore" technique, lesions identified as indeterminate or suspicious on diagnostic MP-MR imaging are being targeted while the patient is in the MR imaging scanner (**Figs. 1** and **2**). Both transrectal and transperineal approaches have been reported using this technique.[12–15] Prebiopsy MP-MR imaging is performed to identify target lesions. Patients are placed in the prone, supine, or decubitus position. Body surface coils are used to improve the signal to noise ratio. Typically, an MR biopsy guide is inserted into the rectum (ie, contrast-filled endorectal needle guide) and multiplanar T2-weighted fast spin echo images are acquired for target localization. The position of the MR biopsy guide is adjusted manually based on the location of the target and automated software calculations, and then the biopsy needle is advanced through the needle guide toward the suspicious lesion. The needle position in relation to the lesion is imaged for confirmation using MR sequences such as T2-weighted fast spin echo, single shot fast spin echo, or TRUE-fast spin echo images. Once the needle position is aligned with the target, the needle is advanced and the biopsy performed. Needle localization may be reconfirmed and tracked by further scanning after tissue sampling.[12] When the robotic device is used for MR-GB, it is fixed typically to the scanner table and the needle guide is inserted into the rectum or perineum. After registration of the robot and the needle guide with localization sequences, the robot is controlled remotely to achieve the

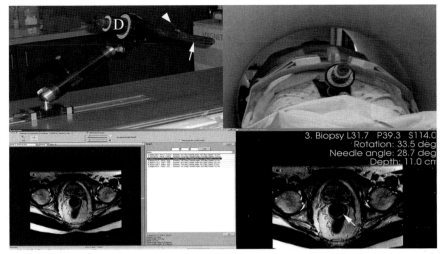

Fig. 1. "In bore" MR imaging–guided prostate biopsy using the endorectal access and MR imaging–compatible biopsy device. The device (*top left*) has an endorectal probe (*arrow*), a needle guide (*arrowhead*), and a set of dials (D) that allow the needle to be directed to the target on the basis of input from the targeting software (*bottom left*). The software provides the necessary angles for probe rotation, needle angulation, and needle depth (*bottom right*). The dials are adjusted manually by the operator on the basis of software calculations derived from prebiopsy targeting MR images. The patient is placed in the prone position (*top right*) with endorectal placement of the biopsy probe (*arrow* at *bottom right*). (*From* Bonekamp D, Jacobs MA, El-Khouli R, et al. Advancements in MR imaging of the prostate: from diagnosis to interventions. Radiographics 2011;31(3):677; with permission.)

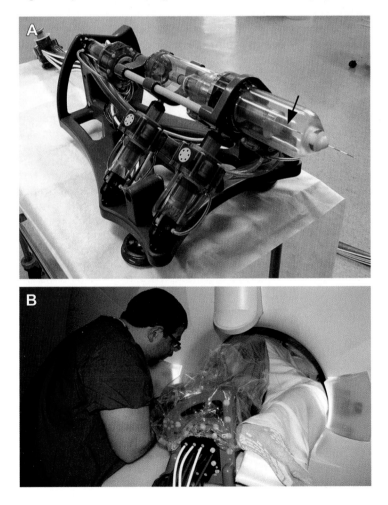

Fig. 2. "In-bore" MR imaging biopsy setup with an MR imaging–compatible stealth prostate intervention robotic device (MR-BOT, an investigational device). (*A*) MR-BOT device is made of MR imaging–compatible materials and uses a pneumatic step motor (PneuStep motor). *Arrow* points to the needle driver which is automatically manipulated with a pneumatic motor. (*B*) The device can operate in the gantry of an MR imaging unit alongside the patient in the decubitus position. Device can be used for transperineal "in-bore" prostate biopsy, as illustrated in this case. ([A] From Bonekamp D, Jacobs MA, El-Khouli R, et al. Advancements in MR imaging of the prostate: from diagnosis to interventions. Radiographics 2011;31(3):677; with permission. [B] *Courtesy of* Dan Stoianovici, PhD, Urology Robotics Program, The Johns Hopkins University, Baltimore, MD.)

desired angulation for inserting the needle to target the suspicious lesion.

Researchers from the National Cancer Institute assessed the accuracy of needle placement and sampling on transrectal MR-GB and reported that 28% of the biopsies had an error of greater than 5 mm, one that may lead to missing CSD defined as a tumor volume more than 0.5 cm³.[13] Further investigations are needed to improve targeting and develop methods to compensate for prostate gland displacements.[13]

Transperineal MR-guided prostate biopsy was introduced initially by researchers from the Brigham and Women's Hospital.[14] Recently, they reported the performance of robotically assisted needle guide placement using transperineal MR-GB and compared that method with the manual placement through the template guide.[15] The robotic device used in this study applied a motorized template to guide the needle with a control resolution of 0.001 mm. The investigators used 3DSlicer (this is the name of open source software http://www.slicer.org/) software for motion control of the robotic device and to optimize the needle placement. T2-weighted images were obtained after each motion of the robotic device to reconfirm the location of the needle. The robotic approach was more accurate than the manual approach in terms of best needle placement attempt. Both mean time per core procedure and whole procedure time were shorter with the robotic method.[15] These robotically assisted techniques require a complex setting, a long time to perform, and specific equipment that is not widely available; in addition, they are costly.

Although MR-GB offers accurate targeting of prostate lesions, these procedures may be subject to the sampling error, inaccurate needle placement secondary to prostate deformation and displacement, and patient movement owing to discomfort. Because no real-time tracking of the prostate location is available during MR-GB, the procedure is lengthened by frequent confirmatory scans that need to be performed to adjust the needle and target alignment.

Magnetic Resonance–Ultrasound Fusion Biopsy

Cognitive registration

Cognitive fusion allows the physician performing the prostate biopsy to use the information from MP-MR imaging that is reviewed before the procedure. Suspicious lesions identified on the MR imaging are targeted with the usual TRUS equipment based on the anatomic location of the lesion. A prospective, multicenter study demonstrated the advantage of cognitive MR-TRUS fusion biopsy compared with systematic TRUS biopsy. A biopsy with cognitive targeting led to a 10% increase in cancer detection and 15% increase in high-grade disease detection.[16]

Software-based registration

To overcome the limitations of cognitive fusion, different software-based image fusion techniques have been developed to assist in registration of real time TRUS images with preprocedure MP-MR imaging, to decrease the procedure time and complexity of equipment, and to allow performance of the targeted biopsy in a standard clinical office.

MP-MR images acquired before the biopsy procedure are analyzed using the postprocessing software, and 3D segmentation of the prostate gland is performed. Additionally, at the time of TRUS, 2-dimensional (2D) images that are acquired are processed by the software and reconstructed into a 3D model. Subsequently, navigational software overlays or fuses MR images to the real-time TRUS images (GE Logiq E9, GE Healthcare, Milwaukee, WI; **Fig. 3**) or performs 3D MR imaging to 3D TRUS datasets registration (UroNav, Philips-Invivo, Gainesville, FL; **Fig. 4**), enabling the operator to target the suspicious lesion on MR imaging as evident on fused images.

MR-TRUS fusion biopsy was shown to improve the risk stratification by reclassifying or upgrading disease. In a study by Siddiqui and colleagues,[17] MR-TRUS fusion biopsy led to tumor upgrading in 32% of patients compared with systematic TRUS biopsy. Accurate targeting of suspicious lesions depends on precise registration of reconstructed 3D prostate models based on MR imaging and TRUS datasets and is limited by prostate deformation during endorectal MR imaging and during TRUS secondary to different pressures applied to the gland by the imaging probe. Two methods have been developed to overcome this issue and achieve better registration of images: (1) elastic registration where gland deformation on a preprocedure MR imaging is taken into account during registration to the 3D model reconstructed from TRUS images,[18] and (2) rigid registration where alignment of 3D models reconstructed from MR and TRUS is achieved by simple rotation and magnification, requiring almost identical models on MR and TRUS images. The optimal registration technique would allow updating of the 3D models and their matching in the real-time mode as the TRUS probe is being moved.

The other component of MR-TRUS fusion systems is a "tracking" mechanism for the location of the needle in relation to the target within the prostate. Methods used for tracking include

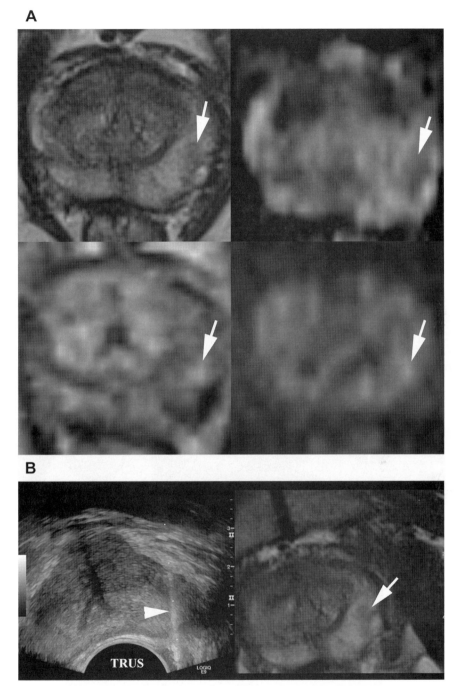

Fig. 3. A 56-year-old man with a prostate-specific antigen level of 5.2 ng/mL and 3 prior negative prostate trans-rectal ultrasound (TRUS) biopsies. Multiparametric prostate MR imaging (MP-MR imaging) showed a dominant suspicious nodule 10 mm in the left mid lateral peripheral zone (ADC 925, dynamic-contrast enhanced–positive with focal early enhancement). MR-TRUS fusion biopsy using GE Logiq E9 system revealed prostatic adenocarci-noma Gleason score of 3 + 3 = 6. Patient underwent radical prostatectomy. (A) Four images from MP-MR imaging show (top left) T2 hypointense nodule (arrows) that has restricted diffusion with low ADC values (top right) and corresponding focal high signal on b 800 image (bottom right) along with focal early enhancement (bottom left). These imaging features indicate PI-RADS assessment category 4 (clinically significant cancer is likely to be pre-sent). (B) TRUS image (left) and MR imaging T2-weighted image (right) are displayed side-by-side after co-registration at the corresponding anatomic level. T2 dark nodule in the left peripheral zone (arrow) is being sampled by 18G biopsy needle (arrowhead) during real-time TRUS.

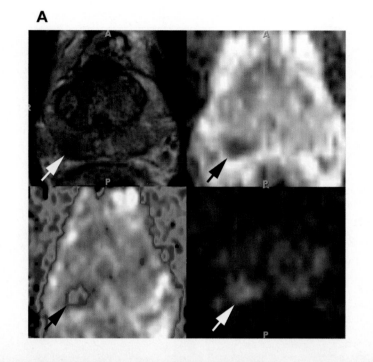

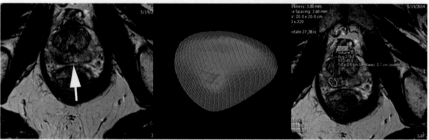

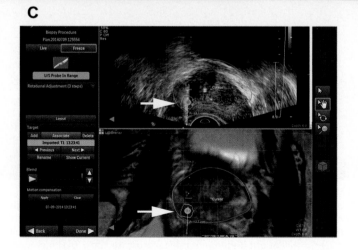

external magnetic field generators, real-time 3D TRUS, and angle-sensing encoders in robotic arms.

A number of devices have been approved by the US Food and Drug Administration for MR-TRUS fusion biopsy. Some devices use the external magnetic field generator for tracking, including the UroNav system (Philips-Invivo), and HI-RVS (Hitachi Real-time Virtual sonography) system (Hitachi Medical Systems, Zug, Switzerland). Both devices use the rigid registration mechanism. Additionally, GE Logiq E9 system (GE Healthcare) uses the electromagnetic field to track motion of the US probe and enables real-time TRUS to be anatomically coregistered with MR imaging.

The UroNav system allows physicians to work in a familiar clinical setting because the equipment set-up is similar to the typical TRUS prostate biopsy system. The magnetic field is generated over the patient's pelvis by a small generator. Sensors are attached to the US probe and they communicate with the magnetic field generator and the navigational software on the UroNav workstation for spatial localization. As the US probe is used to generate TRUS images in real-time, the probe localization in relation to the prostate is tracked. US images are acquired by a freehand probe movement with sweeping from the base to the apex, and a 3D prostate model is created from the TRUS dataset. The reconstructed 3D US model is then registered to the previously acquired MR imaging dataset that is imported to the workstation in the form of a 3D MR imaging–based prostate model with regions of interest representing suspicious lesions that were contoured on MR imaging.

The Urostation 3D TRUS (Koelis, La Tranche, France) is another novel MR-TRUS fusion biopsy device that uses elastic registration and retrospective targeting to record the biopsy needle trajectory during the real-time 3D TRUS imaging. The

workstation has 2 functional modes: the real-time 3D TRUS and MR-TRUS fusion. At the beginning of the procedure, 3D TRUS images are reconstructed from the 3D volume dataset. A reference model is prepared based on 3 registrations, including landmark-based rigid and multipoint-based rigid registrations, as well as algorithmic elastic registration.[19] After needle placement and sampling, the needle is held in place and the biopsy trajectory is recorded on TRUS images, and then transferred to the workstation to correlate with the reference model, a process called retrospective targeting.[18]

The Artemis (Eigen, Grass Valley, CA) is a 3D US-guided biopsy system that also uses MR-TRUS fusion in which MR images are fused to the real-time TRUS images. Lesions are targeted using a mechanical arm equipped with angle-sensing encoders installed on the joints of the mechanical arm. Because the operator is not moving the TRUS probe, this method may be more accurate for targeting lesions; however, the equipment is different from the regular US hardware and additional training is needed. The process of MR-TRUS fusion in this technique includes prostate segmentation of volume data from both MR imaging and TRUS, rigid registration of the segmented gland, surface registration of TRUS and MR images, and elastic registration.[20] In addition, this technique enables the operator to biopsy evenly distributed cores in a systematic TRUS biopsy.[21]

The BiopSee platform (MedCom, Darmstadt, Germany) is a novel transperineal stereotactic biopsy technique. This system includes real-time TRUS, MR-US fusion, and biopsy planning of virtual needle insertion trajectory, which is then used during real-time needle placement. The US probe is placed in a mechanical fixation device called a stepper, and 2 attached encoders track movement and rotation of the US probe. MR images are manually fused to the 3D US dataset

Fig. 4. 68-year-old man with small volume prostate cancer Gleason 3 + 3 = 6 managed in active surveillance (AS). Multiparametric prostate MR imaging (MP-MR imaging) revealed an index lesion in the right mid peripheral zone. MR-guided biopsy using the UroNav platform revealed prostatic adenocarcinoma Gleason 3 + 3 = 6 in 3 of 3 cores obtained from the right mid peripheral zone nodule (60/50/50% core involvement). Patient remains in AS program. (A) Acquisition of MP-MR imaging of the prostate: Four images from MP-MR imaging show (top left) T2 hypointense nodule (arrows) that has restricted diffusion with low ADC values (top right) and color-coded ADC map (bottom left), and corresponding focal high signal on b 1400 image (bottom right). These imaging features indicate prostate imaging reporting and data system (PI-RADS) assessment category 4 (clinically significant cancer is likely to be present). (B) MR imaging data processing: MR images are used subsequently on a separate workstation to define prostate contours (left; arrow) for subsequent segmentation of the 3-dimensional (3D) volumetric model of the prostate (middle). Then, a region of interest (ROI) is outlined on T2 axial images (right). The volumetric prostate 3D model and target ROI are saved and transferred to the UroNav workstation. (C) Biopsy of a target: After the MR–transrectal ultrasound (TRUS) coregistration and fusion, biopsy of the indicated on MR imaging right mid posterior peripheral zone target ROI can be performed, as illustrated (arrow); top image TRUS, bottom image MR imaging; both are coregistered anatomically.

generated after transverse 2D US image acquisition. US images are overlaid by organ and lesion contour, and the planned needle trajectory. Samples are obtained stereotactically with real-time navigation that allows correction of needle deviation from the planned trajectory.[22,23]

CURRENT EVIDENCE OF MAGNETIC RESONANCE-TARGETED BIOPSY PERFORMANCE

There are several clinical circumstances for which MP-MR imaging and targeted biopsies have a role, including men with suspected PCa with no prior biopsy, high PSA but negative biopsy result, and men with low-risk PCa who are candidates for surveillance.

Men with No Prior Biopsy

Early studies showed that prebiopsy MR imaging with targeted biopsy of suspicious lesions detected on MR imaging is a potential approach to the management of men with elevated PSA and no prior biopsy. Haffner and colleagues[24] reported that targeted biopsy using a cognitive technique could decrease the diagnosis of insignificant PCa on random systematic biopsy. Another targeted biopsy study, using either elastic or rigid MR-TRUS image registration techniques, showed detection of significantly more PCa lesions, more high-grade PCa, and diagnosis of fewer low-risk PCa; however, targeted biopsy using the cognitive technique did not improve PCa detection rate compared with that with random TRUS biopsy.[25]

In a prospective multicenter study by Puech and colleagues,[16] the performance of targeted biopsy was compared with that of standard 12-core TRUS biopsy at the initial biopsy of men with elevated PSA. In patients with lesions identified on MR images, 2 cores were obtained using fusion techniques, including cognitive registration and real-time MR-US fusion. Targeted biopsy detected more PCa compared with standard biopsy (69% vs 59%). Moreover, the detection rate of CSD was significantly higher with targeted than with standard biopsy (67% vs 52%). Targeted biopsy led to tumor upgrading in 24% of cancers identified on both systematic and targeted biopsy. The limitation of targeted biopsy was the missing of cancer in 6 of 95 patients (6%) that was detected on standard biopsy, which was CSD in 4 of 6 cases.

Recently, authors from The Netherlands reported results of a prospective study of 226 men with elevated PSA who underwent prebiopsy 3.0 T MP-MR imaging and subsequently were enrolled into 2 cohorts: TRUS biopsy or MR-GB. The authors compared the diagnostic accuracy of random TRUS biopsy with in-bore MR-GB.[26] Cancer detected by MR-GB had a significantly higher proportion of intermediate or high-risk cancers compared with the TRUS random biopsy (93.9% vs 62.7%). A significantly greater proportion of cores sampled by MR-GB were cancerous compared with TRUS biopsy sampled cores (56.4% vs 15%). Moreover, fewer cases of low-risk PCa were diagnosed on MR-GB than TRUS biopsy. It was also revealed that 29 of 226 cases (12.8%) with intermediate or high-risk PCa were either missed on TRUS biopsy (16 cases) or misclassified as low risk (13 cases). On the other hand, 15 patients with intermediate or high-risk PCa detected on TRUS biopsy were either missed on MP-MR imaging (5 cases) or not sampled by targeted biopsy (10 cases).[26]

In a recent study by Mozer and colleagues,[27] the MR-TRUS fusion biopsy using the Urostation (Koelis) was compared with a 12-core standard biopsy. Targeted biopsy revealed significantly higher proportion of CSD in both per-core and per-patient analysis than the standard biopsy protocol. In addition, targeted biopsy detected fewer men with clinically insignificant disease.

A group of authors from the University College, London, assessed the performance of transperineal MR-targeted biopsy using cognitive MR-TRUS fusion in a cohort of 182 men with suspicion of PCa, and compared the results with transperineal template-guided biopsy. Enrolled patients included biopsy-naïve men, men with elevated PSA and negative biopsy, and active surveillance (AS) patients. Overall, MR-targeted biopsy had a similar rate of CSD detection with fewer biopsy cores and similar or lower rate of insignificant disease detection.[28]

Kuru and colleagues[23] reported results of MR-targeted TRUS-guided transperineal fusion biopsy in a large cohort of 347 men with suspicion of PCa at initial (177 men) or repeat biopsy after prior negative biopsy (170 men). Template-guided transperineal biopsy was performed for all patients. In this cohort, 73.5% of men diagnosed with PCa were at intermediate or high risk PCa according to National Comprehensive Cancer Center criteria. PCa was detected in 51% of men with prior negative biopsies, 65% of whom had CSD. The majority of patients (85.1%) with no suspicion of PCa on MP-MR imaging were also negative on systematic template-guided transperineal biopsy.

Men with Prior Negative Biopsies

In a study by Kaufmann and colleagues,[29] 35 men with high or increasing PSA and prior negative biopsy underwent 1.5 T MP-MR imaging and transrectal MR-GB using a portable biopsy device for needle guidance (Invivo GmbH, Schwerin, Germany) followed immediately by systematic TRUS biopsy. The cancer detection rate was significantly higher using targeted biopsy (46%) versus systematic TRUS biopsy (23%). All patients with PCa diagnosed on targeted biopsy harbored CSD.[29] The negative result of targeted biopsy was reassuring; none of the patients with negative targeted biopsy were diagnosed with PCa after a median follow-up of 33 months.

A total of 52 patients with no prior PCa diagnosis underwent transperineal MR-guided prostate biopsy in a prospective clinical observational study by Penzkofer and colleagues.[14] The overall rate of cancer detection was 48.1% (25 of 52 patients) and 80% of cancers were clinically significant in terms of Gleason grade (Gleason score of $\geq 3 + 4$). Anterior targets had the highest rate of PCa detection (58.8%).

Miyagawa and colleagues[30] reported the performance of real-time virtual sonography and MR-TRUS fusion biopsy in men with high PSA and at least 1 prior negative biopsy. The real-time virtual sonography can fuse real-time TRUS images with MR volume data and display them side by side. Real-time biplanar TRUS images were acquired and a transperineal biopsy was performed using this device. The rate of cancer detection per core was significantly higher with targeted than random biopsy (32% vs 9%).

Fiard and colleagues[31] reported the results of an initial clinical experience using the Urostation device for MR-TRUS fusion targeted biopsy in 30 patients with suspected PCa (17 patients with prior negative biopsy). The overall cancer detection rate was higher in targeted than random TRUS biopsies (41% vs 8%, respectively).

Men with Low-Risk Prostate Cancer

MP-MR imaging is still optional in the management algorithm of low-risk PCa; however, it is increasingly used to monitor disease progression in major AS programs.[32]

In a prospective multicenter study of 63 men with low-risk PCa eligible for AS, initial MP-MR imaging and MR-GB were performed at the 3- and 12-month follow-up visits to assess risk reclassification. Surveillance TRUS biopsy could miss 10% of patients with unfavorable risk of disease and misclassify them as AS eligible. Repeat MP-MR imaging and MR-GB helped to avoid misclassification in those patients. MP-MR imaging and MR-GB helped to identify patients harboring higher grade PCa (Gleason grade pattern 4 or 5) earlier. However, the initial MP-MR imaging and

MR-GB failed to identify 14 patients who were risk restratified at 12 months of follow-up.[33]

Penzkofer and colleagues[14] recently published the results of transperineal MR-GB in a small cohort of AS patients. The rate of cancer diagnosis in the AS group was 61.5% (8 of 13). The rate of grade reclassification (Gleason pattern of ≥ 4) was 62.5% (5 of 8).

Authors from the University of California Los Angeles studied the likelihood of disease reclassification in 113 men who qualified for AS based on the Epstein criteria and who had an MR-TRUS fusion targeted biopsy of suspicious lesions on MP-MR imaging using the Artemis system.[34] Confirmatory MR-TRUS fusion biopsy reclassified 36% of men considered as AS eligible based on the Epstein criteria. In another study, they assessed the performance of MR-TRUS fusion biopsy using the Artemis platform to predict tumor grading in reference to final pathology on radical prostatectomy in 54 patients. The per-core cancer detection rate was higher in targeted biopsy (42%) than systematic 12-point grid (mapping biopsy; 20%). The rate of tumor upgrading from fusion biopsy was 17%. Although the fusion biopsy is not perfect for predicting final pathology, it offers an improvement over the conventional TRUS biopsy (81% vs 40%–65%) when combined with a systematic biopsy.[35]

LIMITATIONS OF TARGETED BIOPSY

Small volume high-grade PCa can be missed on MP-MR imaging and some PCa are invisible to MR. Therefore, although promising, the targeted biopsy as the sole strategy for PCa detection and monitoring in different clinical scenarios has not yet been accepted. Further, more centers and more radiologists experienced in prostate MR imaging are needed. Accurate targeting of suspicious lesions detected on MR imaging remains a challenge. If the targeting error is greater than the size threshold of CSD, the chance of missing a CSD will be higher, making it difficult to rely on targeted biopsy alone for patient management. Techniques used for targeted biopsies vary and require specific equipment and expertise that are not yet available widely. Heterogeneous populations of patients enrolled in targeted prostate biopsy studies to date, different platforms used, and different reference standards used make it difficult to compare study results. Therefore, further studies of MR-targeted biopsies are needed to better define criteria of CSD based on the utilization of these emerging techniques.

The interobserver variability in the interpretation of MP-MR imaging is a recognized challenge.

Therefore, a scoring system for levels of suspicion assigned to prostate lesions detected on MP-MR imaging, known as prostate imaging reporting and data system (PI-RADS), has been developed to improve radiologists' consistency in prostate MP-MR imaging analysis and reporting. The revised PI-RADS version 2[36] is now available with the aim of improving detection, localization, and characterization of PCa, and facilitating the use of MR imaging data for targeted biopsy. PI-RADS version 2 assessment uses a 5-point scale based on the likelihood that a combination of MP-MR imaging findings on T2-weighted images, diffusion-weighted imaging, and dynamic-contrast enhanced imaging correlates with the presence of a CSD for each lesion in the prostate gland. The application of standardized reporting schemas and well-defined contemporary biopsy protocols using MR guidance for targeted prostate sampling has the potential to aid in triage of patients to appropriate management and ultimately to improve patient outcomes.

SUMMARY

Prostate tumor characterization and, specifically, assessment of its aggressiveness are crucial for treatment planning and prognostication. MR-detected suspicious lesions in the prostate can be targeted for tissue sampling using a variety of MR imaging–guided biopsy techniques to increase accuracy of the detection of clinically significant PCa and improve patient risk stratification.

REFERENCES

1. Bjurlin MA, Meng X, Le Nobin J, et al. Optimization of prostate biopsy: the role of MRI targeted biopsy in detection, localization, and risk assessment. J Urol 2014;192(3):648–58.
2. Turkbey B, Mani H, Aras O, et al. Prostate cancer: can multiparametric MR imaging help identify patients who are candidates for active surveillance? Radiology 2013;268:144–52.
3. Dianat SS, Carter HB, Pienta KJ, et al. Magnetic resonance-invisible versus magnetic resonance-visible prostate cancer in active surveillance: a preliminary report on disease outcomes. Urology 2015; 85:147–54.
4. Abd-Alazeez M, Ahmed HU, Arya M, et al. The accuracy of multiparametric MRI in men with negative biopsy and elevated PSA level–can it rule out clinically significant prostate cancer? Urol Oncol 2014; 32(45):e17–22.
5. Pepe P, Garufi A, Priolo G, et al. Can 3-Tesla pelvic phased-array multiparametric MRI avoid unnecessary repeat prostate biopsy in patients with PSA < 10 ng/mL? Clin Genitourin Cancer 2014; 13(1):e27–30.
6. Bratan F, Niaf E, Melodelima C, et al. Influence of imaging and histological factors on prostate cancer detection and localisation on multiparametric MRI: a prospective study. Eur Radiol 2013;23:2019–29.
7. Marcus DM, Rossi PJ, Nour SG, et al. The impact of multiparametric pelvic magnetic resonance imaging on risk stratification in patients with localized prostate cancer. Urology 2014;84:132–7.
8. Rastinehad AR, Baccala AA Jr, Chung PH, et al. D'Amico risk stratification correlates with degree of suspicion of prostate cancer on multiparametric magnetic resonance imaging. J Urol 2011;185: 815–20.
9. Macura KJ, Stoianovici D. Advancements in magnetic resonance-guided robotic interventions in the prostate. Top Magn Reson Imaging 2008;19: 297–304.
10. Pondman KM, Futterer JJ, ten Haken B, et al. MR-guided biopsy of the prostate: an overview of techniques and a systematic review. Eur Urol 2008;54: 517–27.
11. Bonekamp D, Jacobs MA, El-Khouli R, et al. Advancements in MR imaging of the prostate: from diagnosis to interventions. Radiographics 2011;31: 677–703.
12. Verma S, Bhavsar AS, Donovan J. MR imaging-guided prostate biopsy techniques. Magn Reson Imaging Clin N Am 2014;22:135–44, v.
13. Xu H, Lasso A, Guion P, et al. Accuracy analysis in MRI-guided robotic prostate biopsy. Int J Comput Assist Radiol Surg 2013;8:937–44.
14. Penzkofer T, Tuncali K, Fedorov A, et al. Transperineal in-bore 3-T MR imaging-guided prostate biopsy: a prospective clinical observational study. Radiology 2015;274(1):170–8.
15. Tilak G, Tuncali K, Song SE, et al. 3T MR-guided in-bore transperineal prostate biopsy: a comparison of robotic and manual needle-guidance templates. J Magn Reson Imaging 2015;42(1):63–71.
16. Puech P, Rouviere O, Renard-Penna R, et al. Prostate cancer diagnosis: multiparametric MR-targeted biopsy with cognitive and transrectal US-MR fusion guidance versus systematic biopsy–prospective multicenter study. Radiology 2013;268:461–9.
17. Siddiqui MM, Rais-Bahrami S, Truong H, et al. Magnetic resonance imaging/ultrasound-fusion biopsy significantly upgrades prostate cancer versus systematic 12-core transrectal ultrasound biopsy. Eur Urol 2013;64:713–9.
18. Ukimura O, Desai MM, Palmer S, et al. 3-Dimensional elastic registration system of prostate biopsy location by real-time 3-dimensional transrectal ultrasound guidance with magnetic resonance/transrectal ultrasound image fusion. J Urol 2012;187: 1080–6.

19. Rothwax JT, George AK, Wood BJ, et al. Multiparametric MRI in biopsy guidance for prostate cancer: fusion-guided. Biomed Res Int 2014; 2014:439171.

20. Natarajan S, Marks LS, Margolis DJ, et al. Clinical application of a 3D ultrasound-guided prostate biopsy system. Urol Oncol 2011;29:334–42.

21. Bax J, Cool D, Gardi L, et al. Mechanically assisted 3D ultrasound guided prostate biopsy system. Med Phys 2008;35:5397–410.

22. Zogal P, Sakas G, Rösch W, et al. BiopSee – transperineal stereotactic navigated prostate biopsy. J Contemp Brachytherapy 2011;3:91–5.

23. Kuru TH, Roethke MC, Seidenader J, et al. Critical evaluation of magnetic resonance imaging targeted, transrectal ultrasound guided transperineal fusion biopsy for detection of prostate cancer. J Urol 2013;190:1380–6.

24. Haffner J, Lemaitre L, Puech P, et al. Role of magnetic resonance imaging before initial biopsy: comparison of magnetic resonance imaging-targeted and systematic biopsy for significant prostate cancer detection. BJU Int 2011;108:E171–8.

25. Delongchamps NB, Peyromaure M, Schull A, et al. Prebiopsy magnetic resonance imaging and prostate cancer detection: comparison of random and targeted biopsies. J Urol 2013;189:493–9.

26. Pokorny MR, de Rooij M, Duncan E, et al. Prospective study of diagnostic accuracy comparing prostate cancer detection by transrectal ultrasound-guided biopsy versus magnetic resonance (MR) imaging with subsequent MR-guided biopsy in men without previous prostate biopsies. Eur Urol 2014;66:22–9.

27. Mozer P, Roupret M, Le Cossec C, et al. First round of targeted biopsies using magnetic resonance imaging/ultrasonography fusion compared with conventional transrectal ultrasonography-guided biopsies for the diagnosis of localised prostate cancer. BJU Int 2015;115:50–7.

28. Kasivisvanathan V, Dufour R, Moore CM, et al. Transperineal magnetic resonance image targeted prostate biopsy versus transperineal template prostate biopsy in the detection of clinically significant prostate cancer. J Urol 2013;189:860–6.

29. Kaufmann S, Kruck S, Kramer U, et al. Direct comparison of targeted MRI-guided biopsy with systematic transrectal ultrasound-guided biopsy in patients with previous negative prostate biopsies. Urol Int 2014;94(3):319–25.

30. Miyagawa T, Ishikawa S, Kimura T, et al. Real-time virtual sonography for navigation during targeted prostate biopsy using magnetic resonance imaging data. Int J Urol 2010;17:855–60.

31. Fiard G, Hohn N, Descotes JL, et al. Targeted MRI-guided prostate biopsies for the detection of prostate cancer: initial clinical experience with real-time 3-dimensional transrectal ultrasound guidance and magnetic resonance/transrectal ultrasound image fusion. Urology 2013;81:1372–8.

32. Dianat SS, Carter HB, Macura KJ. Performance of multiparametric magnetic resonance imaging in the evaluation and management of clinically low-risk prostate cancer. Urol Oncol 2014;32(39):e1–10.

33. Hoeks CM, Somford DM, van Oort IM, et al. Value of 3-T multiparametric magnetic resonance imaging and magnetic resonance-guided biopsy for early risk restratification in active surveillance of low-risk prostate cancer: a prospective multicenter cohort study. Invest Radiol 2014;49:165–72.

34. Hu JC, Chang E, Natarajan S, et al. Targeted prostate biopsy in select men for active surveillance: do the Epstein criteria still apply? J Urol 2014;192: 385–90.

35. Le JD, Stephenson S, Brugger M, et al. Magnetic resonance imaging-ultrasound fusion biopsy for prediction of final prostate pathology. J Urol 2014;192: 1367–73.

36. Available at: http://www.acr.org/~/media/ACR/ Documents/PDF/QualitySafety/Resources/PIRADS/ PIRADS%20V2.pdf. Accessed April 29, 2015.

Magnetic Resonance–Guided Gynecologic Brachytherapy

 CrossMark

Antonio L. Damato, PhD*, Akila N. Viswanathan, MD, MPH

KEYWORDS

- Gynecology • Brachytherapy • MR imaging • Image guidance • Quality assurance

KEY POINTS

- MR imaging guidance is ideal for gynecologic brachytherapy; if access to MR imaging is limited, first-time insertions and patients with large tumors should be given priority.
- MR-compatible brachytherapy equipment is available but needs to be tested for mechanical pull, heating, and image artifact, particularly if greater than 1.5 T is used.
- MR–guided brachytherapy is a multidisciplinary effort involving a radiation oncologist, a radiologist, an imaging physicist, a radiation therapy physicist, nurses, and technical staff.
- New advancements in multiparametric sequencing of MR images allow identification of subregions of interest inside the tumor that may be targeted with brachytherapy.
- Different MR imaging sequences should be used for applicator selection (image quality), insertion guidance (speed of acquisition), and treatment planning (high-resolution, large field of view).

INTRODUCTION

Brachytherapy is a radiotherapy (RT) modality in which the radiation is delivered by positioning radioactive sources directly inside the tumor. Brachytherapy for the treatment of gynecologic malignancies was first proposed in the early 1900s, with an intracavitary radium applicator documented in 1905.[1,2] More than 100 years later, brachytherapy remains the standard of care for a broad range of gynecologic malignancies. The use of brachytherapy to deliver a boost dose to the remaining tumor following external beam RT for the treatment of cervical cancer is the standard of care worldwide because it results in a significantly higher rate of survival than external beam RT alone.[3] During the past decade, a decline in brachytherapy utilization in favor of external beam techniques has been associated with a decrease in the survival rate.[4] In cervical cancer brachytherapy, typically, an applicator composed of a uterine tandem is inserted into the uterine canal and a vaginal component comprising either a ring-shaped applicator (ring) or 2 colpostats (ovoids) is positioned at the top of the vagina against the cervix. Historically, a standard desired-dose distribution, described as pear-shaped (**Fig. 1**), has been used and the dose prescribed to the position referred to as point A. However, this method does not take into account patient-specific information on tumor size and largely disregards information on organs at risk (bladder, rectum, sigmoid, bowel). This practice is still widespread in places without MR–guidance capability, although less by choice than by necessity.[5,6] Whereas ultrasound can assist in the correct identification of the uterine canal during tandem insertion[7,8] and plain radiographs help identify the applicator in relation to landmarks to delineate points representing the bladder and the rectum, neither of these imaging modalities renders the residual tumor visible. Even on computed tomography (CT) scans that

The authors have nothing to disclose.
Department of Radiation Oncology, Brigham and Women's Hospital, LL2, 75 Francis Street, Boston, MA 02115, USA
* Corresponding author.
E-mail address: adamato@partners.org

Magn Reson Imaging Clin N Am 23 (2015) 633–642
http://dx.doi.org/10.1016/j.mric.2015.05.015
1064-9689/15/$ – see front matter © 2015 Elsevier Inc. All rights reserved.

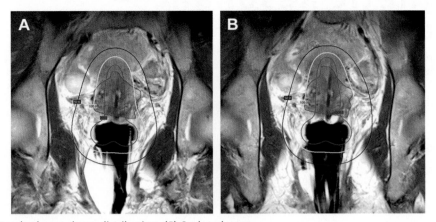

Fig. 1. (*A*) Standard pear-shape distribution. (*B*) Sculpted pear.

enable 3-dimensional (3D) planning and accurate definition of organs at risk,[9,10] cervical tumors are difficult to distinguish from surrounding scar tissue resulting from the external beam treatment that precedes brachytherapy.[11,12] The advent of remote afterloading systems allows the robotic deployment of a high-dose-rate or a pulsed-dose-rate source into the inside of the applicator, with the source resting for varying times at points along the applicator, creating a customized dose distribution. Nevertheless, the technical capability of delivering very precise customized dose distributions has limited value without accurate delineation of the gross tumor volume (GTV) and the surrounding areas likely containing microscopic disease (clinical target volume [CTV]).

The utility of MR imaging for cervical cancer delineation to assist with brachytherapy planning was first recognized in the early 1990s.[13] With increased availability of MR scanners for use with RT, a growing interest in MR–guided insertions and planning resulted in a period of intense exploration of MR–guided cervical-cancer brachytherapy both in Europe, with publications as early as 1992, and in the United States, with the first prospective trial starting in 2004.[13–15] The variability in MR scanner characteristics; MR sequences; applicator material and configuration; tumor-contouring methodologies; and dose prescription, planning, and reporting require careful interpretation of the data from many clinics. A task force was set up by the Group Européen de Curiethérapie–European Society for Therapeutic Radiology and Oncology (GEC-ESTRO) to promote and standardize the use of MR imaging for cervical cancer brachytherapy. This effort culminated in a series of guidelines in Europe[16–19] and in the United States (through the American Brachytherapy Society).[6,20–22] The combination of tumor visibility on

MR images and flexibility in dose planning shifted dose distributions from a standard pear-shape configuration to a sculpted-pear configuration (see **Fig. 1**).[23] Clinical[24–27] and physics[23,28–31] investigations have since shown that customized planning provides better dosimetry, which translates into superior clinical outcomes. An international research effort to collect and analyze treatment data for cervical-cancer brachytherapy delivered according to the GEC-ESTRO guidelines is underway with the EMBRACE research trial (www.embracestudy.dk).

Technological advances and economic factors have increased the availability of MR scanners for brachytherapy procedures, especially high-field-strength scanners. Although the number of centers performing MR–guided insertions continues to grow, MR imaging planning based on a post facto scan (ie, a scan acquired after the insertion is completed and after patient transfer from the operating room) is already performed in a wide variety of centers. Guidelines on which MR imaging sequences should be used have been published[16,19] and validated[32,33]; however, the fast pace of technological change may result in a separation between current imaging practices and available guidelines. For instance, 3 T MR is becoming more available and its use is expected to improve image quality and available resolution. Concerns regarding the applicability of existing contouring guidelines,[12] image deformation, heating of the brachytherapy equipment, and image artifacts have been raised by some investigators.[19] Experience in some major centers, notably in the Advanced Multimodality Image Guided Operating (AMIGO) suite at the Brigham and Women's Hospital in Boston, has proven the feasibility of 3 T MR-based brachytherapy.[27,34]

This article focuses on the state of the art and recent innovations in the use of MR guidance for gynecologic brachytherapy. The analysis is subdivided by thematic areas. First, the intraoperative role of MR imaging in the practice of gynecologic brachytherapy, allowing for the interactive adjustment of applicator positioning, is discussed. Second, the practical aspects of MR–guided gynecologic brachytherapy, with the presentation of recent innovations in the field, are discussed. Finally, some radiation therapy physics considerations regarding treatment planning and quality assurance are introduced.

INTRAOPERATIVE USE OF MR IMAGING FOR GYNECOLOGIC CANCER

The availability of MR imaging at the time of applicator insertion increases the likelihood of proper source placement inside the tumor. Optimization during planning is a poor substitute for less than ideal applicator positioning due to the potential for overdosing normal tissue proximal to the applicator when a curative dose needs to be projected into areas distant from the sources. Real-time image guidance during insertion of a brachytherapy applicator has historically been performed with ultrasound.[35] Real-time ultrasound guidance is used as an instantaneous feedback for the attending physician. This form of continuous visualization is optimal for intraoperative procedures because it allows immediate corrections when departures from the ideal insertion path are noticed. A combination of real-time guidance, as is provided by ultrasound, and the superior imaging capabilities of MR would be ideal. Unfortunately, an MR-compatible ultrasound is not readily available. Real-time MR guidance has proven elusive in clinical practice. One example was the MR–guided interstitial therapy (MRT) experience at Brigham and Women's Hospital.[15,36] An open 0.5 T MR scanner, installed in 1994, was used between 2002 and 2006 for MR-guided gynecologic brachytherapy interventions.[37] The MRT was a modified design to allow intervention in an open low-field scanner. Closed-bore MR scanners have the disadvantages of constraining access to the patient and causing

logistical difficulty in obtaining real-time visualization. An alternative form of iterative MR guidance is delayed-feedback guidance in which a preliminary insertion is performed in the MR room, a scan is then obtained, and adjustments are performed. The process is repeated until the applicator position is considered satisfactory (**Fig. 2**). This delayed feedback workflow requires optimization of MR sequences to provide time-effective information during and at the end of the insertion.[34]

In addition to MR imaging safety concerns typical of all MR imaging use, specific safety procedures need to be established in regard to ferromagnetic characteristics of brachytherapy applicators and equipment, and attention paid to training of personnel for the joint application of MR-specific safety rules and brachytherapy quality-assurance practices. A team that includes radiation oncologists, radiologists, radiation therapy and MR imaging physicists, radiation therapists, MR imaging technologists, and nurses is advisable. Once a process map of the procedure is established, optimization of the process,[38] safety analysis, and dry-runs should be performed. This section discusses areas directly related to the use of MR imaging as the gynecologic insertion is occurring (see later discussion of MR-based planning that can also be performed with an MR image acquired post facto). The topics covered in this section are (1) how to best use potentially limited MR imaging access by prioritizing the insertions for which MR imaging is most useful, (2) brachytherapy-specific considerations relating to MR imaging safety and treatment quality, (3) practical considerations for set-up and sequence selection, and (4) maximizing visibility of tumor and of the brachytherapy applicator.

PRIORITIZING MR GUIDANCE IN ENVIRONMENTS WITH LIMITED MR IMAGING ACCESS

The utility of MR guidance varies from patient to patient. In departments in which MR access is limited and needs to be negotiated with other interventional and diagnostic services, it is important to identify cases that would benefit most from MR

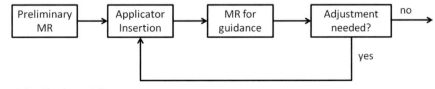

Fig. 2. Delayed-feedback workflow.

imaging use. An intracavitary applicator can be positioned effectively without MR guidance. Nevertheless, with such an approach there is no or limited visibility of the residual tumor to be treated, which then must be approximated by clinical examination at the time of applicator insertion.[11] Lack of direct tumor visibility introduces uncertainty in the targeting of the radiation. Therefore, acquisition of an MR scan following at least the first applicator insertion is advised. If the use of MR imaging is not possible for subsequent insertions, use of CT, clinical examination, and radiographs combined with information from the first insertion MR imaging can be considered.[39] If MR is not used during applicator insertion, the transfer of the patient to an MR scanner would probably substantially increase procedure time and use of clinic resources, potentially resulting in longer anesthesia time. Moreover, repeated transfer of a patient with applicator in situ increases the possibility of dislocation of the applicator from the inserted position.

Applicator selection is usually based on clinical examination at the time of the insertion, and on MR scans typically acquired before external beam RT. Because tumor response during external beam RT can vary considerably among patients, applicator selection can be suboptimal without the availability of an MR scan at the time of brachytherapy. This is of particular importance for patients with large residual tumors or asymmetric tumors. In these cases, a standard intracavitary applicator may not be sufficient to achieve good source distribution geometry due to the great distance between the uterine canal and the border of the tumor (**Fig. 3**). The addition of needles has been shown to allow increased dose to the tumor while maintaining low toxicities for the organs at risk.[40,41] Clear visibility of the tumor at the time of insertion is essential to the proper positioning of the needles inside tissue. MR–guided insertions provide maximum

advantage for cases with large and/or asymmetric residual tumors, and for cases with tumors extending into the vagina with a significant paravaginal component.

In summary, MR-guided insertions for gynecologic brachytherapy are preferable. If access to the MR scanner is limited, scheduling an MR imaging before or after the first insertion is a reasonable strategy to maximize the advantage associated with the use of MR imaging. The first-insertion MR can be fused, based on applicator placement, onto subsequent insertion CT scans and used for further guidance in tumor contouring. If not all first-time insertions can be scheduled under MR guidance, preference should be given to patients with large tumors at the time of the MR scans before external beam RT and to patients requiring interstitial insertions.

MR SAFETY AND QUALITY ASSURANCE FOR GYNECOLOGIC BRACHYTHERAPY

MR-compatible and CT-compatible applicators are commercially available from multiple vendors and are fabricated in either plastic or titanium. Each clinic must validate both the absence of mechanical pull from the magnetic field and the heating characteristics of the applicator during imaging. Concerns for heating of titanium devices, especially when used in 3 T scanners, have been raised as a reason to prefer 1.5 T MR.[19] All brachytherapy equipment should be tested, including stylets that may be used to assist with needle insertions, templates and vaginal obturators, applicator immobilization devices, and vaginal packing equipment. The general principle of testing all equipment under all possible clinical configurations and using all possible clinical sequences applies. Quality-assurance practices to ensure the safe delivery of the brachytherapy should be maintained in MR-guided workflows. For instance, immobilization and identification of

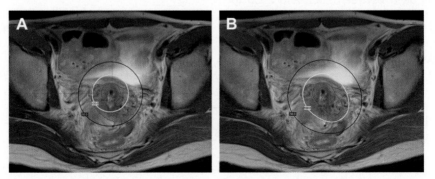

Fig. 3. (*A*) Axial image of a dose distribution from a tandem, showing under-coverage of the distal region of the CTV (*in red*). (*B*) The addition of an interstitial needle permits an increase in coverage of the cervix.

the various components of a brachytherapy applicator must, in some cases, occur at the time of implantation.

In summary, MR safety and treatment quality assurance are critical elements of MR-guided procedures. A joint radiology and radiation oncology team should establish dedicated workflows and a quality management program. The primary risk for a potential safety hazard lies in the introduction of brachytherapy equipment that may be magnetic and/or heat up during MR imaging procedures. Particular care should be taken with nonplastic equipment and when field strengths greater than 1.5 T are used.

THE PRACTICE OF MR–GUIDED GYNECOLOGIC BRACHYTHERAPY INSERTIONS

Many practical aspects should be considered when designing an MR-guided gynecologic brachytherapy practice. MR scanner configuration and field strength are important considerations in the design of a facility for MR-guided insertions. Open-geometry scanners have the advantage of easy access to the patient, which make this geometry preferable for interventions in the pelvic area. Despite the geometric advantage, open MR scanners are usually limited in field strength (<1 T), which has a negative impact on signal-to-noise ratio and resolution. Closed-bore MR scanners are the most commonly used for interventional imaging. Their use in gynecologic brachytherapy is limited by bore size and accessibility of the peritoneal area for the insertion. Wide-bore (70 cm) magnets are available in field strengths up to 3 T, and are currently the best compromise between geometric requirements and resolution. Patient setup inside the MR room should be carefully designed and validated through testing and practice runs. Transport of brachytherapy patients out of the room must be done with care to minimize the possibility of applicator displacement or needle shift.[42] Staff should be trained to handle patients with applicators in place. There should be visual verification of the applicator immediately before and after movement of the patient from the MR table to the transportation stretcher. For access to the perineal area, positioning of the patient's pelvis at the edge of the MR table is optimal but often impractical. This may be due to the presence of an obstructive bar or of bulky electronics obstructing access to the table edge. Moreover, limited table travel may not allow the table's edge to reach the scanner's isocenter. Workflows involving less than ideal access to the perineal area may be required. Successful MR–guided brachytherapy insertion programs have been established in many centers despite these difficulties.[24,28,35,43] With increased visibility of the tumor on MR imaging compared with CT, the use of fiducial markers implanted in the tumor to enhance its visibility is, in most cases, unnecessary. Fiducial markers should be used in gynecologic brachytherapy when registration of MR with CT images is needed for planning or treatment verification. In these cases, identification of the fiducial markers on MR imaging will be required for registration. Imaging characteristics of gold fiducials depend on their shape and their orientation with the magnetic field.[44] It is, therefore, necessary to commission the use of fiducials inside the MR scanner with clinical sequences and with various fiducial orientations.

Choice and optimization of MR sequences should be performed by a multidisciplinary team comprising the attending physician, a radiologist, an MR physicist, and a radiation therapy physicist. Three sets of sequences should be developed: the first performed immediately before implantation for final applicator selection and evaluation of tumor response to external beam RT; the second performed during implantation, allowing for relatively quick adjustments and reverification of applicator position; and the third performed at completion of implantation for planning purposes. The intraprocedure sequence should focus on the visibility of the tumor while allowing enough visibility of the applicator to verify its positioning relative to the targeted area. In general, these scans are not used for precise tumor contouring or for applicator digitization. Therefore, speed may be optimized by restricting the field of view to the region of the implant under current investigation, using a slice thickness of 5 mm or more, and scanning in a single orientation. Visibility of the tandem, ovoids, and ring applicator on T2 MR imaging is usually sufficient for guidance purposes (**Fig. 4**). Visibility of needles must be sufficient both to distinguish between a needle and the surrounding vasculature and for identification of the needle to allow for the correction of its position, if needed. This is challenging when many needles, with possibly intersecting paths, are inserted. The use of dummy markers inserted into the applicator and needles to increase their visibility has been reported. Although these techniques may be useful for better visualizing the internal lumen of an applicator,[43,45] this approach may have limited success for 6F-sized needles, due to the small volumes available.

Three alternative approaches have been explored for increasing the visibility of

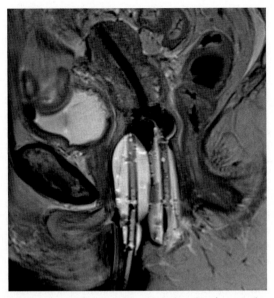

Fig. 4. View of a tandem insertion in the uterine canal.

brachytherapy needles for interstitial insertions. One possibility is to increase the artifact around the needle's metallic components (e.g., selecting a needle made of titanium or using metallic stylets surrounded by plastic catheters) with dedicated MR sequences (e.g., balanced steady-state free precession sequences).[34] Another approach for enhancing the visibility of needles is through post-processing. Encouraging results have been presented[46] but clinical applicability has not yet been achieved. A third approach is the use of active tracking of needles using smart stylets containing one or more coils relaying their location in the MR scanner frame of reference to an external computer system. This approach was recently described[47] and has the dual advantages of allowing the automatic identification of the coordinates of the needles in the image and increased visibility of the needles. This approach is similar to the recent proposal to use an RF coil to identify brachytherapy needles in ultrasound- and CT-based insertions.[48,49]

Although speed of insertion is important for maximizing the efficient use of resources and minimizing anesthesia time for the patient, the use of additional imaging should be considered when more information about the CTV is requested. The use of diffusion-weighted imaging and associated apparent diffusion coefficient maps to contour the GTV inside the CTV has been recently discussed,[50] along with possible implications for radiation therapy.

In summary, many practical considerations need to be taken into account in the design of an

MR-guided brachytherapy program. The design is, therefore, a multidisciplinary effort[51] involving a radiation oncologist, a radiologist, an imaging physicist, a radiation therapy physicist, nurses, technical staff, and, potentially, engineers. MR safety considerations, solutions for patient positioning that allow imaging and accessibility to the pelvic area, and selection of MR imaging sequences and technologies allowing sufficient visualization of the tumor and of the applicator components (including needles) should be considered. Advancements are underway in active needle visualization and in the use of MR imaging to identify subregions of interest inside the tumor.

TREATMENT PLANNING AND QUALITY ASSURANCE FOR MR–GUIDED GYNECOLOGIC BRACHYTHERAPY

Following implantation, treatment planning occurs. A physicist imports the 3D images (MR CT) of a patient and identifies, in the scan, the lumens inside the applicators and inside the needles. With the coordinates of possible source location identified, the planning system can display the dose resulting from possible loading of the sources, overlaid directly on the images. In the planning system, as the physician delineates the organs at risk (bladder, sigmoid, rectum, bowel) and the tumor, aggregate measures of the dose to each organ (dose metrics) are calculated. Correlations between dose metrics and tumor control probability and between dose metrics and normal-tissue complication probability have been explored clinically. A system of automatic checks for complex procedures such as MR–guided brachytherapy has been shown to decrease the chance of errors in planning[52] and should be encouraged. Three causes of uncertainty related to MR imaging use exist: applicator reconstruction, contouring, and delivery. Many investigators have discussed the role of applicator reconstruction in MR imaging.[43,53–55] It was reported that direct reconstruction is feasible for plastic applicators using the availability of digital models that describe the location of the internal lumen and the outline of the applicator.[34] By fusing the external outline of the model with the visible shape of the applicator on MR imaging, a reconstruction of the location of the internal lumen of the applicator not visible on MR imaging is possible (**Fig. 5**). If a model is not available from the vendor, or if the general shape of the applicator is not visible on T2 MR, as is sometimes the case with titanium applicators, T1 with CuSO4 dummy markers[23] inside the internal lumen or T2 with a saline dummy[27] can be used as has been reported. An alternative approach is

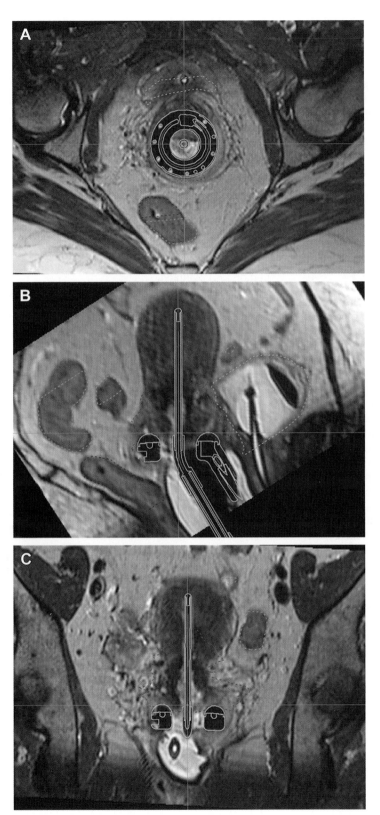

Fig. 5. Paraxial (*A*), parasagittal (*B*), and paracoronal (*C*) views of a T2 scan of a patient with a tandem and ring insertion. Applicator lumen is not visible; however, dark applicator outline allows registration with a digital applicator model (*in green*).

to obtain a postimplant CT and use a CT-MR image fusion to perform applicator digitization. This method requires the transfer of the patient to a CT scanner, exposure to ionizing radiation, and increased use of clinic resources (additional imaging, image fusion). Moreover, uncertainties related to imperfect image fusion may be introduced. This approach should be used only when other approaches are not viable, such as for interstitial implantation in which visibility of the needles may not be sufficient.[34] Registration should be based only on the applicator and needles. Misalignment of anatomy resulting from the fusion should be evaluated and, potentially, MR imaging contours may be adjusted based on CT information. Dose distribution, overlaid both on MR and CT, should be analyzed. Information from active tracking during MR-guided insertions[47] or electromagnetic tracking post facto[49] can be used to aid digitization. To ensure proper reconstruction, a planning MR scan at a slice thickness less than 3 mm should be acquired when feasible. 3D "SPACE" scans (sampling perfection with application-optimized contrasts using different flip angle evolutions) can be acquired to allow verification of the reconstruction in 3D. Scan field of view should include all the relevant applicator components, allowing reconstruction and identification of channel assignment and all relevant anatomy. The planning scan can take substantially more acquisition time than other scans. Contouring uncertainties have been explored.[56,57] The dose metric effect of uncertainties can be substantial and care should be taken that only properly trained staff contour brachytherapy applications. Finally, delivery uncertainties should be considered. These can be effects of applicator and needle shifts or anatomic deformations that occurred between the time of the planning MR imaging and the time of treatment.[45] To avoid applicator and needle displacement, the patient should be properly immobilized at the time of the MR scan and care should be taken to not disturb the implant area during transport. Markings and clinical photography can be used to help identify shifts; additional imaging can be considered in some cases. Anatomic changes due to differences in bladder filling can be controlled with bladder-filling protocols; rectal filling control through a rectal tube can be considered in some cases.

In summary, a planning MR scan, with a field of view including all relevant anatomy and applicator components, should be acquired when implantation is complete. Fusion of MR and CT images to aid with reconstruction should be considered only in cases in which MR imaging alone is not sufficient. Quality assurance practices must ensure that the geometry captured during MR imaging is replicated at treatment.

SUMMARY

MR imaging enhances the visibility of gynecologic tumors compared with imaging by CT and ultrasound. It has emerged as the preferred modality for image-guided gynecologic brachytherapy in centers equipped with an MR scanner. When a dedicated MR equipped operating room is not available, strategies for patient selection are possible to maximize the benefit of MR imaging use. Multiparametric MR imaging should be considered to achieve ideal tumor visibility and brachytherapy catheter reconstruction during insertion and planning.

ACKNOWLEDGMENTS

Thank you to Barbara Silver for reviewing this article.

REFERENCES

1. Abbe R. The use of radium in malignant disease. Lancet 1913;2:524–7.
2. Mould RF. Invited review: the early years of radiotherapy with emphasis on X-ray and radium apparatus. Br J Radiol 1995;68:567–82.
3. Han K, Milosevic M, Fyles A, et al. Trends in the utilization of brachytherapy in cervical cancer in the United States. Int J Radiat Oncol Biol Phys 2013; 87:111–9.
4. Gill BS, Lin JF, Krivak TC, et al. National cancer data base analysis of radiation therapy consolidation modality for cervical cancer: the impact of new technological advancements. Int J Radiat Oncol Biol Phys 2014;90:1083–90.
5. Viswanathan AN, Creutzberg CL, Craighead P, et al. International brachytherapy practice patterns: a survey of the Gynecologic Cancer Intergroup (GCIG). Int J Radiat Oncol Biol Phys 2010;82(1):250–5.
6. Viswanathan AN, Thomadsen B. American Brachytherapy Society consensus guidelines for locally advanced carcinoma of the cervix. Part I: general principles. Brachytherapy 2012;11:33–46.
7. Van Dyk S, Narayan K, Fisher R, et al. Conformal brachytherapy planning for cervical cancer using transabdominal ultrasound. Int J Radiat Oncol Biol Phys 2009;75:64–70.
8. van Dyk S, Schneider M, Kondalsamy-Chennakesavan S, et al. Ultrasound use in gynecologic brachytherapy: time to focus the beam. Brachytherapy 2015;14(3):390–400.

9. Erickson B. CT guidance assists brachytherapy for gynecologic disease. Diagn Imaging (San Franc) 2000;22:167–71, 91.

10. Viswanathan AN. The Frank Ellis memorial lecture: the use of three-dimensional imaging in gynaecological radiation therapy. Clin Oncol (R Coll Radiol) 2008;20:1–5.

11. Viswanathan AN, Dimopoulos J, Kirisits C, et al. Computed tomography versus magnetic resonance imaging-based contouring in cervical cancer brachytherapy: results of a prospective trial and preliminary guidelines for standardized contours. Int J Radiat Oncol Biol Phys 2007;68:491–8.

12. Viswanathan AN, Erickson B, Gaffney DK, et al. Comparison and consensus guidelines for delineation of clinical target volume for CT- and MR-based brachytherapy in locally advanced cervical cancer. Int J Radiat Oncol Biol Phys 2014;90:320–8.

13. Schoeppel SL, Ellis JH, LaVigne ML, et al. Magnetic resonance imaging during intracavitary gynecologic brachytherapy. Int J Radiat Oncol Biol Phys 1992;23:169–74.

14. Wachter-Gerstner N, Wachter S, Reinstadler E, et al. The impact of sectional imaging on dose escalation in endocavitary HDR-brachytherapy of cervical cancer: results of a prospective comparative trial. Radiother Oncol 2003;68:51–9.

15. Viswanathan AN, Szymonifka J, Tempany-Afdhal CM, et al. A prospective trial of real-time magnetic resonance-guided catheter placement in interstitial gynecologic brachytherapy. Brachytherapy 2013;12:240–7.

16. Haie-Meder C, Potter R, Van Limbergen E, et al. Recommendations from Gynaecological (GYN) GEC-ESTRO Working Group (I): concepts and terms in 3D image based 3D treatment planning in cervix cancer brachytherapy with emphasis on MRI assessment of GTV and CTV. Radiother Oncol 2005;74:235–45.

17. Potter R, Haie-Meder C, Van Limbergen E, et al. Recommendations from gynaecological (GYN) GEC ESTRO working group (II): concepts and terms in 3D image-based treatment planning in cervix cancer brachytherapy-3D dose volume parameters and aspects of 3D image-based anatomy, radiation physics, radiobiology. Radiother Oncol 2006;78:67–77.

18. Hellebust TP, Kirisits C, Berger D, et al. Recommendations from Gynaecological (GYN) GEC-ESTRO Working Group: considerations and pitfalls in commissioning and applicator reconstruction in 3D image-based treatment planning of cervix cancer brachytherapy. Radiother Oncol 2010;96:153–60.

19. Dimopoulos JC, Petrow P, Tanderup K, et al. Recommendations from Gynaecological (GYN) GEC-ESTRO Working Group (IV): Basic principles and parameters for MR imaging within the frame of image based adaptive cervix cancer brachytherapy. Radiother Oncol 2012;103:113–22.

20. Viswanathan AN, Beriwal S, De Los Santos JF, et al. American Brachytherapy Society consensus guidelines for locally advanced carcinoma of the cervix. Part II: high-dose-rate brachytherapy. Brachytherapy 2012;11:47–52.

21. Lee LJ, Das IJ, Higgins SA, et al. American Brachytherapy Society consensus guidelines for locally advanced carcinoma of the cervix. Part III: low-dose-rate and pulsed-dose-rate brachytherapy. Brachytherapy 2012;11:53–7.

22. Nag S, Ellis RJ, Merrick GS, et al. American Brachytherapy Society recommendations for reporting morbidity after prostate brachytherapy. Int J Radiat Oncol Biol Phys 2002;54:462–70.

23. Tanderup K, Nielsen SK, Nyvang GB, et al. From point A to the sculpted pear: MR image guidance significantly improves tumour dose and sparing of organs at risk in brachytherapy of cervical cancer. Radiother Oncol 2010;94:173–80.

24. Potter R, Georg P, Dimopoulos JC, et al. Clinical outcome of protocol based image (MRI) guided adaptive brachytherapy combined with 3D conformal radiotherapy with or without chemotherapy in patients with locally advanced cervical cancer. Radiother Oncol 2011;100:116–23.

25. Charra-Brunaud C, Harter V, Delannes M, et al. Impact of 3D image-based PDR brachytherapy on outcome of patients treated for cervix carcinoma in France: results of the French STIC prospective study. Radiother Oncol 2012;103:305–13.

26. Chargari C, Magne N, Dumas I, et al. Physics contributions and clinical outcome with 3D-MRI-based pulsed-dose-rate intracavitary brachytherapy in cervical cancer patients. Int J Radiat Oncol Biol Phys 2009;74:133–9.

27. Kharofa J, Morrow N, Kelly T, et al. 3-T MRI-based adaptive brachytherapy for cervix cancer: treatment technique and initial clinical outcomes. Brachytherapy 2014;13:319–25.

28. Kirisits C, Potter R, Lang S, et al. Dose and volume parameters for MRI-based treatment planning in intracavitary brachytherapy for cervical cancer. Int J Radiat Oncol Biol Phys 2005;62:901–11.

29. Jurgenliemk-Schulz IM, Lang S, Tanderup K, et al. Variation of treatment planning parameters (D90 HR-CTV, D 2cc for OAR) for cervical cancer tandem ring brachytherapy in a multicentre setting: comparison of standard planning and 3D image guided optimisation based on a joint protocol for dose-volume constraints. Radiother Oncol 2010;94:339–45.

30. Lindegaard JC, Tanderup K, Nielsen SK, et al. MRI-guided 3D optimization significantly improves DVH parameters of pulsed-dose-rate brachytherapy in locally advanced cervical cancer. Int J Radiat Oncol Biol Phys 2008;71:756–64.

31. De Brabandere M, Mousa AG, Nulens A, et al. Potential of dose optimisation in MRI-based PDR brachytherapy of cervix carcinoma. Radiother Oncol 2008;88:217–26.

32. Lang S, Nulens A, Briot E, et al. Intercomparison of treatment concepts for MR image assisted brachytherapy of cervical carcinoma based on GYN GEC-ESTRO recommendations. Radiother Oncol 2006;78:185–93.

33. Dimopoulos JC, De Vos V, Berger D, et al. Interobserver comparison of target delineation for MRI-assisted cervical cancer brachytherapy: application of the GYN GEC-ESTRO recommendations. Radiother Oncol 2009;91:166–72.

34. Kapur T, Egger J, Damato A, et al. 3-T MR-guided brachytherapy for gynecologic malignancies. Magn Reson Imaging 2012;30:1279–90.

35. Davidson MT, Yuen J, D'Souza DP, et al. Optimization of high-dose-rate cervix brachytherapy applicator placement: the benefits of intraoperative ultrasound guidance. Brachytherapy 2008;7:248–53.

36. Viswanathan AN, Cormack R, Holloway CL, et al. Magnetic resonance-guided interstitial therapy for vaginal recurrence of endometrial cancer. Int J Radiat Oncol Biol Phys 2006;66:91–9.

37. Viswanathan A, Kirisits C, Erickson B, et al. Gynecologic radiation therapy. New York: Springer; 2011.

38. Damato AL, Lee LJ, Bhagwat MS, et al. Redesign of process map to increase efficiency: reducing procedure time in cervical cancer brachytherapy. Brachytherapy 2015;14:471–80.

39. Kirisits C, Lang S, Dimopoulos J, et al. Uncertainties when using only one MRI-based treatment plan for subsequent high-dose-rate tandem and ring applications in brachytherapy of cervix cancer. Radiother Oncol 2006;81:269–75.

40. Kirisits C, Lang S, Dimopoulos J, et al. The Vienna applicator for combined intracavitary and interstitial brachytherapy of cervical cancer: design, application, treatment planning, and dosimetric results. Int J Radiat Oncol Biol Phys 2006;65:624–30.

41. Jurgenliemk-Schulz IM, Tersteeg RJ, Roesink JM, et al. MRI-guided treatment-planning optimisation in intracavitary or combined intracavitary/interstitial PDR brachytherapy using tandem ovoid applicators in locally advanced cervical cancer. Radiother Oncol 2009;93:322–30.

42. Damato AL, Cormack RA, Viswanathan AN. Characterization of implant displacement and deformation in gynecologic interstitial brachytherapy. Brachytherapy 2014;13:100–9.

43. De Leeuw AA, Moerland MA, Nomden C, et al. Applicator reconstruction and applicator shifts in 3D MR-based PDR brachytherapy of cervical cancer. Radiother Oncol 2009;93:341–6.

44. Jonsson JH, Garpebring A, Karlsson MG, et al. Internal fiducial markers and susceptibility effects in MRI-simulation and measurement of spatial accuracy. Int J Radiat Oncol Biol Phys 2012;82:1612–8.

45. Haack S, Nielsen SK, Lindegaard JC, et al. Applicator reconstruction in MRI 3D image-based dose planning of brachytherapy for cervical cancer. Radiother Oncol 2009;91:187–93.

46. Pernelle G, Mehrtash A, Barber L, et al. Validation of catheter segmentation for MR-guided gynecologic cancer brachytherapy. Med Image Comput Comput Assist Interv 2013;16:380–7.

47. Wang W, Dumoulin CL, Viswanathan AN, et al. Real-time active MR-tracking of metallic stylets in MR-guided radiation therapy. Magn Reson Med 2014;73(5):1803–11.

48. Mehrtash A, Damato A, Pernelle G, et al. EM-navigated catheter placement for gynecologic brachytherapy: an accuracy study. Proc SPIE Int Soc Opt Eng 2014;9036:90361F.

49. Damato AL, Viswanathan AN, Don SM, et al. A system to use electromagnetic tracking for the quality assurance of brachytherapy catheter digitization. Med Phys 2014;41:101702.

50. Dyk P, Jiang N, Sun B, et al. Cervical gross tumor volume dose predicts local control using magnetic resonance imaging/diffusion-weighted imaging-guided high-dose-rate and positron emission tomography/computed tomography-guided intensity modulated radiation therapy. Int J Radiat Oncol Biol Phys 2014;90:794–801.

51. Tanderup K, Viswanathan AN, Kirisits C, et al. Magnetic resonance image guided brachytherapy. Semin Radiat Oncol 2014;24:181–91.

52. Damato AL, Devlin PM, Bhagwat MS, et al. Independent brachytherapy plan verification software: improving efficacy and efficiency. Radiother Oncol 2014;113:420–4.

53. Berger D, Dimopoulos J, Potter R, et al. Direct reconstruction of the Vienna applicator on MR images. Radiother Oncol 2009;93:347–51.

54. Wills R, Lowe G, Inchley D, et al. Applicator reconstruction for HDR cervix treatment planning using images from 0.35 T open MR scanner. Radiother Oncol 2010;94:346–52.

55. Petit S, Wielopolski P, Rijnsdorp R, et al. MR guided applicator reconstruction for brachytherapy of cervical cancer using the novel titanium Rotterdam applicator. Radiother Oncol 2013;107:88–92.

56. Damato AL, Townamchai K, Albert M, et al. Dosimetric consequences of interobserver variability in delineating the organs at risk in gynecologic interstitial brachytherapy. Int J Radiat Oncol Biol Phys 2014;89:674–81.

57. Hellebust TP, Tanderup K, Lervag C, et al. Dosimetric impact of interobserver variability in MRI-based delineation for cervical cancer brachytherapy. Radiother Oncol 2013;107:13–9.

Magnetic Resonance-Guided Drug Delivery

Andrew S. Mikhail, PhD[a], Ari Partanen, PhD[a,b], Pavel Yarmolenko, PhD[c],
Aradhana M. Venkatesan, MD[d], Bradford J. Wood, MD[a,*]

KEYWORDS

- MR imaging • Drug delivery • Tumor targeting • Nanomedicine • Cancer
- Thermosensitive liposome • High-intensity focused ultrasound • Imaging guidance

KEY POINTS

- MR imaging can enable planning, monitoring, real-time control, and posttherapy assessment of tumor-targeted drug delivery.
- Use of MR imaging to guide the combination of hyperthermia and thermosensitive drug delivery systems constitutes an effective approach for enhancing drug delivery to tumors.
- MR-guided high intensity focused ultrasound (MR-HIFU) is a particularly promising technique for improving delivery of systemically administered therapies and potential modulation of the tumor microenvironment.

ADVANCED DRUG DELIVERY SYSTEMS

Targeted drug delivery, whereby therapeutic agents are transported from the site of administration specifically to diseased tissues, remains a "holy grail" of pharmaceutical research. This concept has significant potential in oncology, since side effects from chemotherapeutic drugs with narrow therapeutic windows (the range between effective and toxic doses) can limit the dose and compromise the efficacy of treatment. Recent progress in pharmaceutical nanotechnology has led to the development of a variety of advanced drug delivery systems (DDS) with the capacity to transport small-molecule drugs to tumors, resulting in reduced systemic toxicity and improved treatment outcomes.

In general, DDS-based drug formulations possess several advantages over their conventional counterparts, including (1) enhanced tumor targeting, (2) extended systemic circulation, and (3) controlled drug release. Careful design of DDS can exploit these characteristics to dramatically increase the safety margin of cytotoxic drugs with traditionally narrow therapeutic windows. Examples of DDS used for this purpose include polymeric micelles,[1] liposomes,[2] polymer-drug conjugates,[3] and antibody-targeted therapies (Fig. 1).[4] To date, liposomes have achieved significant success, with several formulations receiving clinical approval and many others, including temperature-sensitive liposomes (TSLs), are in clinical trials.[2]

This work was supported by the Center for Interventional Oncology in the Intramural Research Program of the National Institutes of Health (NIH). NIH and Celsion Corp. have a Cooperative Research and Development Agreement (CRADA). NIH and Philips Healthcare have a CRADA supported by NIH Grant # Z1A CL040015-06. Dr A. Partanen is a paid employee of Philips Healthcare. The content of this article does not necessarily reflect the views or policies of the Department of Health and Human Services, nor does mention of trade names, commercial products, or organizations imply endorsement by the US Government.

[a] Center for Interventional Oncology, Department of Radiology and Imaging Sciences, Clinical Center, National Institutes of Health, 10 Center Drive, Bethesda, MD 20892, USA; [b] Philips Healthcare, 3000 Minuteman Road, Andover, MA 01810, USA; [c] The Sheikh Zayed Institute for Pediatric Surgical Innovation, Children's National Medical Center, 111 Michigan Avenue, Washington, DC 20010, USA; [d] Section of Abdominal Imaging, Department of Diagnostic Radiology, M.D. Anderson Cancer Center, 1515 Holcombe Blvd, Houston, TX 77030-4009, USA
* Corresponding author.
E-mail address: bwood@nih.gov

mri.theclinics.com

CrossMark

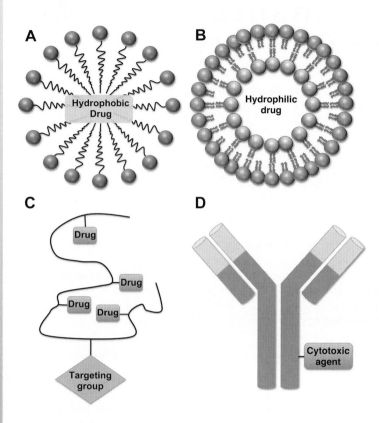

Fig. 1. Examples of drug delivery systems: micelles (*A*), liposomes (*B*), polymer-drug conjugates (*C*), and antibody conjugates (*D*).

DDS may be "passively" targeted by exploiting features of the tumor microenvironment to enhance drug accumulation, and/or "actively" targeted by binding of DDS to cancer cells or endothelium via specific chemical affinity. Tumor accumulation via passive targeting is achieved because of the characteristically hyperporous blood vessels of neoplasms (resulting in increased extravasation of macromolecules and nanoparticles) and dysfunctional lymphatic drainage, a phenomenon referred to as the enhanced permeability and retention (EPR) effect.[5] Active tumor targeting exploits the specific molecular affinity of bioactive ligands, such as peptides and antibodies, for cellular receptors preferentially expressed in malignant tissues to enhance tumor localization, retention, and cellular uptake.[6]

Barriers to Effective Drug Delivery

Following successful tumor targeting, stable DDS tend to be confined to perivascular tissues because of their limited penetration into the tumor interstitium.[7–9] If the drug remains bound to or encapsulated by the carrier, concentrations deep within the interstitium and in regions of low vascular density or high interstitial pressure will be limited. Recent efforts to improve drug delivery have focused on increasing both the amount and bioavailability of drugs delivered to a tumor by incorporating external release stimuli into the drug delivery paradigm. Drug release may be triggered by endogenous stimuli such as tissue pH[10] and redox reactions[11] associated with the microenvironment of tumors, or by application of exogenous triggers such as alternating magnetic fields,[12] heat,[13] and light.[14] Unlike endogenous stimuli, the spatiotemporal application of exogenous triggers can be controlled, providing a means for modulating drug release.

Insufficient dosing of tumors during chemotherapy resulting from poor intratumoral drug distribution and penetration is regarded as a major limitation of intravenous drug delivery. Many factors present barriers to drug delivery at the intratumoral level, including inefficient angiogenic vessels, the spatial heterogeneity of the tumor vasculature network, high cellular and stromal density, and elevated interstitial fluid pressure, among others.[1,15–17] Indeed, numerous studies have demonstrated the limited penetration of both conventional and DDS-based chemotherapy from tumor blood vessels into the interstitium.[8,9,18] These regions, deep within the interstitial space, are prone to transport-mediated and hypoxia-mediated drug resistance, and are a cause of tumor recurrence.[17] Identifying and mitigating transport barriers by means of chemical,[15] thermal, or mechanical alteration[19] of the tumor microenvironment, and by enhanced guidance of drug delivery, are active areas of research.

Image-Guided Drug Delivery

In the emerging era of personalized medicine, the ability to provide optimal treatment to the "right patient at the right dose at the right time" is a central tenet. However, new tools are required to facilitate better customization of therapy based on the specific needs of individual patients. Recently, image-guided drug delivery, which leverages clinical imaging modalities for guidance of DDS, has emerged as a viable strategy for enhancement of targeted, personalized drug therapies. In this drug delivery paradigm, imaging may be used to identify target and nontarget anatomy or for screening, planning, monitoring, and postprocedural assessment of treatment outcome (**Fig. 2**).

MR imaging is particularly well suited for the purpose of image-guided drug delivery because of its ability to acquire images and quantitative measurements with high spatiotemporal resolution during therapy. MR imaging–guided drug delivery may facilitate or augment existing minimally invasive image-guided therapies, with the eventual goals of improving efficacy or expanding the indications beyond existing local and regional paradigms. The remainder of this article reviews the current state of MR imaging–guided drug delivery, with a focus on hyperthermia-mediated drug delivery and potential future applications.

Hyperthermia-Mediated Drug Delivery

Hyperthermia, in the context of drug delivery and thermal therapy, refers to the application of heat resulting in tissue temperatures greater than normal physiologic temperature. In general, hyperthermia can be divided into mild ($\sim 40°$–$45°C$) and ablative ($\sim 50°$–$100°C$) regimes in which bioeffects are governed by a time-temperature Arrhenius continuum (thermal dose). Commonly used methods for generating local hyperthermia include the use of radiofrequency,[20] microwaves,[21] laser,[22] or superficial hot water applicators.[23] Temperature-sensitive DDS can be used as an adjuvant to thermal ablation to reduce the potential for tumor regrowth in regions of sublethal thermal damage such as at the ablation margin.[24] In addition, mild hyperthermia can be used to trigger drug release[25] within heated tissue and may be used just before subablative or ablative temperature elevation, potentially resulting in a "drug depot" effect whereby drug is concentrated in target tissues following local vascular shutdown.[26,27] Mild hyperthermia and ablation can also be combined to treat large or conjoined tumors, or geographically distributed tumors that might not otherwise have local or regional interventional oncology options (ie, because of size, number, or distribution).

HIGH-INTENSITY FOCUSED ULTRASOUND

High-intensity focused ultrasound (HIFU) represents a noninvasive alternative to more traditional hyperthermia applications by tightly focusing ultrasonic waves from an external transducer to generate localized temperature elevation in target tissues (**Fig. 3**). The use of HIFU to generate heat in target tissues is particularly advantageous, as it can be focused deep within the body and can achieve both mild and ablative hyperthermia. The interaction of propagating ultrasound waves with tissue can result in thermal and mechanical bioeffects[28–30] that can enhance extravasation, uptake, or stimulate drug release from temperature-sensitive or pressure-sensitive DDS.[31] Both thermal and mechanical bioeffects can also be used to enhance intracellular drug delivery and tissue permeability.[32] Furthermore, HIFU-mediated bioeffects can be tuned and controlled by adjusting the device power, frequency, duty cycle, timing, and other settings.

The use of MR imaging for image guidance of HIFU therapy, referred to as MR-HIFU, provides high-resolution anatomic imaging, and the ability to monitor HIFU-mediated temperature changes and tissue displacement. To date, MR-HIFU has been primarily used for the ablation of symptomatic uterine leiomyomata.[33,34] However, it is currently under investigation for several oncologic applications including treatment of benign breast fibroadenomas,[35] malignant breast carcinoma,[36] and prostate cancer,[37] palliative treatment of painful osseous metastases,[38] and ablation of brain tumors.[39] Moreover, MR-HIFU is being investigated as a treatment for neurologic disorders (eg, epilepsy, essential tremor, neuropathic pain, and

Screening, diagnosis and staging > Therapy planning > Therapy monitoring and guidance > Therapy assessment > Post-therapy surveillance

Fig. 2. MR imaging as part of drug delivery paradigm.

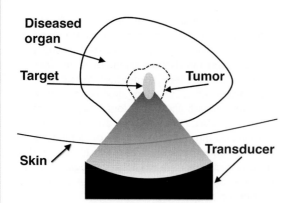

Fig. 3. Schematic of high-intensity focused ultrasound producing localized, elevated temperatures deep within the body, without heating or damaging surrounding tissues.

Parkinson disease),[40–42] and as an immunomodulator to inhibit local tumor recurrence and metastases following ablation.[43] MR-HIFU has also been shown to improve drug delivery to the brain by modulation of the blood-brain barrier (BBB).[44]

Temperature-Sensitive Liposomes

Developments in ultrasound applicators and delivery techniques and in MR imaging–based temperature monitoring and control methods[45–48] have made MR-HIFU–mediated mild hyperthermia an intriguing modality for noninvasive hyperthermia therapies in combination with drug delivery. A particularly attractive strategy for facilitating tumor-localized drug delivery consists of applying mild hyperthermia in combination with intravenous administration of TSLs.[49–51] When heat is applied to the tumor, circulating TSLs in transit through the tumor vasculature rapidly release the drug, resulting in high intravascular drug concentrations that promote extravasation and penetration into the tumor interstitium (**Fig. 4**).[7]

TSLs optimized for drug release at mild hyperthermic temperatures between 39.5°C and 41°C are known as low-temperature–sensitive liposomes (LTSLs). Various preclinical studies have demonstrated substantial reductions in tumor volume using LTSLs in combination with mild hyperthermia when compared with conventional therapy or nonthermally sensitive liposomes.[50,52,53] Recently, an LTSL formulation containing doxorubicin underwent a phase III clinical trial for the treatment of hepatocellular carcinoma in combination with radiofrequency ablation (RFA).[54]

MR-GUIDED DRUG DELIVERY

MR imaging offers several advantages over other imaging techniques, such as ultrasonography and computed tomography, which make it ideal for guidance of drug delivery. First, variation between tissue-specific MR parameters enables excellent contrast between soft tissues, and between normal and abnormal morphology/pathology, enhancing precision of the treatment plan. However, MR imaging is devoid of ionizing radiation, which is of particular importance because repeated imaging is usually necessary to monitor and guide drug delivery and to assess tumor progression. Furthermore, MR imaging can be used to obtain anatomic, functional, and metabolic information via volumetric and multiplanar imaging. Recently, MR imaging has been used in the planning, monitoring, and posttreatment assessment phases of LTSL drug delivery in combination with HIFU.[55] **Fig. 5** depicts the use of MR-HIFU in combination with LTSLs.

Treatment Planning

Treatment planning for hyperthermia-mediated drug delivery can be performed using MR images displayed within a graphical user interface (GUI)

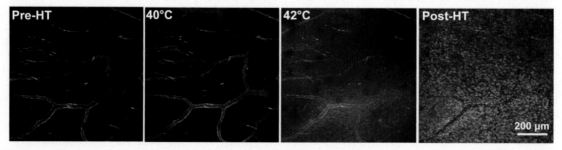

Fig. 4. In vivo release of doxorubicin from TSLs using intravital fluorescence microscopy in a murine sarcoma window chamber model. Endothelial cells are shown in green and doxorubicin in red. HT, hyperthermia. (*Adapted from* Li L, Ten Hagen TL, Hossann M, et al. Mild hyperthermia triggered doxorubicin release from optimized stealth thermosensitive liposomes improves intratumoral drug delivery and efficacy. J Control Release 2013;168:147; with permission.)

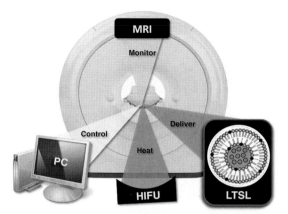

Fig. 5. MR-HIFU in combination with LTSLs. A combination of MR imaging, HIFU heating, and software-based automated temperature feedback control is used to plan, monitor, and control the treatment in real time. LTSLs are used to deliver the drug at the target location.

real-time progress, allowing for intraprocedural adjustments in response to changing conditions or new information acquired during the procedure.

Planning can also involve coregistration and fusion of multiple imaging modalities that best depict the tumor margin or relevant anatomy in relation to the treatment plan. For example, ultrasonography or PET can be combined with MR imaging to perform simultaneous multimodality imaging to enhance tumor detection or margin delineation with fused therapy guidance.[56] An example of therapy planning for MR-guided drug delivery is depicted in **Fig. 7**.

Monitoring and Real-Time Guidance

To account for intrapatient and interpatient variability in intratumoral drug accumulation and distribution, direct imaging of drug delivery or an appropriate surrogate marker may be used to guide therapy adjustments in real time. For example, MR imaging can be used to monitor heat deposition, tissue perfusion, or tissue displacement, and other bioeffects that direct and also predict drug distribution from triggered DDS. Moreover, a suitable surrogate of drug delivery, such as a contrast agent coloaded inside the DDS, can allow for a spatiotemporal estimate of drug release and intratumoral

that provides tools for precise delineation of the target tissue (**Fig. 6**). The treatment plan is directly overlaid on the anatomic images, defining, for example, lower and upper temperature thresholds at targeted locations. The GUI provides comprehensive visualization of the therapy plan and

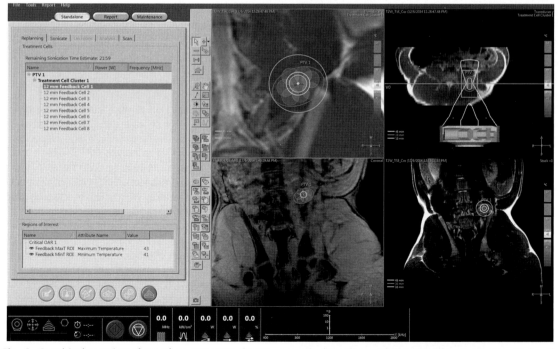

Fig. 6. Graphical user interface of an MR-HIFU therapy console (Sonalleve, Philips Healthcare, Vantaa, Finland), demonstrating delineation of target tissue for MR-guided, hyperthermia-mediated drug delivery. The treatment plan is overlaid on the anatomic MR images and includes definition of lower and upper temperature limits for automated temperature feedback control. The blue and green circular overlays indicate therapy targets and the currently active target, respectively.

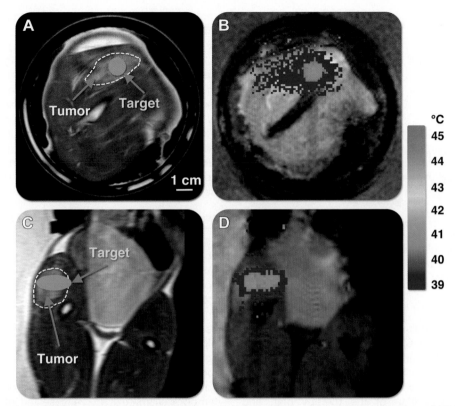

Fig. 7. Planning and temperature mapping for hyperthermia-mediated drug delivery. (*A, C*) a rabbit Vx2 tumor (hyperintense) identified (*white dashed line*) on planning MR imaging. A target (green overlay) selected for therapy is shown. (*B, D*) Temperature maps (color scale) overlaid on dynamic magnitude images (gray scale) during hyperthermia-mediated drug delivery. Mild hyperthermic temperatures were maintained in the target region using a temperature feedback control algorithm. *A* and *B* depict the coronal imaging plane; *C* and *D* depict the sagittal imaging plane. (*Adapted from* Partanen A, Yarmolenko PS, Viitala A, et al. Mild hyperthermia with magnetic resonance-guided high-intensity focused ultrasound for applications in drug delivery. Int J Hyperthermia 2012;28:324; with permission.)

distribution.[51,57] Whether these imaging parameters can serve as effective surrogates for drug distribution remains an open question.

MR Thermometry

Tissue temperature can be measured using MR imaging, providing important feedback for the guidance and adjustment of parameters or locations of hyperthermia treatment. Several MR parameters are temperature sensitive, including the T_1 and T_2 relaxation constants and water proton resonance frequency.[46] The proton resonance frequency shift (PRFS) method[58] has been shown to deliver the best temperature sensitivity, providing a temperature standard deviation of less than 1°C at a temporal resolution less than 1 second and a spatial resolution of roughly 2 mm.[59] In addition, the PRFS method is almost independent of tissue type and has excellent linearity of temperature dependency in nonadipose tissues.[46,59] On the other hand, the PRFS of adipose tissue does

not linearly depend on temperature. Fat suppression or spectrally selective excitation techniques can be applied to preferentially image water protons,[60,61] allowing for accurate PRFS-based thermometry in tissues containing both fat and water protons.[62] An example of PRFS-based temperature monitoring during MR-HIFU mediated drug delivery in an animal model is depicted in **Fig. 7**.

Other MR thermometry methods may be used instead of, or in addition to, PRFS-based methods to further enhance the accuracy of the temperature measurements, or perform thermometry in adipose tissues.[46,63,64] Although tissue motion also may affect temperature measurements, exact measurements may not always be a practical requirement.

Tissue Displacement

In addition to mild hyperthermia and thermal ablation, HIFU can also be used in a pulsed mode to produce mechanical bioeffects without significant heat deposition.[65] For instance, acoustic cavitation and acoustic radiation forces may be produced that induce tissue displacement, and can be used as stimuli for targeted drug delivery.[32] Additional potential bioeffects include alterations to endothelial gaps, extravasation, interstitial pressures, membrane permeability, or even nuclear uptake and transfection. How best to optimally combine these differing mechanisms for MR-HIFU drug delivery remains speculative and of intense interest.

As certain MR imaging methods are sensitive to tissue displacement on the order of micrometers, MR imaging can be used to monitor HIFU-induced spatiotemporal pressure variations in tissue. This technique is known as MR-guided acoustic radiation force imaging (MR-ARFI).[66] One advantage of MR-ARFI is the ability to localize and characterize the HIFU focal spot in situ using relatively low energy deposition and without causing any irreversible tissue changes. Thus, it can be used as a "test shot" to ensure the accuracy of spatial targeting,[67] or adjust the targeting or calibration, to assess and improve the HIFU focusing quality,[68] and estimate the acoustic pressures and intensities within the target location.[44] This information may be useful in calibrating target or treatment location, and the amount of deposited drug or MR imaging contrast agent.

Drug Release

Few methods exist for the in vivo assessment of drug release, dosing, and distribution at the intratumoral level. However, MR contrast agents may be used as drug surrogates when encapsulated in liposomes. These imageable LTSLs (iLTSLs) can provide information regarding the location of drug release, drug coverage of the tumor, and drug concentration following hyperthermia-mediated delivery. In this approach the desired drug dose and spatial distribution are prescribed, and an image-guided applicator manipulates heat in the target region to achieve the desired drug dose coverage. This technique exploits the interactions between MR contrast agent and water that determine T1 shortening and signal enhancement to identify membrane disruption and drug/contrast release from iLTSLs.[57,69] HIFU[70] and other heating modalities[71] have been used to precisely regulate the spatiotemporal distribution of heat and, consequently, direct and adjust drug delivery. This process, whereby heat is used to selectively distribute a drug within a tumor under MR imaging guidance, is referred to as "drug dose painting."[57,69] Precise observation of drug distribution can help to identify undertreated areas and allow for adjustments to be made to the treatment plan, including the addition of other ablative approaches.

For mild hyperthermia-mediated drug delivery with iLTSLs, MR imaging can be used to evaluate T1-weighted signal intensity before and after iLTSL injection, and to capture contrast agent release in real time or during and after each HIFU exposure. An example of the use of this technique is depicted in **Fig. 8**. At present, the magnetic susceptibility effects of iLTSLs on PRFS-based MR thermometry and the theoretic risks of toxicity attributable to contrast agent dechelation[72] with hyperthermia pose challenges for drug dose painting.[73] However, mild hyperthermia-induced release of LTSL-encapsulated doxorubicin without contrast is under investigation in preclinical and phase I trials.[74]

Posttherapy Assessment and Optimization

Standard T1-weighted and T2-weighted MR imaging methods, with or without the use of contrast agents, can provide volumetric assessment of posttherapy tumor regression or growth.[55] Additional MR imaging methods can be used to examine posttherapy changes in tumor vascularization or tumor blood volume. For example, diffusion-weighted (DW) imaging can be used to evaluate changes in tumor diffusion and heat-induced tissue damage. Similarly, contrast-enhanced (CE) imaging can be used to locate and characterize the extent of nonperfused volumes or volumes of lower perfusion following drug delivery therapies that exploit, for example, ablative hyperthermia or the drug depot effect (**Fig. 9**). The thermal lesions induced by ablative hyperthermia appear as hypointense (nonenhancing) regions in T1-weighted CE imaging because of the reduced delivery of contrast agent to these nonperfused regions (see **Fig. 8**).[75–78] Good correlation has been shown between histologic and CE imaging assessments of regions of thermal coagulation.[75,76]

Dynamic contrast-enhanced MR (DCE-MR) imaging can be performed to acquire a series of MR images before, during, and after the administration of an intravascular MR contrast agent such as Gd-DTPA (gadopentetic acid). DCE-MR imaging depicts the wash-in and wash-out contrast kinetics within tumor extravascular and intravascular compartments, and provides important insight into bulk tissue properties that may be used to guide additional therapy planning.

PRECLINICAL WORK AND FUTURE CLINICAL APPLICATIONS

Significant preclinical work in recent years has been dedicated to elucidating potential clinical

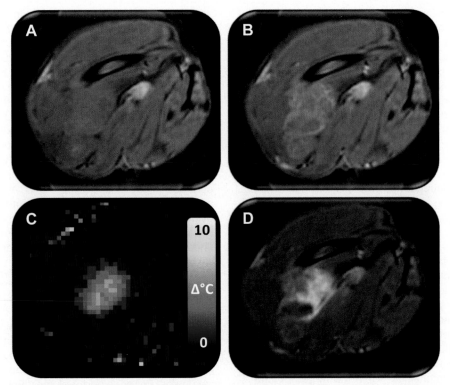

Fig. 8. MR signal intensity before and after iLTSL injection and MR-HIFU heating. Signal intensity (*A*) before, and (*B*) after iLTSL injection. (*C*) A temperature elevation map during heating. (*D*) Signal intensity after 40 minutes of heating. Contrast agent release is limited to the heated region. *A, B,* and *D* depict T1-weighted MR images. (*From* Partanen A. Magnetic resonance-guided high intensity focused ultrasound mediated mild hyperthermia and drug delivery. Helsinki (Finland): University of Helsinki; 2013. p. 36; with permission.)

applications of MR-guided drug delivery, including mild hyperthermia-mediated drug delivery to solid tumors and using HIFU as a means for enabling reversible opening of the BBB to enable drug delivery to cerebral tissues.

Hyperthermia and Tumor Drug Delivery

Heat-mediated drug release from TSLs has been the subject of several recent clinical trials. A phase I dose-escalation clinical trial evaluated the safety and feasibility of doxorubicin-loaded TSLs in combination with RFA in patients with primary and metastatic liver cancer.[79] This paradigm was further examined to define the impact and indications for this combined therapy in a phase III trial with more than 700 patients.[54]

More recent preclinical studies aim to determine whether MR-HIFU–mediated hyperthermia with imageable heat-sensitive liposomes may serve as an effective noninvasive means for delivering chemotherapeutic agents to solid tumors while enabling real-time monitoring and temporospatial control of drug release.[51,80,81] Many outstanding questions remain to be addressed concerning the feasibility, efficacy, and applicability of MR-

HIFU–mediated hyperthermia for tumor drug delivery, such as: the optimal means for loading a range of tumor specific chemotherapeutic agents within liposomes; whether there may be drug-specific heating algorithms to ensure maximal drug release and concentration within solid tumors; whether repeated treatments are safe and feasible in patients with cancer; and identification of the enduring systemic consequences of systemic liposomal administration. The long-term goal may be to expand the indications for patients with locally dominant disease for whom there are currently few or no ablative treatment options. Drugs limited by narrow therapeutic windows may be reevaluated if MR-HIFU can improve tumor localization and distribution, serving to improve therapeutic efficacy while minimizing systemic toxicities. Whether MR-HIFU hyperthermia radiation sensitization may play a role in combination therapies also remains speculative.

Blood-Brain Barrier Disruption

MR-guided, pulsed HIFU (pHIFU)-mediated BBB disruption shows promise for drug delivery in the brain.[44,82] For example, following pHIFU

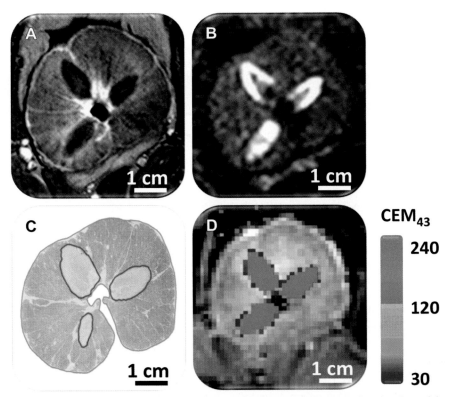

Fig. 9. Transurethral prostate HIFU in animal model shows (*A*) CE imaging of nonperfused regions, (*B*) DW imaging with diffusion changes in ablated regions, (*C*) cytokeratin-8–stained tissue with areas of nonviable tissue, and (*D*) real-time cumulative thermal dose estimates. (*From* Partanen A, Yerram NK, Trivedi H, et al. Magnetic resonance imaging (MRI)-guided transurethral ultrasound therapy of the prostate: a preclinical study with radiological and pathological correlation using customised MRI-based molds. BJU Int 2013;112(4):512; with permission.)

treatment, BBB disruption was detected in F98 glioma-bearing rats using intravenously injected Evans blue dye (EB).[82] This study demonstrated an enhanced tumor-to-contralateral brain ratio of EB, suggesting that pHIFU exposure may increase drug delivery to brain tumors.[82] The effect of pHIFU on microvascular disruption was studied in greater detail by Marty and colleagues,[44] using

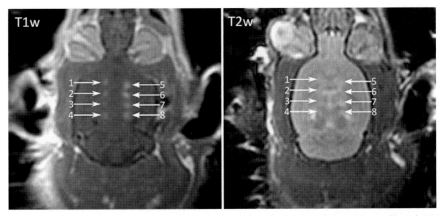

Fig. 10. (*Left*) Contrast-enhanced T1-weighted MR image of a rat brain after HIFU-mediated BBB disruption. (*Right*) T2-weighted MR image of the same rat brain showing enhancement, indicating edema at the sonicated locations. *Arrows* indicate sonication locations. *Numbers* indicate different delays between cycles: (1) 300 μs; (2) 600 μs; (3) 1 s; (4) 60 μs, (5-8) 6 μs. (*From* O'Reilly MA, Waspe AC, Ganguly M, et al. Focused-ultrasound disruption of the blood-brain barrier using closely timed short pulses: influence of sonication parameters and injection rate. Ultrasound Med Biol 2011;37(4):590; with permission.)

MR contrast agents of different hydrodynamic diameters. These investigators estimated the molecular size cutoff and duration of BBB opening following HIFU-mediated BBB disruption as a basis for potential optimization of nanoparticle design and delivery. Similar measurements were made by O'Reilly and colleagues[83] using an MR imaging contrast agent and variable sonication parameters along with the Definity microbubble contrast agent. This study showed that even very short ultrasound bursts (3 μs) and low burst repetition rates (1–2 Hz) were capable of disrupting the BBB (**Fig. 10**).

Research concerning the role of pHIFU in disruption of the BBB, with or without coadministration of microbubbles, is ongoing. Continuing investigation aims to control the release of microbubbles and their associated risks (eg, unstable cavitation) when deployed in proximity to the cerebrovasculature, and to time BBB disruption in relation to drug administration for maximal concentration of drug in the central nervous system.

SUMMARY

MR imaging–guided drug delivery is a promising strategy for facilitating or augmenting targeted drug delivery to solid tumors. MR imaging may be used for screening, planning, monitoring, or postprocedural assessment of treatment outcome. MR-guided HIFU is a particularly promising technique for augmentation of drug delivery in certain patients with cancer with unmet clinical needs and without availability of other local image-guided minimally invasive treatment options because of the size, scope, or distribution of disease. However, further research is needed to clarify HIFU drug delivery mechanisms, optimize HIFU parameters and MR imaging methods, and define roles and timing in combination therapies with other ablative energies, chemoembolization, or radiation. Similarly, the effects of mechanical or hyperthermic HIFU on drug release, transit time, wash-out, and extravasation are poorly defined, and present a fertile ground for research into the bioeffects of HIFU. The benefits of MR-HIFU–mediated local drug delivery for avoidance of systemic toxicities could define a clear pathway toward routine clinical use for many patients with cancer. In addition, although speculative, MR-HIFU-mediated, noninvasive drug delivery (the "drug paintbrush") could open a new door to a novel interdisciplinary therapy for designated patients with cancer. MR imaging–guided drug delivery therapies are also being investigated for treatment of difficult-to-treat anatomies by modulation of the tumor microenvironment or by improved delivery of systemically administered therapies (eg, via opening of the BBB). Along with other emerging MR imaging–guided treatment strategies, this may enable customization of therapy to better account for tumor heterogeneity and circumvent common barriers to effective drug delivery.

REFERENCES

1. Mikhail AS, Allen C. Block copolymer micelles for delivery of cancer therapy: transport at the whole body, tissue and cellular levels. J Control Release 2009;138:214–23.
2. Allen TM, Cullis PR. Liposomal drug delivery systems: from concept to clinical applications. Adv Drug Deliv Rev 2013;65(1):36–48.
3. Kopecek J. Polymer-drug conjugates: origins, progress to date and future directions. Adv Drug Deliv Rev 2013;65(1):49–59.
4. Chari RV, Miller ML, Widdison WC. Antibody-drug conjugates: an emerging concept in cancer therapy. Angew Chem Int Ed Engl 2014;53(15):3796–827.
5. Maeda H. Tumor-selective delivery of macromolecular drugs via the EPR effect: background and future prospects. Bioconjug Chem 2010;21:797–802.
6. Bazak R, Houri M, El Achy S, et al. Cancer active targeting by nanoparticles: a comprehensive review of literature. J Cancer Res Clin Oncol 2015;141(5):769–84.
7. Manzoor AA, Lindner LH, Landon CD, et al. Overcoming limitations in nanoparticle drug delivery: triggered, intravascular release to improve drug penetration into tumors. Cancer Res 2012;72:5566–75.
8. Dreher MR, Liu W, Michelich CR, et al. Tumor vascular permeability, accumulation, and penetration of macromolecular drug carriers. J Natl Cancer Inst 2006;98:335–44.
9. Yuan F, Leunig M, Huang SK, et al. Microvascular permeability and interstitial penetration of sterically stabilized (stealth) liposomes in a human tumor xenograft. Cancer Res 1994;54:3352–6.
10. Gao W, Chan JM, Farokhzad OC. pH-Responsive nanoparticles for drug delivery. Mol Pharm 2010;7(6):1913–20.
11. McCarley RL. Redox-responsive delivery systems. Annu Rev Anal Chem (Palo Alto Calif) 2012;5:391–411.
12. Kumar CS, Mohammad F. Magnetic nanomaterials for hyperthermia-based therapy and controlled drug delivery. Adv Drug Deliv Rev 2011;63:789–808.
13. Dicheva BM, Koning GA. Targeted thermosensitive liposomes: an attractive novel approach for increased drug delivery to solid tumors. Expert Opin Drug Deliv 2014;11(1):83–100.
14. Spratt T, Bondurant B, O'Brien DF. Rapid release of liposomal contents upon photoinitiated destabilization

with UV exposure. Biochim Biophys Acta 2003; 1611(1–2):35–43.

15. Chauhan VP, Stylianopoulos T, Boucher Y, et al. Delivery of molecular and nanoscale medicine to tumors: transport barriers and strategies. Annu Rev Chem Biomol Eng 2011;2:281–98.

16. Jain RK, Stylianopoulos T. Delivering nanomedicine to solid tumors. Nat Rev Clin Oncol 2010;7:653–64.

17. Minchinton AI, Tannock IF. Drug penetration in solid tumours. Nat Rev Cancer 2006;6:583–92.

18. Mikhail AS, Eetezadi S, Ekdawi SN, et al. Image-based analysis of the size- and time-dependent penetration of polymeric micelles in multicellular tumor spheroids and tumor xenografts. Int J Pharm 2014;464:168–77.

19. Lai CY, Fite BZ, Ferrara KW. Ultrasonic enhancement of drug penetration in solid tumors. Front Oncol 2013;3:204.

20. Fatehi D, van der Zee J, de Bruijne M, et al. RF-power and temperature data analysis of 444 patients with primary cervical cancer: deep hyperthermia using the Sigma-60 applicator is reproducible. Int J Hyperthermia 2007;23(8):623–43.

21. Juang T, Stauffer PR, Neuman DG, et al. Multilayer conformal applicator for microwave heating and brachytherapy treatment of superficial tissue disease. Int J Hyperthermia 2006;22(7):527–44.

22. McNichols RJ, Kangasniemi M, Gowda A, et al. Technical developments for cerebral thermal treatment: water-cooled diffusing laser fibre tips and temperature-sensitive MRI using intersecting image planes. Int J Hyperthermia 2004;20(1):45–56.

23. Boreham DR, Gasmann HC, Mitchel RE. Water bath hyperthermia is a simple therapy for psoriasis and also stimulates skin tanning in response to sunlight. Int J Hyperthermia 1995;11(6):745–54.

24. Ahmed M, Moussa M, Goldberg SN. Synergy in cancer treatment between liposomal chemotherapeutics and thermal ablation. Chem Phys Lipids 2012;165:424–37.

25. Ranjan A, Jacobs GC, Woods DL, et al. Image-guided drug delivery with magnetic resonance guided high intensity focused ultrasound and temperature sensitive liposomes in a rabbit Vx2 tumor model. J Control Release 2012;158:487–94.

26. Gasselhuber A, Dreher MR, Partanen A, et al. Targeted drug delivery by high intensity focused ultrasound mediated hyperthermia combined with temperature-sensitive liposomes: computational modelling and preliminary in vivo validation. Int J Hyperthermia 2012;28:337–48.

27. Hijnen NM, de Smet M, Heijman E, et al. Hyperthermia mediated drug delivery combined with ablation improves therapeutic efficacy of MR-HIFU thermal therapy. FUS Symposium. Bethesda (MD), October 12-16, 2014.

28. Fry WJ, Wulff VJ, Tucker D, et al. Physical factors involved in ultrasonically induced changes in living

systems: I. identification of non-temperature effects. J Acoust Soc Am 1950;22(6):867–76.

29. Hill CR, Bamber JC, ter Haar GR. Physical principles of medical ultrasonics. 2nd edition. West Sussex, England: John Wiley & Sons Ltd; 2004.

30. Bailey M, Khokhlova V, Sapozhnikov O, et al. Physical mechanisms of the therapeutic effect of ultrasound (a review). Acoust Phys 2003;49(4):369–88.

31. Bibi S, Lattmann E, Mohammed AR, et al. Trigger release liposome systems: local and remote controlled delivery? J Microencapsul 2012;29(3):262–76.

32. Gourevich D, Dogadkin O, Volovick A, et al. Ultrasound-mediated targeted drug delivery with a novel cyclodextrin-based drug carrier by mechanical and thermal mechanisms. J Control Release 2013; 170(3):316–24.

33. Tempany CM, Stewart EA, McDannold N, et al. MR imaging-guided focused ultrasound surgery of uterine leiomyomas: a feasibility study. Radiology 2003; 226(3):897–905.

34. Kim YS, Keserci B, Partanen A, et al. Volumetric MR-HIFU ablation of uterine fibroids: role of treatment cell size in the improvement of energy efficiency. Eur J Radiol 2012;81(11):3652–9.

35. Hynynen K, Pomeroy O, Smith DN, et al. MR imaging-guided focused ultrasound surgery of fibroadenomas in the breast: a feasibility study. Radiology 2001;219(1):176–85.

36. Furusawa H, Namba K, Nakahara H, et al. The evolving non-surgical ablation of breast cancer: MR guided focused ultrasound (MRgFUS). Breast Cancer 2007;14(1):55–8.

37. Chopra R, Colquhoun A, Burtnyk M, et al. MR imaging-controlled transurethral ultrasound therapy for conformal treatment of prostate tissue: initial feasibility in humans. Radiology 2012;265(1):303–13.

38. Liberman B, Gianfelice D, Inbar Y, et al. Pain palliation in patients with bone metastases using MR-guided focused ultrasound surgery: a multicenter study. Ann Surg Oncol 2009;16(1):140–6.

39. McDannold N, Clement GT, Black P, et al. Transcranial magnetic resonance imaging-guided focused ultrasound surgery of brain tumors: initial findings in 3 patients. Neurosurgery 2010;66(2):323–32.

40. Martin E, Jeanmonod D, Morel A, et al. High-intensity focused ultrasound for noninvasive functional neurosurgery. Ann Neurol 2009;66(6):858–61.

41. Jeanmonod D, Werner B, Morel A, et al. Transcranial magnetic resonance imaging-guided focused ultrasound: noninvasive central lateral thalamotomy for chronic neuropathic pain. Neurosurg Focus 2012; 32(1):E1.

42. Tyler WJ, Tufail Y, Pati S. Pain: noninvasive functional neurosurgery using ultrasound. Nat Rev Neurol 2010;6(1):13–4.

43. Haen SP, Pereira PL, Salih HR, et al. More than just tumor destruction: immunomodulation by thermal

ablation of cancer. Clin Dev Immunol 2011;2011: 160250.

44. Marty B, Larrat B, Van Landeghem M, et al. Dynamic study of blood-brain barrier closure after its disruption using ultrasound: a quantitative analysis. J Cereb Blood Flow Metab 2012;32:1948–58.

45. Mougenot C, Quesson B, de Senneville BD, et al. Three-dimensional spatial and temporal temperature control with MR thermometry-guided focused ultrasound (MRgHIFU). Magn Reson Med 2009;61(3): 603–14.

46. Denis de Senneville B, Quesson B, Moonen CT. Magnetic resonance temperature imaging. Int J Hyperthermia 2005;21(6):515–31.

47. Köhler MO, Mougenot C, Quesson B, et al. Volumetric HIFU ablation under 3D guidance of rapid MRI thermometry. Med Phys 2009;36(8):3521–35.

48. Enholm JK, Köhler MO, Quesson B, et al. Improved volumetric MR-HIFU ablation by robust binary feedback control. IEEE Trans Biomed Eng 2010;57(1): 103–13.

49. Yatvin M, Weinstein J, Dennis W, et al. Design of liposomes for enhanced local release of drugs by hyperthermia. Science 1978;202:1290–3.

50. Needham D, Anyarambhatla G, Kong G. A new temperature-sensitive liposome for use with mild hyperthermia: characterization and testing in a human tumor xenograft model. Cancer Res 2000;60(5): 1197–201.

51. Negussie AH, Yarmolenko PS, Partanen A, et al. Formulation and characterisation of magnetic resonance imageable thermally sensitive liposomes for use with magnetic resonance-guided high intensity focused ultrasound. Int J Hyperthermia 2011;27: 140–55.

52. Kong G, Anyarambhatla G, Petros WP, et al. Efficacy of liposomes and hyperthermia in a human tumor xenograft model: importance of triggered drug release. Cancer Res 2000;60(24):6950–7.

53. Yarmolenko PS, Zhao Y, Landon CD, et al. Comparative effects of thermosensitive doxorubicin-containing liposomes and hyperthermia in human and murine tumours. Int J Hyperthermia 2010;26:485–98.

54. Celsion. Phase 3 study of ThermoDox with radiofrequency ablation (RFA) in treatment of hepatocellular carcinoma (HCC) In: ClinicalTrials.gov [Internet]. Available at: https://clinicaltrials.gov/ct2/show/NCT00617981. Accessed February 1, 2015.

55. Staruch RM, Hynynen K, Chopra R. Hyperthermia-mediated doxorubicin release from thermosensitive liposomes using MR-HIFU: therapeutic effect in rabbit Vx2 tumours. Int J Hyperthermia 2015;31(2): 118–33.

56. Curiel L, Chopra R, Hynynen K. Progress in multimodality imaging: truly simultaneous ultrasound and magnetic resonance imaging. IEEE Trans Med Imaging 2007;26(12):1740–6.

57. Ponce AM, Viglianti BL, Yu D, et al. Magnetic resonance imaging of temperature-sensitive liposome release: drug dose painting and antitumor effects. J Natl Cancer Inst 2007;99(1):53–63.

58. Ishihara Y, Calderon A, Watanabe H, et al. A precise and fast temperature mapping using water proton chemical shift. Magn Reson Med 1995;34(6):814–23.

59. Quesson B, de Zwart JA, Moonen CT. Magnetic resonance temperature imaging for guidance of thermotherapy. J Magn Reson Imaging 2000;12(4): 525–33.

60. Delfaut EM, Beltran J, Johnson G, et al. Fat suppression in MR imaging: techniques and pitfalls. Radiographics 1999;19(2):373–82.

61. Schick F, Forster J, Machann J, et al. Highly selective water and fat imaging applying multislice sequences without sensitivity to B1 field inhomogeneities. Magn Reson Med 1997;38(2):269–74.

62. de Zwart JA, Vimeux FC, Delalande C, et al. Fast lipid-suppressed MR temperature mapping with echo-shifted gradient-echo imaging and spectral-spatial excitation. Magn Reson Med 1999;42(1): 53–9.

63. Winter P, Lanier M, Partanen A, et al. MRI guided HIFU of visceral fat: effect of heating on T2 relaxation of fat. Milan (Italy): ISMRM; 2014.

64. Waspe AC, Mougenot C, Pichardo S, et al. Simultaneous PRF and T1-mapping based MR thermometry for monitoring high-intensity focused ultrasound ablation of primary bone tumors. Salt Lake City (UT): ISMRM; 2013.

65. Larrat B, Pernot M, Aubry JF, et al. MR-guided transcranial brain HIFU in small animal models. Phys Med Biol 2010;55(2):365–88.

66. McDannold N, Maier SE. Magnetic resonance acoustic radiation force imaging. Med Phys 2008; 35(8):3748–58.

67. Kaye EA, Chen J, Pauly KB. Rapid MR-ARFI method for focal spot localization during focused ultrasound therapy. Magn Reson Med 2011;65(3):738–43.

68. Vyas U, Kaye E, Pauly KB. Transcranial phase aberration correction using beam simulations and MR-ARFI. Med Phys 2014;41(3):032901.

69. Viglianti BL, Abraham SA, Michelich CR, et al. In vivo monitoring of tissue pharmacokinetics of liposome/drug using MRI: illustration of targeted delivery. Magn Reson Med 2004;51(6):1153–62.

70. Grüll H, Langereis S. Hyperthermia-triggered drug delivery from temperature-sensitive liposomes using MRI-guided high intensity focused ultrasound. J Control Release 2012;161:317–27.

71. Needham D, Ponce AM. Nanoscale drug delivery vehicles for solid tumors: a new paradigm for localized drug delivery using temperature sensitive liposomes. In: Group TF, editor. Nanotechnology for Cancer Therapy. Boca Raton, FL: CRC Press; 2007. p. 678–719.

72. Port M, Idee JM, Medina C, et al. Efficiency, thermodynamic and kinetic stability of marketed gadolinium chelates and their possible clinical consequences: a critical review. Biometals 2008;21(4):469–90.

73. Hijnen N, Elevelt A, Pikkemaat J, et al. The magnetic susceptibility effect of gadolinium-based contrast agents on PRFS-based MR thermometry during thermal interventions. J Ther Ultrasound 2013;1(1):8.

74. University of Oxford. Targeted chemotherapy using focused ultrasound for liver metastases (TARDOX). 2015. Available at: https://clinicaltrials.gov/ct2/show/NCT02181075. Accessed February 1, 2015.

75. Hazle JD, Stafford RJ, Price RE. Magnetic resonance imaging-guided focused ultrasound thermal therapy in experimental animal models: correlation of ablation volumes with pathology in rabbit muscle and VX2 tumors. J Magn Reson Imaging 2002;15(2):185–94.

76. Cheng HL, Purcell CM, Bilbao JM, et al. Prediction of subtle thermal histopathological change using a novel analysis of Gd-DTPA kinetics. J Magn Reson Imaging 2003;18(5):585–98.

77. Rowland IJ, Rivens I, Chen L, et al. MRI study of hepatic tumours following high intensity focused ultrasound surgery. Br J Radiol 1997;70:144–53.

78. Köhler MO, Denis de Senneville B, Quesson B, et al. Spectrally selective pencil-beam navigator for motion compensation of MR-guided high-intensity focused ultrasound therapy of abdominal organs. Magn Reson Med 2011;66(1):102–11.

79. Wood BJ, Poon RT, Locklin JK, et al. Phase I study of heat-deployed liposomal doxorubicin during radiofrequency ablation for hepatic malignancies. J Vasc Interv Radiol 2012;23:248–55.

80. de Smet M, Heijman E, Langereis S, et al. Magnetic resonance imaging of high intensity focused ultrasound mediated drug delivery from temperature-sensitive liposomes: an in vivo proof-of-concept study. J Control Release 2011;150:102–10.

81. de Smet M, Langereis S, van den Bosch S, et al. Temperature-sensitive liposomes for doxorubicin delivery under MRI guidance. J Control Release 2010;143:120–7.

82. Yang FY, Lin GL, Horng SC, et al. Pulsed high-intensity focused ultrasound enhances the relative permeability of the blood-tumor barrier in a glioma-bearing rat model. IEEE Trans Ultrason Ferroelectr Freq Control 2011;58(5):964–70.

83. O'Reilly MA, Waspe AC, Ganguly M, et al. Focused-ultrasound disruption of the blood-brain barrier using closely-timed short pulses: influence of sonication parameters and injection rate. Ultrasound Med Biol 2011;37(4):587–94.

Update on Clinical Magnetic Resonance–Guided Focused Ultrasound Applications

Thiele Kobus, PhD[a,b,*], Nathan McDannold, PhD[a]

KEYWORDS

- MR imaging • Focused ultrasound • Thermal ablation prostate cancer • Uterine fibroids
- Bone metastasis pain management • Breast cancer • Brain disease

KEY POINTS

- Thousands of patients with uterine fibroid have successfully been treated with magnetic resonance (MR)-guided focused ultrasound (FUS), leading to technical improvements and increased experience to further improve clinical outcome.
- MR-guided FUS has been approved to bring thermal damage to the periosteal nerves, which leads to pain relief from bone metastases and other bone diseases.
- Thermal ablation of specific parts of the thalamus with transcranial MR-guided FUS can lead to symptom relief in several neurologic disorders.
- MR-guided FUS can be used for more clinical applications (eg, breast and prostate cancer), but clinical trials are needed to prove its potential.

FOCUSED ULTRASOUND

Ultrasound is well known for its application as an imaging modality. To obtain an image, a transducer transmits acoustic waves through the body and receives their reflections at tissue interfaces. Another property of these acoustic waves is that the tissue through which they propagate absorbs their energy. This mechanism is the basis for thermal ablation by focused ultrasound (FUS). By focusing high-intensity acoustic waves, the temperature in the focus increases as a result of energy absorption by the tissue. At a temperature of approximately 56°C for 1 second, irreversible cell death by coagulative necrosis occurs.

Furthermore, blood in small vessels can coagulate and stop the blood perfusion.[1] To reach these temperatures, usually an equal amount of ultrasound energy is applied continuously. Because the energy absorption in the ultrasound beam path is lower, the surrounding tissue is spared.

In addition to thermal effects, the tissue can also be damaged through inertial cavitation. Ultrasound waves cause compression and rarefaction of the tissue, and during the latter, gas can be drawn out of solution and bubbles can be created. These microbubbles are compressed and expanded by the ultrasound and can collapse (inertial cavitation), leading to cell damage. Nucleation of such microbubbles can enhance the

---

The authors have nothing to disclose.
[a] Department of Radiology, Brigham and Women's Hospital, Harvard Medical School, 221 Longwood Avenue, #521, Boston, MA 02115, USA; [b] Department of Radiology and Nuclear Medicine, Radboud University Medical Center, Geert Grooteplein 10, 6500 HB, Nijmegen, Netherlands
* Corresponding author. Department of Radiology, Brigham and Women's Hospital, Harvard Medical School, 221 Longwood Avenue, #521, Boston, MA 02115.
E-mail address: tkobus@partners.org

Magn Reson Imaging Clin N Am 23 (2015) 657–667
http://dx.doi.org/10.1016/j.mric.2015.05.013
1064-9689/15/$ – see front matter © 2015 Elsevier Inc. All rights reserved.

energy absorption and heating in the focus, a mechanism called enhanced sonication. During an enhanced sonication protocol, short bursts at a very high power are used to form microbubbles in the focus. These microbubbles interact with the acoustic waves, which increases the absorption of energy in the target.[2] Thermal ablation is the primary clinical application for FUS.

MAGNETIC RESONANCE GUIDANCE

By performing FUS under image guidance, the target (eg, tumor) can be localized, and the ultrasound focus can be aimed at this target. Two techniques that enable image guidance are ultrasound and MR imaging. The initial FUS treatments were performed under ultrasound guidance, because this technique is inexpensive and has a high temporal resolution. However, the options for treatment planning and monitoring are limited. MR imaging has excellent soft tissue contrast, allowing for three-dimensional treatment planning. Furthermore, real-time temperature information can be obtained, enabling monitoring of thermal damage to ensure coagulative necrosis. After the sonication, MR imaging can be used to assess treatment response, for example, with contrast-enhanced T1-weighted imaging. The contrast agent, gadolinium, does not reach the necrotic tissue, because the blood vessels are damaged. In contrast to well-perfused tissue, no increase in signal intensity on postcontrast T1-weighted images is observed in the necrotic tissue. The percentage of nonperfused volume (NPV) of the target volume can be determined, which can be an indication of the success of the treatment. In this review, the current clinical applications of MR-guided FUS are updated.

UTERINE FIBROIDS

Uterine fibroids are common benign tumors in the uterus that can cause abnormal uterine bleeding, pelvic pain, and infertility but are usually symptomless.[3] The ExAblate 2000 (InSightec, Tirat Carmel, Israel) has received both the CE mark (2002) and US Food and Drug Administration (FDA) approval (2004) for the treatment of uterine fibroids. In 2009, Sonalleve (Phillips Healthcare, Vantaa, Finland) received the CE mark. Both FUS systems consist of extracorporeal multielement phased-array transducers, which are built into a special MR table. They operate at a frequency between 0.95 and 1.35 MHz (ExAblate) and 1.2 and 1.5 MHz (Sonalleve) and can be used in combination with 1.5-T and 3.0-T MR scanners.

Since the FDA approval in 2004, thousands of patients have been treated, and several follow-up studies have been performed.[4–6] The success of treatment has been evaluated based on the volume change of the fibroids, improvement of symptoms, and the reintervention rate. For patients with a higher NPV after the treatment, a lower risk of additional treatment was observed within 1 to 5 years after treatment.[5–7] The same holds true for older patients, who have a lower risk for reinterventions.[5,6,8] Based on pretreatment T2-weighted MR imaging, fibroids can be classified into 3 types: (1) fibroids that appear hypointense, (2) fibroids that are isointense, and (3) fibroids that are hyperintense in relation to skeletal muscle.[4–6,9] The NPV of patients with type 3 uterine fibroids was lower than type 1 and 2 fibroids,[4] and these patients required reintervention significantly more often than types 1 and 2.[5,6] An example of a successful treatment of a type 1 uterine fibroid is shown in **Fig. 1**. FUS therapy may not be suitable for type 3 fibroids and MR screening can be used to exclude these patients from FUS treatment. Patients who received neoadjuvant therapy with gonadotropin-releasing hormone agonist, a therapy that decreases the vascularity of the fibroids,[10] had significantly larger NPV at the same applied energy[11] and a lower risk for additional therapy.[5] In a 5-year follow-up study,[5] an overall reintervention rate of 58.6% was reported. When only patients with an NPV larger than 50% were included, the reintervention rate decreased to 50%. Insights and experience from the initial treatments have led to adaptation in patient selection and improvements in the FUS system, with the expectation that long-term outcomes should improve accordingly.

In the initial treatments, long cooling periods between sonications were used to prevent thermal build-up along the ultrasound beam path for multiple overlapping sonications. A new strategy to reduce the cooling period to 22 seconds[12] is the interleave mode, in which the overlap between sonications is minimized by changing the order of the sonications so that the energy absorption in the beam path is decreased.[13] In the new-generation ExAblate system, the transducer can be elevated to minimize the distance from the abdominal wall. This strategy leads to an increase in the maximum energy in the focus and reduces the energy absorption in the near and far field. To limit adverse effects in the beam path, selective transducer elements are automatically disabled if vital structures such as the bowels, bladder, or sciatic nerves are detected in the beam path.[14] In a recent study with 115 patients,[14] these technical improvements, increased experience, and

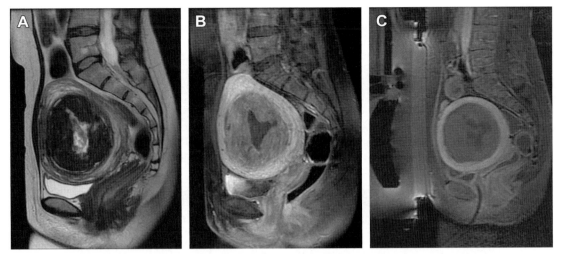

Fig. 1. A 45-year-old woman with a 418-cm³ fibroid experiencing gradually worsening pelvic pressure and hypermenorrhea. (*A*) Sagittal T2-weighted MR image obtained before treatment shows predominantly hypointense fibroid (type 1). (*B*) Sagittal contrast-enhanced fat-suppressed MR image before treatment shows homogeneous enhancement of vital fibroid tissue. (*C*) Sagittal contrast-enhanced fat-suppressed MR image acquired immediately after treatment shows completely nonperfused fibroid tissue. (*From* Trumm CG, Stahl R, Clevert D-A, et al. Magnetic resonance imaging–guided focused ultrasound treatment of symptomatic uterine fibroids: impact of technology advancement on ablation volumes in 115 patients. Invest Radiol 2013;48(6):362; with permission.)

the use of a screening MR imaging examination have improved the NPV to an average of 88%, but follow-up data are not yet available. In this study, patients with hyperintense fibroids on T2-weighted imaging (type 3) were excluded.

An early limitation of MR-guided FUS for fibroids was the long treatment time, often several hours. Both the ExAblate and Sonalleve systems use phased arrays to electronically steer the beam to enlarge the ablated volume during each sonication. The Sonalleve device also has closed-loop feedback, which modulates the power output based on real-time temperature measurements so as to optimize treatment delivery. The technique, along with the interleave mode used with the ExAblate system, has increased the treatment rate and reduced treatment times.

In general, the adverse effects after treatment are minor (eg, transient abdominal pain, mild skin burns, back pain, nausea, and nerve irritation).[5–7,15,16] In a few cases, serious complications were observed: skin burn requiring repair, fibroid expulsion, persistent neuropathy, and abdominal burn.[5,17] An area that requires more research is the effect of FUS on fertility. Several studies report successful pregnancies after MR-guided FUS treatment,[18–20] but there has been no study evaluating the effect on fertility of different treatments for uterine fibroids. A clinical trial will compare the safety and effectiveness of MR-guided FUS and uterine artery embolization (NCT00995878-

clinicaltrials.gov). Two additional ongoing clinical trials are NCT01142791-clinicaltrials.gov, which is investigating the use of enhanced sonication to improve clinical outcome, and a multicenter phase 2 and 3 study using the Sonalleve system (NCT01504308-clinicaltrials.gov).

BONE METASTASES–RELATED PAIN MANAGEMENT

The second MR-guided FUS application that received both CE and FDA approval is bone metastases–related pain management. For this treatment, the ExAblate and Sonalleve (only CE mark) systems can be used. Because cortical bone has high acoustic impedance, a great deal of energy is absorbed by the bone. Therefore, lower energies are applied compared with that used in uterine fibroid treatments. Two mechanisms for FUS-mediated pain relief are suggested. The temperature increase in the cortical bone leads to heating of the periosteal surface, which results in thermal damage to the periosteal nerves, which are responsible for pain perception.[21] The second mechanism is tumor debulking caused by thermal ablation, which diminishes the pressure on the adjacent tissue. The observed pain relief immediately after sonication advocates for the first mechanism, but there is increasing evidence that tumor debulking also plays a role.[21–23]

Several hundred patients have been treated who have exhausted, declined, or are unsuitable for other pain palliation methods. The success of the treatment can be evaluated based on changes in the pain scores, quality of life scores, and decrease in pain medication usage. A secondary measure is change in tumor size. In 2 multicenter trials, significant improvements in the pain scores without an increase in the pain medication were observed 3 months after sonication in 64% of 112[24] and 72% of 25 patients.[25] In 67% of the patients, the dosage of pain medication was decreased.[25] In addition to pain relief, necrosis and increase in the bone density were observed 3 months after FUS treatment.[22,23] Fig. 2 shows the imaging data of a patient whose treatment led to complete pain relief and reduction in tumor size. There were small areas of NPV seen on post-contrast T1-weighted imaging after the treatment. The use of NPV to evaluate the success of treatment is limited,[23] and more research in the predictive value of this measure is needed. Generally,

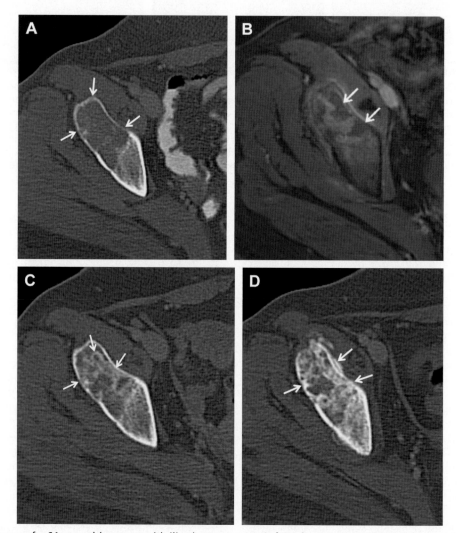

Fig. 2. Images of a 64-year-old woman with iliac bone metastasis from breast cancer. (*A*) Axial computed tomography (CT) image shows the presence of a wide lytic lesion located in the right anterior superior iliac spine (*arrows*), with evidence of focal cortical erosion causing severe pain (pain severity score, 10). (*B*) Axial T1-weighted sequence acquired after contrast agent injection at the end of the MR-guided FUS treatment shows the presence of some small areas of NPV (*arrows*) inside the lesion and at the periosteal margin. (*C*) At the 2-month follow-up, axial CT identified the presence of some focal areas of de novo mineralization inside the treated tissue with partial restoration of cortical borders (*arrows*). (*D*) At 3 months after treatment, the lesion showed further de novo remineralization of the ablated tissue (*arrows*). (*From* Napoli A, Anzidei M, Marincola BC, et al. Primary pain palliation and local tumor control in bone metastases treated with magnetic resonance-guided focused ultrasound. Invest Radiol 2013;48(6):354; with permission.)

no[21–23,25] or minor[24] adverse events are observed. Observed adverse events included skin burns, sonication pain, fractures, neuropathy, posttreatment fatigue, and skin numbness.[24]

MR-guided FUS also shows promise for pain relief in other bone diseases. In 2 studies,[26,27] patients with osteoid osteoma were treated and in 90% to 100% of the patients symptoms were completely resolved at a 6-month to 12-month follow-up. Eighteen patients with facet joint osteoarthritis were successfully treated, and a decrease in pain was observed, together with an improvement in disability.[28] Pain relief from osteoarthritis was also observed in 6 of 8 patients who were treated with MR-guided FUS for medial knee pain.[29] No adverse events were observed in any of these studies, supporting the use of MR-guided FUS for bone pain management in a range of bone diseases.

BRAIN DISEASE

FUS has great potential for treating brain disease, because the technique could be used to ablate targeted tissue without injuring the normal brain. In contrast, during conventional neurosurgery, damage to normal brain tissue is usually inevitable, especially when deep-seated brain structures are involved. The challenge for FUS in the brain is the high acoustical impedance of the skull. The high impedance leads to absorption of a great part of the applied energy, resulting in heating of the skull. This situation may, in turn, increase the temperature in the brain tissue adjacent to the skull. To minimize skull heating, a hemispherical design for the transducer is chosen, so that the applied energy is distributed over a larger area.[30] A lower operating frequency reduces absorption in the bone, at the cost of an increase focal size. It was determined that a frequency of approximately 700 kHz is optimal for transcranial FUS.[30] Another issue concerning the acoustic impedance of the skull is the large difference between the impedance of the skull and that of brain tissue. This difference leads to refraction of the acoustic waves and distortion of the focus. The focus can be restored by using many transducer elements, each with an optimized phase.[31] The required phase corrections can be calculated from radiograph-computed tomography, from which the spatial distribution of the skull thickness and density can be determined. Thermal ablation using FUS in the brain should be performed under MR guidance, because high-resolution anatomic images are a prerequisite for proper treatment planning. The ExAblate Neuro system (InSightec) consists of a hemispherical

1024-element phased-array transducer, which operates at 650 kHz. This device has received CE mark for targets in the thalamus, subthalamus, and pallidum.

A precursor of this system (ExAblate 3000, 512 elements, 670 kHz) was used to show, for the first time, the ability to focus therapeutic ultrasound through the skull into the brain[32] (Fig. 3). In 3 male patients with glioblastoma, with tumors located deep and central in the brain, it was shown that the target tissue can be heated, and significant heating in the tissue close to the skull was prevented. Because the researchers were limited by the power of the device (650–800 W), it was estimated that they did not achieve coagulative necrosis. Extrapolation of their results suggests that this treatment should be possible without overheating the tissue at the brain surface. However, the targetable regions may be limited to deep, central locations in the brain. This factor makes transcranial MR-guided FUS particularly suitable for treating neurologic disorders such as essential tremor, Parkinson disease, and neuropathic pain. Ablation of specific parts of the thalamus can result in relief of the symptoms in these diseases.

The feasibility of transcranial MR-guided FUS has been shown for several neurologic disorders. The relief of symptoms and targeting accuracy were used to evaluate the success of the treatments. The lesions were highly visible 24 to 48 hours after the treatment as a hyperintense region on T2-weighted imaging. By superimposing the stereotactic atlas of the human thalamus of Morel[33] on the T2-weighted images, the accuracy of the treatment can be determined.[34] Eleven patients were treated for neuropathic pain by ablating the posterior part of the central lateral thalamic nucleus with MR-guided FUS.[35,36] The lesions were within a millimeter from the targeted region for all 3 planes. The pain relief 1 year after treatment was 56.9% (8 patients in follow-up). In another study,[37] the ventral intermediate nucleus of the thalamus was ablated in 15 patients with severe, medication-refractory essential tremor. In all patients, this treatment resulted in an improvement of the hand tremor score, the disability scores, and quality of life in a 12-month follow-up. A large, randomized multicenter trial to investigate the use of transcranial MR-guided FUS for the treatment of essential tremor is being undertaken (NCT01304758-clinicaltrials.gov).

In 13 patients with therapy-resistant Parkinson disease, the fiber tract between the pallidum to the thalamus was ablated.[38] In these patients, each target had to be heated 4 or 5 times to the targeted temperature to have relief of symptoms.

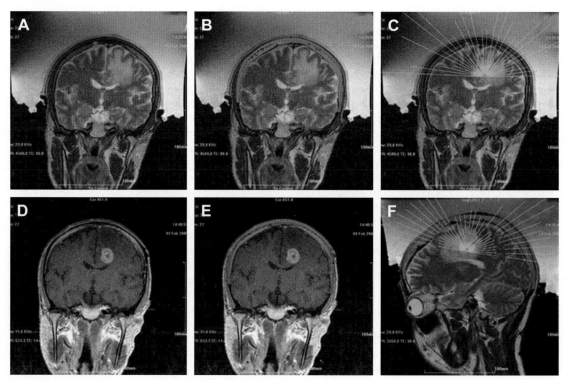

Fig. 3. Screenshots from transcranial MR-guided FUS treatment planning workstation. (*A*) Coronal T2-weighted images of the patient in the transcranial MR-guided FUS device. The target of the current sonication is indicated by the blue rectangle. The water filling the space between the patient's shaved head and the transducer can be seen. (*B*) Pretreatment computed tomography (CT) scan data of the cranium is registered to the intratreatment MR imaging scans. The cranium is automatically segmented from the CT scan and shown as a green region on top of the MR images used for treatment planning. Any registration errors can be seen on these images and corrected by the user by using a graphic tool. MR tracking coils integrated into the transducer are used to register the transcranial MR-guided FUS system coordinates with the imaging coordinates. Acoustic models taking into account the patient-specific cranium geometry and density are used to correct for aberrations to the ultrasound beam. (*C*) The beam paths for each phased-array element are superimposed on the images, allowing the user to verify that no beams pass through undesired structures. (*D*, *E*) Pretreatment contrast-enhanced T1-weighted images, which can be useful for defining tumor margins, acquired the day before treatment can also be registered to the intratreatment images. Axial and sagittal images are also acquired, allowing for treatment planning in 3 dimensions. (*F*) Sagittal T2-weighted image. (*From* McDannold N, Clement GT, Black P, et al. Transcranial magnetic resonance imaging-guided focused ultrasound surgery of brain tumors: initial findings in 3 patients. Neurosurgery. 2010;66(2):326. [discussion: 332]; with permission.)

In 9 patients, a reduction of 61% in the Unified Parkinson Disease Rating Scale was observed after 3 months. Although it was sufficient for the targets in the nuclei (gray matter) to reach the targeted temperature once for successful coagulative necrosis,[35,37] the fiber tracts, consisting of axons protected by myelin sheaths, may need a stronger thermal ablation.[38]

Compared with other techniques for ablating thalamic nuclei, MR-guided FUS has no risk of intracranial infection and is not limited by trajectory constraints for reaching the target. In general, the adverse events were minor and transient (eg, paresthesia of the lip, tongue, or finger, ataxia, and an unsteady feeling). In 4 patients,

the paresthesia was still present after 12 months.[37] In 1 patient, a bleed with ischemia occurred in the motor thalamus resulting in dysmetria, which gradually decreased over time.[35] Jeanmonod and colleagues[35] recommend the installation of a cavitation detector and the use of sonication temperatures less than 60°C to prevent future bleedings. This detector is now implemented in every treatment.

In addition to symptom relief in Parkinson disease, essential tremor, and neuropathic pain, other applications are conceivable as well, such as epilepsy, trigeminal neuralgia, and psychosurgery.[39] The treatment of glioblastoma may not be the best clinical application, because of its infiltrative nature,[32] but tumors with well-defined margins such as metastases might be. However, use for tumor ablation is limited based on the treatment time and limitations on which brain regions can be targeted for thermal ablation. Only central targets within the brain can be safely sonicated without overheating the skull.

Another approach to treating brain tumors and other brain diseases is the use of transcranial MR-guided FUS to disrupt the blood-brain barrier. This barrier prevents delivery of almost all therapeutic agents to the brain. Low-intensity FUS in combination with circulating microbubbles can temporarily ($\sim$4 hours) disrupt the blood-brain barrier without apparent damage to the brain. Large molecules, such as antibodies, have been successfully delivered in animal models,[40,41] and a 1024-element ExAblate system operating at 220 kHz has been used successfully in rhesus monkeys to disrupt the blood-brain barrier.[42] Another application for transcranial FUS is neuromodulation. In volunteers, a 0.5-MHz transducer was used to stimulate the primary somatosensory cortex. This strategy resulted in significant attenuation of the somatosensory evoked potentials and enhanced performance of sensory discrimination tasks.[43] Future research will show the clinical applicability of MR-guided FUS for neuromodulation, blood-brain barrier disruption, and a variety of brain diseases. Such treatments use lower-intensity sonications and will be able to target a larger portion of the brain.

PROSTATE CANCER

FUS under ultrasound guidance has been used for many years to treat prostate cancer. However, the ability to visualize the tumor with ultrasound is limited, and considerable variability in the occurrence of adverse events has been reported.[44] MR imaging is the method of choice for depicting prostate lesions, and a multiparametric approach is recommended.[45] There is increasing interest in performing prostate cancer thermal ablation under MR guidance, because of the superiority of MR in tumor localization and thermometry. The location of the prostate in the body makes it approachable from 2 body cavities, leading to a transrectal and a transurethral approach. There is no CE or FDA approval for these methods, but their clinical use is being investigated in several centers.

For the transrectal approach, the ExAblate 2100 system can be used with a 990-element rectal transducer. After placement of the transducer in the rectum, the probe is filled with degassed water at 12°C to cool the rectal wall and eliminate air between the rectum and the transducer. In 2012, the

first case report[46] described the treatment of a low-risk tumor without any adverse events 1 month after treatment. Napoli and colleagues[47] treated 5 patients before a radical prostatectomy. They showed good correlation between the region of thermal damage (based on MR thermometry) and the nonperfused region based on contrast-enhanced T1-weighted imaging (**Fig. 4**). Furthermore, on histopathologic sections, extensive coagulative necrosis was observed in the treated region surrounded by a rim of inflamed tissue. However, in all patients, additional tumors (either significant or nonsignificant) that were not evident on the pretreatment MR imaging were present outside the treated area.

In-house built[48,49] and the PAD-105 (Profound Medical, Toronto, ON, Canada) transducers have been used for the intraurethral approach. Transurethral ultrasound ablation uses high-intensity unfocused ultrasound. A probe with multiple small transducers is inserted into the urethra and can be rotated 360° at a variable rate to treat the desired region in the prostate. Degassed water runs through the transducer for cooling and coupling, and a cooling device is placed in the rectum. In a feasibility study of 8 patients, a 180° angular target around the urethra was sonicated (at 8 MHz) before a radical prostatectomy.[49] A spatial temperature feedback algorithm[50] was used to ensure that a temperature of 55°C was reached at the boundary of the target. A challenge for MR thermometry in the prostate is not only the movement of the bowels but also motion of air in the bowels, which can affect the local magnetic susceptibility. Preliminary results from a phase 1 clinical trial with the PAD-105 in which the entire prostate was sonicated showed a high correlation between the NPV and spatial temperature maps.[51] No cases of incontinence, fistulas, or rectal injury were reported in these 16 patients after a 1-month follow-up. The advantage of treating the entire prostate is that it deals with the heterogeneous and multifocal nature of prostate cancer.

Both the transurethral and transrectal approaches show high correlation between the thermal damage based on MR thermometry and the observed histopathologic effects.[47,49] These initial results make MR-guided FUS a promising method for a noninvasive treatment of prostate cancer.

BREAST CANCER

Breast tumors are well suited for MR-guided FUS treatment, because they are superficial and can be accessed easily through the skin. The tumors are well defined on contrast-enhanced T1-weighted imaging. In 2001, the first MR-guided

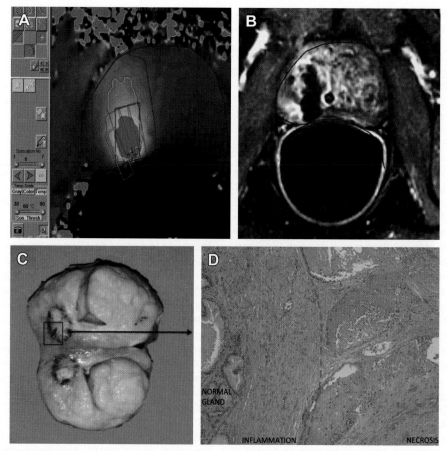

Fig. 4. (*A*) Color-coded MR thermometry acquired during real-time MR-guided FUS treatment shows a definite area of temperature increase corresponding to greater than 60°C (*red area*). (*B*) A contrast-enhanced MR imaging scan acquired immediately after treatment shows an area of NPV in the exact location of the delivered sonication. The control MR imaging also shows the absence of rectal wall injuries or unexpected side effects. (*C*) This macroscopic section after radical prostatectomy shows an extensive coagulative necrosis at the site of sonication. (*D*) This microscopic image (hematoxylin-eosin stained) shows tissue necrosis with a peripheral layer of inflammatory infiltrates. (*From* Napoli A, Anzidei M, De Nunzio C, et al. Real-time magnetic resonance–guided high-intensity focused ultrasound focal therapy for localised prostate cancer: preliminary experience. Eur Urol. 2013;63(2):397; with permission.)

FUS ablation of breast fibroadenomas[52] and invasive ductal carcinoma[53] took place. Since then, several hundred patients have been treated. In many of the patients, FUS treatment was followed by surgery,[53–56] and the effect of the treatment could be evaluated based on histopathology. The success of the treatment was variable, with complete necrosis of the tumor in 16.7% to 54% of the patients.[54–58] Best results were obtained when the contrast-enhanced MR imaging to outline the tumor was acquired immediately before the start of the treatment[58] instead of during a separate MR examination. Retrospective analysis showed that in some cases of incomplete tumor necrosis, not all recommended treatment margins were treated. This situation can be prevented by ensuring that the entire tumor is sonicated with

an additional 5-mm safety margin.[58] In other patients, the success of the treatment was evaluated by follow-up MR imaging [52,59] or biopsy.[60] The treated region is dark and nonenhancing on contrast-enhanced T1-weighted imaging (**Fig. 5**). A high correlation between several parameters from dynamic contrast-enhanced MR imaging and the percentage of viable tumor was observed.[54] When contrast-enhanced MR imaging was used to evaluate the treatment, one should be aware that immediately after treatment, an enhancing rim around the treated area could be observed (see **Fig. 5**). This edema disappeared several days after treatment.[58] In 20 of 21 patients treated with MR-guided FUS, no recurrence was observed on MR imaging or ultrasound 3 to 26 months after treatment.[59]

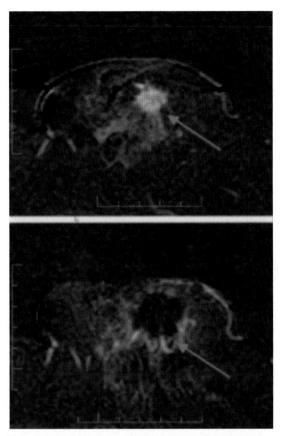

Fig. 5. T1-weighted contrast-enhanced subtraction image before treatment (*top*) and after treatment (*bottom*). In the top image, the tumor (*arrow*) is clearly identified. In the bottom image, the tumor (*arrow*) is nonenhancing. The hyperintense areas in the edges of the treated region are hyperemia. (*From* Furusawa H, Namba K, Thomsen S, et al. Magnetic resonance–guided focused ultrasound surgery of breast cancer: reliability and effectiveness. J Am Coll Surg 2006;203(1):56; with permission.)

Severe and minor adverse events have been reported, including third-degree skin burns, allergic reaction to the plastic material, sonication-related pain, and posture-related pain.[58]

For the initial studies, a focused transducer operating at 1.5 or 1.7 MHz was used and moved with a positioning system to treat the tumor.[52,53] It is expected that in the near future, the ExAblate 2000 system can be used with a multielement phased-array transducer to steer the focus.[55] A transducer in which the ultrasound beams target the breast from the lateral sides, potentially diminishing heating in critical structures such as the ribs, heart, and lungs, has been developed for the Sonalleve system, but no clinical data have been published.[61] These systems do not yet have FDA or CE approval for treating breast cancer. Clinical

trials (eg, NCT01620359-clinicaltrials.gov) are expected to show the clinical value of MR-guided FUS for breast tumors.

SUMMARY

MR-guided FUS has FDA and CE approval for the treatment of uterine fibroids and pain management for bone metastases and the CE mark for transcranial MR-guided FUS for targets in the thalamus, subthalamus, and pallidum. There is promise for thermal ablation of breast and prostate tumors; however, the excellent soft tissue contrast of MR, the availability of MR thermometry, and the noninvasiveness of the treatment make MR-guided FUS a potential treatment of many more diseases. Multicenter trials and long follow-up studies have shown the effectiveness and safety of MR-guided FUS to treat uterine fibroids, and this has led to improvements in the system, treatments, and patient selection. For other applications, these trials are ongoing or need to be initiated to optimize treatments. The clinical value of developments such as targeted drug delivery by blood-brain barrier disruption, enhanced sonication, and neuromodulation needs to be shown.

REFERENCES

1. Hynynen K, Darkazanli A, Damianou CA, et al. The usefulness of a contrast agent and gradient-recalled acquisition in a steady-state imaging sequence for magnetic resonance imaging-guided noninvasive ultrasound surgery. Invest Radiol 1994;29(10):897–903.
2. Kopelman D, Inbar Y, Hanannel A, et al. Magnetic resonance-guided focused ultrasound surgery using an enhanced sonication technique in a pig muscle model. Eur J Radiol 2006;59(2):190–7.
3. Stewart EA. Uterine fibroids. The Lancet 2001; 357(9252):293–8.
4. Funaki K, Fukunishi H, Sawada K. Clinical outcomes of magnetic resonance-guided focused ultrasound surgery for uterine myomas: 24-month follow-up. Ultrasound Obstet Gynecol Off J Int Soc Ultrasound Obstet Gynecol 2009;34(5):584–9.
5. Quinn SD, Vedelago J, Gedroyc W, et al. Safety and five-year re-intervention following magnetic resonance-guided focused ultrasound (MRgFUS) for uterine fibroids. Eur J Obstet Gynecol Reprod Biol 2014;182:247–51.
6. Gorny KR, Borah BJ, Brown DL, et al. Incidence of additional treatments in women treated with MR-guided focused us for symptomatic uterine fibroids: review of 138 patients with an average follow-up of 2.8 years. J Vasc Interv Radiol 2014;25(10): 1506–12.

7. Stewart EA, Gostout B, Rabinovici J, et al. Sustained relief of leiomyoma symptoms by using focused ultrasound surgery. Obstet Gynecol 2007;110(2, Part 1): 279–87.

8. Machtinger R, Inbar Y, Cohen-Eylon S, et al. MR-guided focus ultrasound (MRgFUS) for symptomatic uterine fibroids: predictors of treatment success. Hum Reprod 2012;27(12):3425–31.

9. Funaki K, Fukunishi H, Funaki T, et al. Magnetic resonance-guided focused ultrasound surgery for uterine fibroids: relationship between the therapeutic effects and signal intensity of preexisting T2-weighted magnetic resonance images. Am J Obstet Gynecol 2007;196(2):184.e1–6.

10. Di Lieto A, De Falco M, Staibano S, et al. Effects of gonadotropin-releasing hormone agonists on uterine volume and vasculature and on the immunohistochemical expression of basic fibroblast growth factor (bFGF) in uterine leiomyomas. Int J Gynecol Pathol Off J Int Soc Gynecol Pathol 2003;22(4):353–8.

11. Smart OC, Hindley JT, Regan L, et al. Magnetic resonance guided focused ultrasound surgery of uterine fibroids–the tissue effects of GnRH agonist pre-treatment. Eur J Radiol 2006;59(2):163–7.

12. Shen S-H, Fennessy F, McDannold N, et al. Image-guided thermal therapy of uterine fibroids. Semin Ultrasound CT MRI 2009;30(2):91–104.

13. Tempany CMC, McDannold NJ, Hynynen K, et al. Focused ultrasound surgery in oncology: overview and principles. Radiology 2011;259(1):39–56.

14. Trumm CG, Stahl R, Clevert D-A, et al. Magnetic resonance imaging–guided focused ultrasound treatment of symptomatic uterine fibroids: impact of technology advancement on ablation volumes in 115 patients. Invest Radiol 2013;48(6):359–65.

15. Fennessy FM, Tempany CM, McDannold NJ, et al. Uterine leiomyomas: MR imaging–guided focused ultrasound surgery—results of different treatment protocols. Radiology 2007;243(3):885–93.

16. Morita Y, Ito N, Hikida H, et al. Non-invasive magnetic resonance imaging-guided focused ultrasound treatment for uterine fibroids–early experience. Eur J Obstet Gynecol Reprod Biol 2008;139(2):199–203.

17. Leon-Villapalos J, Kaniorou-Larai M, Dziewulski P. Full thickness abdominal burn following magnetic resonance guided focused ultrasound therapy. Burns 2005;31(8):1054–5.

18. Morita Y, Ito N, Ohashi H. Pregnancy following MR-guided focused ultrasound surgery for a uterine fibroid. Int J Gynecol Obstet 2007;99(1):56–7.

19. Gavrilova-Jordan LP, Rose CH, Traynor KD, et al. Successful term pregnancy following MR-guided focused ultrasound treatment of uterine leiomyoma. J Perinatol 2007;27(1):59–61.

20. Rabinovici J, David M, Fukunishi H, et al. Pregnancy outcome after magnetic resonance–guided focused ultrasound surgery (MRgFUS) for conservative treatment of uterine fibroids. Fertil Steril 2010;93(1): 199–209.

21. Catane R, Beck A, Inbar Y, et al. MR-guided focused ultrasound surgery (MRgFUS) for the palliation of pain in patients with bone metastases–preliminary clinical experience. Ann Oncol 2007;18(1):163–7.

22. Gianfelice D, Gupta C, Kucharczyk W, et al. Palliative treatment of painful bone metastases with MR imaging–guided focused ultrasound. Radiology 2008;249(1):355–63.

23. Napoli A, Anzidei M, Marincola BC, et al. Primary pain palliation and local tumor control in bone metastases treated with magnetic resonance-guided focused ultrasound. Invest Radiol 2013;48(6):351–8.

24. Hurwitz MD, Ghanouni P, Kanaev SV, et al. Magnetic resonance–guided focused ultrasound for patients with painful bone metastases: phase III trial results. J Natl Cancer Inst 2014;106(5):dju082.

25. Liberman B, Gianfelice D, Inbar Y, et al. Pain palliation in patients with bone metastases using MR-guided focused ultrasound surgery: a multicenter study. Ann Surg Oncol 2009;16(1):140–6.

26. Geiger D, Napoli A, Conchiglia A, et al. MR-guided focused ultrasound (MRgFUS) ablation for the treatment of nonspinal osteoid osteoma. J Bone Jt Surg 2014;96(9):743–51.

27. Napoli A, Mastantuono M, Cavallo Marincola B, et al. Osteoid osteoma: MR-guided focused ultrasound for entirely noninvasive treatment. Radiology 2013; 267(2):514–21.

28. Weeks EM, Platt MW, Gedroyc W. MRI-guided focused ultrasound (MRgFUS) to treat facet joint osteoarthritis low back pain–case series of an innovative new technique. Eur Radiol 2012;22(12):2822–35.

29. Izumi M, Ikeuchi M, Kawasaki M, et al. MR-guided focused ultrasound for the novel and innovative management of osteoarthritic knee pain. BMC Musculoskelet Disord 2013;14(1):267.

30. Clement GT, Sun J, Giesecke T, et al. A hemisphere array for non-invasive ultrasound brain therapy and surgery. Phys Med Biol 2000;45(12):3707.

31. Hynynen K, Jolesz FA. Demonstration of potential noninvasive ultrasound brain therapy through an intact skull. Ultrasound Med Biol 1998;24(2):275–83.

32. McDannold N, Clement GT, Black P, et al. Transcranial magnetic resonance imaging- guided focused ultrasound surgery of brain tumors: initial findings in 3 patients. Neurosurgery 2010;66(2):323–32 [discussion: 332].

33. Morel A. Stereotactic atlas of the human thalamus and basal ganglia. New York: CRC Press; 2007.

34. Moser D, Zadicario E, Schiff G, et al. Measurement of targeting accuracy in focused ultrasound functional neurosurgery. Neurosurg Focus 2012;32(1):E2.

35. Jeanmonod D, Werner B, Morel A, et al. Transcranial magnetic resonance imaging-guided focused ultrasound: noninvasive central lateral thalamotomy for

chronic neuropathic pain. Neurosurg Focus 2012; 32(1):E1.

36. Martin E, Jeanmonod D, Morel A, et al. High-intensity focused ultrasound for noninvasive functional neurosurgery. Ann Neurol 2009;66(6):858–61.

37. Elias WJ, Huss D, Voss T, et al. A pilot study of focused ultrasound thalamotomy for essential tremor. N Engl J Med 2013;369(7):640–8.

38. Magara A, Bühler R, Moser D, et al. First experience with MR-guided focused ultrasound in the treatment of Parkinson's disease. J Ther Ultrasound 2014;2(1):1–8.

39. Monteith S, Sheehan J, Medel R, et al. Potential intracranial applications of magnetic resonance–guided focused ultrasound surgery. J Neurosurg 2013;118(2):215–21.

40. Park E-J, Zhang Y-Z, Vykhodtseva N, et al. Ultrasound-mediated blood–brain/blood-tumor barrier disruption improves outcomes with trastuzumab in a breast cancer brain metastasis model. J Controlled Release 2012;163(3):277–84.

41. Kinoshita M, McDannold N, Jolesz FA, et al. Noninvasive localized delivery of Herceptin to the mouse brain by MRI-guided focused ultrasound-induced blood-brain barrier disruption. Proc Natl Acad Sci U S A 2006;103(31):11719–23.

42. McDannold N, Arvanitis CD, Vykhodtseva N, et al. Temporary disruption of the blood–brain barrier by use of ultrasound and microbubbles: safety and efficacy evaluation in rhesus macaques. Cancer Res 2012;72(14):3652–63.

43. Legon W, Sato TF, Opitz A, et al. Transcranial focused ultrasound modulates the activity of primary somatosensory cortex in humans. Nat Neurosci 2014;17(2):322–9.

44. Warmuth M, Johansson T, Mad P. Systematic review of the efficacy and safety of high-intensity focussed ultrasound for the primary and salvage treatment of prostate cancer. Eur Urol 2010;58(6): 803–15.

45. Hoeks CMA, Barentsz JO, Hambrock T, et al. Prostate cancer: multiparametric MR imaging for detection, localization, and staging. Radiology 2011; 261(1):46–66.

46. Lindner U, Ghai S, Spensieri P, et al. Focal magnetic resonance guided focused ultrasound for prostate cancer: initial North American experience. Can Urol Assoc J 2012;6(6):E283–6.

47. Napoli A, Anzidei M, De Nunzio C, et al. Real-time magnetic resonance–guided high-intensity focused ultrasound focal therapy for localised prostate cancer: preliminary experience. Eur Urol 2013;63(2): 395–8.

48. Chopra R, Baker N, Choy V, et al. MRI-compatible transurethral ultrasound system for the treatment of localized prostate cancer using rotational control. Med Phys 2008;35(4):1346–57.

49. Chopra R, Colquhoun A, Burtnyk M, et al. MR imaging–controlled transurethral ultrasound therapy for conformal treatment of prostate tissue: initial feasibility in humans. Radiology 2012;265(1):303–13.

50. Chopra R, Burtnyk M, Haider MA, et al. Method for MRI-guided conformal thermal therapy of prostate with planar transurethral ultrasound heating applicators. Phys Med Biol 2005;50(21):4957.

51. Roethke M, Burtnyk M, Kuru T, et al. Whole-gland MRI-guided transurethral ultrasound ablation of low-risk prostate cancer: preliminary results from a multicenter phase I clinical trial. In: Proceedings of the 22nd Meeting of the International Society for Magnetic Resonance in Medicine. Milan, Italy, May 10-16, 2014.

52. Hynynen K, Pomeroy O, Smith DN, et al. MR imaging-guided focused ultrasound surgery of fibroadenomas in the breast: a feasibility study. Radiology 2001;219(1):176–85.

53. Huber PE, Jenne JW, Rastert R, et al. A new noninvasive approach in breast cancer therapy using magnetic resonance imaging-guided focused ultrasound surgery. Cancer Res 2001;61(23):8441–7.

54. Gianfelice D, Khiat A, Amara M, et al. MR imaging-guided focused ultrasound surgery of breast cancer: correlation of dynamic contrast-enhanced MRI with histopathologic findings. Breast Cancer Res Treat 2003;82(2):93–101.

55. Gianfelice D, Khiat A, Amara M, et al. MR imaging-guided focused US ablation of breast cancer: histopathologic assessment of effectiveness–initial experience. Radiology 2003;227(3):849–55.

56. Zippel DB, Papa MZ. The use of MR imaging guided focused ultrasound in breast cancer patients: a preliminary phase one study and review. Breast Cancer 2005;12(1):32–8.

57. Khiat A, Gianfelice D, Amara M, et al. Influence of post-treatment delay on the evaluation of the response to focused ultrasound surgery of breast cancer by dynamic contrast enhanced MRI. Br J Radiol 2006;79(940):308–14.

58. Furusawa H, Namba K, Thomsen S, et al. Magnetic resonance–guided focused ultrasound surgery of breast cancer: reliability and effectiveness. J Am Coll Surg 2006;203(1):54–63.

59. Furusawa H, Namba K, Nakahara H, et al. The evolving non-surgical ablation of breast cancer: MR guided focused ultrasound (MRgFUS). Breast Cancer 2007;14(1):55–8.

60. Gianfelice D, Khiat A, Boulanger Y, et al. Feasibility of magnetic resonance imaging–guided focused ultrasound surgery as an adjunct to tamoxifen therapy in high-risk surgical patients with breast carcinoma. J Vasc Interv Radiol 2003;14(10):1275–82.

61. Merckel LG, Bartels LW, Köhler MO, et al. MR-guided high-intensity focused ultrasound ablation of breast cancer with a dedicated breast platform. Cardiovasc Intervent Radiol 2013;36(2):292–301.

Magnetic Resonance Sequences and Rapid Acquisition for MR-Guided Interventions

Adrienne E. Campbell-Washburn, PhD[a],*, Anthony Z. Faranesh, PhD[b],
Robert J. Lederman, MD[b], Michael S. Hansen, PhD[a]

KEYWORDS

- Real-time MR imaging • MR image reconstruction • Parallel imaging • Non-Cartesian imaging

KEY POINTS

- Interventional MR imaging requires a specialized environment and work-flow.
- Rapid image acquisition and rapid image reconstruction are a prerequisite for all MR-guided interventions.
- High frame-rate real-time imaging can be achieved for dynamic procedural guidance.
- Imaging can be accelerated using parallel imaging or efficient k-space trajectories.
- MR imaging can enable simultaneous device and tissue visualization.

▶ This article includes a video of real-time imaging in an interactive environment at http://www.mri.theclinics.com/

INTRODUCTION

Interventional MR imaging is valuable for real-time dynamic procedural guidance and intraprocedural imaging during diagnostic or therapeutic procedures, including surgery, tissue biopsy, ablation therapy, endovascular procedures, and device placement. The flexibility of MR image contrast is appealing for procedural guidance; however, the demands of MR-guided interventions are unique and require a specialized environment.

Diagnostic MR imaging is well established in the clinic to provide high-resolution images with excellent soft-tissue contrast, designed to assess pathologic tissue and derive quantitative metrics. Typically diagnostic MR imaging uses long scan times to generate the desired image contrast, and may require offline image reconstruction or processing.

Interventional MR imaging, on the other hand, demands much faster image acquisition, reconstruction, and processing. Furthermore, procedural guidance uses interactive parameter control and requires the simultaneous visualization of tissue and interventional devices (eg, biopsy needles, guide wires, catheters, stents, occluders, forceps). **Table 1** summarizes the differing demands of diagnostic and interventional MR imaging.

The authors disclose that this work was supported by the National Heart, Lung, and Blood Institute Division of Intramural Research (Z01-HL006039, Z01-HL005062). The National Heart, Lung, and Blood Institute and Siemens Medical Systems have a Cooperative Research and Development Agreement (CRADA).

[a] Cardiovascular and Pulmonary Branch, Division of Intramural Research, National Heart, Lung, and Blood Institute, National Institutes of Health, 9000 Rockville Pike, Building 10, Room B1D416, Bethesda, MD 20892, USA; [b] Cardiovascular and Pulmonary Branch, Division of Intramural Research, National Heart, Lung, and Blood Institute, National Institutes of Health, 9000 Rockville Pike, Building 10, Room 2C713, Bethesda, MD 20892, USA

* Corresponding author.
E-mail address: adrienne.campbell@nih.gov

Magn Reson Imaging Clin N Am 23 (2015) 669–679
http://dx.doi.org/10.1016/j.mric.2015.05.006
1064-9689/15/$ – see front matter Published by Elsevier Inc.

Table 1
Differences between diagnostic and interventional MR imaging

Diagnostic MR Imaging	Interventional MR Imaging
Scans run in batch mode	Interactive environments are used to modify real-time imaging on-the-fly
Long scan times	Short scan times
Offline reconstruction and postprocessing is possible	Reconstruction and processing must be performed with low latency
Image quality is of utmost importance	Imaging speed is of utmost importance
Used for anatomic imaging	Used for anatomic imaging and device imaging
Cardiac and respiratory gating and/or breath-holding can be used to compensate for motion	Real-time imaging is not gated or breath held

IMAGING PROTOCOLS

Interventional MR imaging encompasses preprocedural imaging for planning, intraprocedural imaging to assess progress, and real-time imaging for dynamic procedural guidance. The preprocedural and intraprocedural imaging is used to assess anatomy, physiology, or pathology relevant to the procedure. This article focuses primarily on the technical details of the rapid real-time imaging used during dynamic procedural guidance.

Real-Time Imaging

Imaging efficiency is crucial during MR-guided interventions, especially when competing against established interventional modalities such as radiography and ultrasonography. Radiography generates approximately 15 frames/s with a pixel matrix of 1024 × 1024. In comparison, 5 to 10 frames/s are used for MR imaging during procedural guidance with a much smaller pixel matrix of 128 × 128 or 144 × 192. Real-time imaging is not gated nor breath held, and the entire image is acquired in a single shot. **Fig. 1** shows the single-shot real-time image acquisition running continuously, with multiple slices updating in rapid succession. Throughout an interventional procedure, slice geometry and image contrast are interactively controlled, either by interventionists in the MR suite or by operators in the control room.

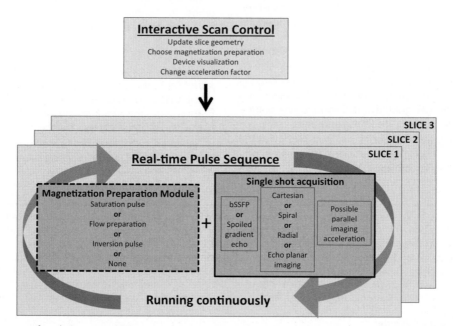

Fig. 1. Diagram of real-time acquisition running continuously with multiple slices updating in rapid succession. Image contrast is changed using an optional magnetization preparation module and interactive parameter control. bSSFP, balanced steady-state free precession.

For real-time procedural guidance, the challenge is to generate adequate tissue contrast and sufficient image quality in terms of signal-to-noise ratio (SNR) and artifact, while also maintaining short imaging times. Typically, balanced steady-state free precession (bSSFP) imaging is used to accomplish this.[1,2] bSSFP uses magnetization efficiently to provide high SNR with short repetition times, and the resulting images have T2/T1-weighted contrast with bright blood and fat signal, and darker muscle tissue. Fully sampled bSSFP images can achieve a temporal resolution of 377 milliseconds per image or 2.6 frames/s (echo time [TE]/repetition time [TR] = 1.27/2.62 milliseconds, matrix = 192 × 144). Using parallel imaging, the temporal resolution can be pushed to 94 milliseconds per image or 10.6 frames/s (acceleration factor 4, see Parallel Imaging section). Banding artifacts in bSSFP are not usually a concern for these short TR sequences; however, real-time bSSFP does suffer from undesirable bright signal from fat. If needed, fat suppression for bSSFP can be accomplished using radiofrequency (RF) cycling and TR alternation.[3–5] Real-time imaging can also be achieved using spoiled gradient echo sequences,[6] although these are used less frequently because of the lower SNR.

A magnetization preparation module can be programmed into the pulse sequence such that it is toggled on/off interactively while the single-shot acquisition runs continuously. For example, nonselective saturation prepulses can be added to the sequence to enhance gadolinium contrast while suppressing tissue signal (see Device Visualization section). Furthermore, flow-sensitive saturation preparations can produce dark-blood images to enhance the gadolinium contrast and preserve tissue signal.[7] Inversion pulses can be inserted into the real-time pulse sequence for infarct imaging.[8] Interactive color-flow MR imaging using phase contrast has been implemented to rapidly visualize cardiac and vascular flow.[9] Virtual dye angiography uses volume-selective saturation pulses that can be turned on/off interactively to provide flow visualization, mimicking contrast angiography during endovascular procedures[10] (**Fig. 2**). These interactive magnetization preparation modules modify image contrast, as needed, throughout the procedure.

Parallel Imaging

Parallel imaging can be used to accelerate real-time imaging by skipping some phase-encoding lines throughout the acquisition and exploiting multichannel signal receiver arrays during reconstruction for added spatial encoding. By eliminating some phase-encoding steps, the resulting images are aliased. Parallel imaging describes a family of reconstruction techniques that allows recovery of images from the aliased ones. The 2 most common methods used in the clinic are SENSE[11] and GRAPPA.[12] Excellent reviews of parallel imaging techniques are available.[13,14]

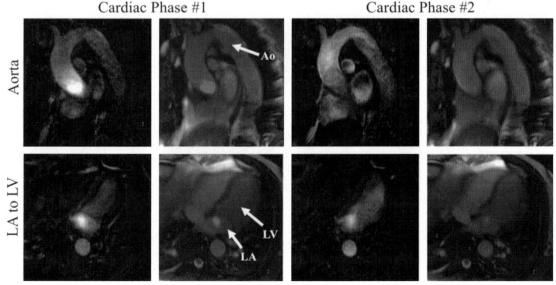

Fig. 2. Virtual dye angiography uses volume selective-saturation pulses to saturated blood signal locally. The difference images between saturation off/on (black and white images) are used to produce a color-flow map. Ao, aorta; LA, left atrium; LV, left ventricle. (*From* George AK, Faranesh AZ, Ratnayaka K, et al. Virtual dye angiography: flow visualization for MRI-guided interventions. Magn Reson Med 2012;67(4):1019; with permission.)

Each point in an aliased single-coil image is a linear signal superposition with weights according to the coil sensitivity profile (**Fig. 3**). SENSE reconstruction unambiguously unfolds aliased images by solving a linear system using knowledge of coil sensitivity maps calibrated at the beginning of the examination. TSENSE[15] is an alternative algorithm, which uses interleaved undersampling to integrate the coil sensitivity maps with the image acquisition. TSENSE is specifically designed for dynamic imaging and is critical for high frame-rate imaging.

GRAPPA aims to regenerate the missing phase-encoding lines from the raw k-space data using information about a given data point contained within the neighboring points in k-space. GRAPPA requires a fully sampled region of k-space known as the autocalibration signal that is used to calculate a kernel to regenerate all missing k-space points. GRAPPA is robust in cases where sensitivity maps are difficult to generate, for example, when the prescribed field of view is too small for the imaged object and there are regions with aliasing in the calibration data.

In general, acceleration rates of 4 are robustly used in a clinical setting, and both SENSE and GRAPPA reconstructions are available with vendor-supplied reconstruction software.

Compressed sensing algorithms show potential for further accelerating image acquisition,[16] but are currently limited in their application to interventional MR imaging by prohibitively long reconstruction times.

Efficient k-Space Trajectories

More efficient k-space trajectories can also be used to speed up image acquisitions (**Fig. 4**). Echo planar imaging (EPI) is an accelerated Cartesian acquisition whereby multiple phase-encoding steps are acquired following an RF pulse. Using single-shot EPI the entire image can be acquired following a single RF pulse. EPI has found clinical utility for interventional and real-time applications.[17–20]

Spiral imaging[21] and radial imaging[22] are examples of non-Cartesian acquisitions used for MR-guided interventions.[23–26] Spiral imaging is particularly attractive for high frame-rate applications in the interventional MR imaging environment. Oversampling of the k-space center in non-Cartesian sampling patterns results in flow and motion insensitivity and robustness to aliasing artifacts. Either spoiled gradient echo or bSSFP contrast can be achieved with spiral and radial trajectories.

Spiral and radial k-space trajectories do not lie on a Cartesian grid and, therefore, require samples to be interpolated onto a grid during image reconstruction in a process called regridding.[27] Typically regridding uses a Kaiser-Bessel kernel[28] or, in the case of nonuniform fast Fourier transformation,[29] using least-squares design of interpolation coefficients. Because sampling density is nonuniform over k-space, density compensation is applied before regridding.[30] Alternatively, radial acquisitions can be reconstructed using back-projection methods originally designed for computed tomography reconstruction.

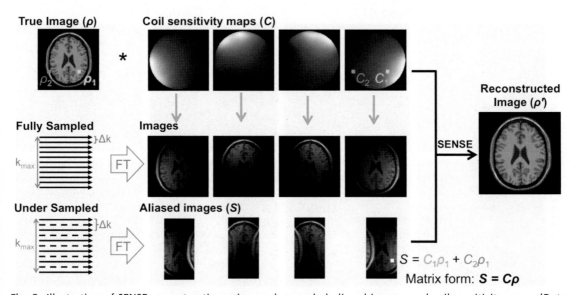

Fig. 3. Illustration of SENSE reconstruction using undersampled aliased images and coil sensitivity maps. (*Data from* Collins DL, Zijdenbos AP, Kollokian V, et al. Design and construction of a realistic digital brain phantom. IEEE Trans Med Imaging 1998;17(3):463–8; and BrainWeb: Simulated Brain Database. Available at: http://brainweb.bic.mni.mcgill.ca/brainweb/.)

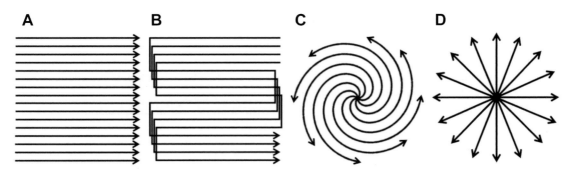

Fig. 4. Spin warp Cartesian imaging (*A*) compared with more efficient k-space trajectories: echo planar imaging (*B*), spiral (*C*), and radial k-space trajectories (*D*).

Parallel imaging can be combined with non-Cartesian acquisitions. Undersampling is achieved by omitting spiral interleaves or radial projections from the acquisition. For non-Cartesian trajectories, the resulting aliasing is irregular and classic SENSE unfolding is impossible. Instead, an iterative method, namely, conjugate gradient SENSE,[31,32] is used to solve the linear system. GRAPPA reconstruction can also be performed with undersampled non-Cartesian data sets[33–37]; however, non-Cartesian GRAPPA schemes are currently incompatible with the interventional environment because of the large number of fully sampled calibration frames required. Approaches to reduce the number of calibration scans are under development.[38] Readers are directed to reviews on non-Cartesian imaging for further details.[39,40]

Keyhole Imaging

Keyhole imaging increases apparent frame rate by reconstructing consecutive images combining newly acquired data with data acquired from previous frames.[23,41,42] Non-Cartesian sampling patterns are better suited to keyhole reconstruction because the center of k-space is reacquired with each interleaf/projection, and a full range of spatial frequencies is contained in both new and old data.

Fast Reconstruction

For interventional applications, fast acquisition is only valuable if it is paired with fast reconstruction. MR system vendors provide the capability to reconstruct Cartesian images with standard parallel imaging in real time. However, for more complicated reconstructions (eg, non-Cartesian imaging, complex parallel imaging schemes, or iterative reconstructions), additional reconstruction tools are necessary.

Imaging with large coil arrays is computationally costly. Several algorithms have been proposed for coil selection[43–45] to choose the most suitable subset of coils for reconstruction, and array compression[46–49] to combine channels for reducing reconstruction time. Most notably, principal component analysis has been used for array compression without the need for coil sensitivity maps.[47]

Graphics processing unit (GPU) accelerated computing has been used for significant improvements in reconstruction speed, has been applied to advanced 3-dimensional reconstructions,[50] parallel imaging,[51,52] and nonuniform FFT.[53] An 85-fold acceleration compared with a state-of-the-art 64-bit central processing unit has been reported.[53] GPU-accelerated computing requires additional hardware that may not be available on the vendor-supplied reconstruction system.

An open-source software package (Gadgetron, http://gadgetron.github.io[54]) for medical image reconstruction has recently been made available. The software contains standard reconstruction tools, iterative solvers, and GPU components; it is designed to run on either the local MR computer, an external workstation, or multiple nodes in a distributed computing environment.[55] Images may be piped directly to the host computer for on-line display. This framework permits complicated reconstructions in a reasonable time frame, with image display on the MR imaging host computer.

Device Visualization

Real-time device visualization is also necessary during MR imaging–guided interventions. Passive visualization uses the intrinsic material properties. For example, metallic devices (eg, biopsy needles, guide wires, stents, occluders) create a signal void on real-time MR images because they distort the local magnetic field, leading to local signal dephasing.[56] Signal voids can be emphasized using long TE gradient echo sequences. Alternatively, positive contrast techniques whereby the metallic device appears bright compared with the background signal can be used for real-time visualization.[57,58] Nonmetallic devices, such as plastic catheters, can be made visible on real-time imaging by filling the lumen with gadolinium,[59,60] although it restricts use of the lumen to deliver other devices or agents. Balloon catheters filled with air, gadolinium, or carbon dioxide have been used to guide right heart catheterization under MR-guidance.[61,62] Saturation prepulse modules are used to enhance gadolinium contrast of catheter devices (**Fig. 5**).

Active visualization involves the embedding of receiver electronics into the device such that a unique device signal can be collected separately from the other receiver coils. This unique signature can be overlaid in color onto anatomic images in real time.[63] Alternatively, device tracking uses fast device localization and graphically represents the device position on previously acquired images[64] (**Fig. 6**). Point source coils can be localized rapidly using 3 orthogonal echoes,[65] whereas spatially extensive coils can be localized using 3 orthogonal projection images (non–slice-selective). The unique signature of active devices can also be exploited for automatic repositioning of the imaging slice when the tip moves out of plane.[66,67] Accurate localization of devices is essential for effective procedural guidance.

Interactive Environments

Interactive environments permit graphical control for real-time imaging, allowing flexibility to modify imaging parameters according to the needs of the procedure without stopping to change the pulse sequences or imaging protocol.[68] The entire infrastructure of the MR imaging system, reconstruction pipeline, and interactive control is outlined in **Fig. 7**. Features found in interactive environments are:

- Graphical slice positioning
- Multislice display
- Real-time modification of scan parameters (eg, slice thickness, acceleration factor, magnetization preparation modules)

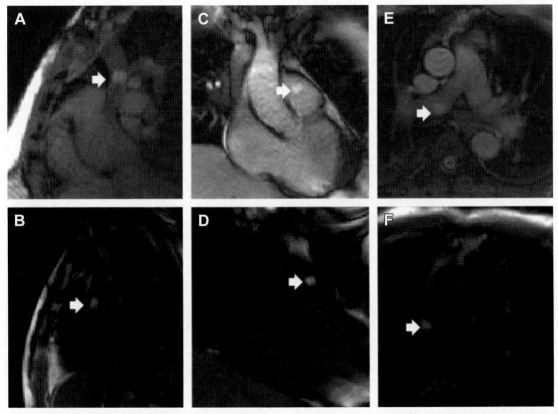

Fig. 5. Right heart catheterization using real-time MR imaging to navigate a gadolinium-filled balloon (*arrows*) between cardiac chambers. Standard real-time bSSFP (*A, C, E*) and real-time bSSFP with saturation prepulses (*B, D, F*) are depicted. Saturation prepulses are used to isolate the gadolinium-filled balloon signal. (*From* Ratnayaka K, Faranesh AZ, Hansen MS, et al. Real-time MRI-guided right heart catheterization in adults using passive catheters. Eur Heart J 2013;34(5):380–9; with permission.)

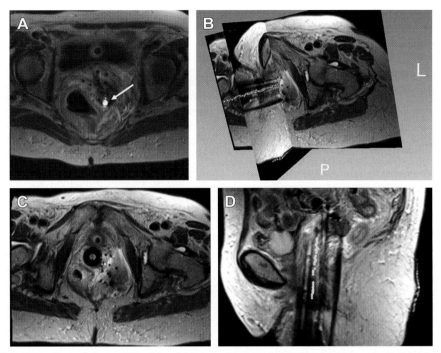

Fig. 6. (*A–D*) Active microcoil (*arrow*) tracking of brachytherapy stylet. The trajectory (*yellow points*) represents consecutive tracking positions overlaid on previously acquired images. (*From* Wang W, Dumoulin CL, Viswanathan AN, et al. Real-time active MR-tracking of metallic stylets in MR-guided radiation therapy. Magn Reson Med 2015;73(5):1810; with permission.)

- Roadmap visualization in combination with real-time imaging or device tracking
- Color visualization of device channels and device tracking

Video 1 demonstrates the modification of imaging parameters in an interactive environment. Interactive imaging environments are available from each of the major MR system vendors: Siemens Medical Solutions offers the Interactive Front End (Siemens Corporate Research, Princeton, NJ, USA) for investigational use; General Electric Medical Systems (Waukesha, WI, USA) offers MR Echo; and Philips Healthcare (Best, Netherlands) offers eXTernal Control (XTC).[69] In addition, third-party software can provide interactive imaging and visualization. RT Hawk (HeartVista, Menlo Park, CA, USA)[70] runs from a "stub" pulse sequence and offers dynamic switching between pulse sequences and reconstruction algorithms. Vurtigo (Sunnybrook Health Sciences Center, Toronto, ON, Canada)[71,72] is open-source software for visualization of interventional procedures.

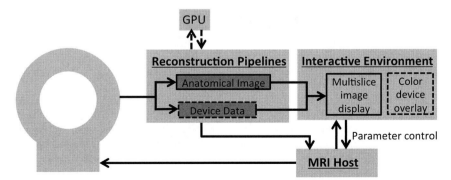

Fig. 7. Overview of the imaging infrastructure that could be used in the interventional MR imaging environment. The device data can be isolated during reconstruction to permit the color overlay of the device signal in the interactive environment. Dashed lines represent optional components. GPU, graphics processing unit.

Furthermore, automatic device-scanner interaction has been demonstrated, whereby temporal resolution and field of view are automatically increased when fast device motion is detected.[73] Automatic slice positioning for device visualization can also be incorporated in the interactive environments.[66,67]

PEARLS, PITFALLS, AND VARIANTS
Artifacts

Pushing the limits of temporal resolution can result in unwelcome artifacts in images. Parallel imaging acceleration comes at the expense of a loss in image SNR:

$$SNR_{parallel\ imaging} = \frac{SNR}{g\sqrt{R}}$$

where R is the acceleration factor and g ($g \geq 1$) is the coil geometry factor (or g-factor) related to the properties of the coil receiver array. The coil geometry in relation to the slice position is constantly changing throughout an MR-guided intervention; therefore, it is useful to interactively modify the acceleration factor to trade off image quality and imaging speed for a given slice geometry.

EPI, spiral imaging, and radial imaging methods are also susceptible to image artifacts. Specifically, ghosting artifacts are common in EPI images caused by system imperfection, which result in the misalignment of odd and even echoes during the bipolar readout. Standard reference lines are used to correct this by default, but users should be aware of the potential for residual ghosting. EPI is also susceptible to distortions caused by magnetic field inhomogeneity.

Off-resonance manifests as blurring in non-Cartesian images that can be eliminated in a composite image from multifrequency reconstruction.[74] Non-Cartesian k-space trajectories are also sensitive to distortions caused by errors in gradient waveforms. Several methods have been developed to retrospectively measure the true spiral k-space trajectories for distortion correction during image reconstruction.[75,76] Similarly, gradient delays can be measured and compensated for within the pulse sequence for correction of radial images.[77] Unfortunately, these additional measurements are impractical in the interventional MR imaging setting. Recently, the gradient system impulse response function (GIRF) has been demonstrated for predicting true gradient waveforms from the nominal waveforms prescribed in the pulse sequence,[78] and a real-time framework using GIRF trajectory correction and interactive off-resonance reconstruction for deblurring has been applied for distortion correction of spiral images.[79]

RF-Induced Heating

Device safety can also be a concern in the interventional MR imaging environment. Energy deposited by the RF pulses used for imaging can cause heating in conductive devices that may lead to tissue damage. Eddy currents in conductive devices will create slight heating.[80] Resonating RF waves along long metallic guide wires can generate dangerous levels of heating (up to 70°C).[81–84] RF-induced heating is inversely proportional to TR and is proportional to the square of the flip angle. bSSFP imaging uses flip angles of 40° to 60° and short TRs. Gradient echo (low flip angle) and non-Cartesian (long TR) imaging methods use lower RF energy. Patient safety must be considered when using metallic devices in the MR imaging environment.

POINTS FOR THE REFERRING PHYSICIAN

Interventional MR imaging is different from diagnostic MR imaging, and the successful implementation of MR-guided interventions requires a highly specialized environment and trained staff beyond that requisite for a standard diagnostic MR imaging.[85] Features found in the interventional MR imaging environment are:

- A real-time interactive scanning environment
- Devices that are visible and safe with MR imaging
- In-room image display used during dynamic procedural guidance
- Audio communication between interventionists and scanner control room
- Physiology and hemodynamic monitoring (higher quality than that used for diagnostic MR imaging) to monitor the patient throughout the procedure
- An emergency patient bailout strategy (usually to an adjoining suite using an intermodality transfer table)

SUMMARY

A wide variety of different pulse sequences may be used during an MR-guided interventions. The choice among these is dictated by pathologic factors and the type of procedure. One common requirement for all MR-guided interventions is that both imaging and reconstruction must be rapid. The capability now exists to perform very fast imaging with interactive control, permitting real-time procedural guidance with MR imaging.

With the technology in place, many more clinical applications of this promising tool can be expected in the future.

SUPPLEMENTARY DATA

Supplementary data related to this article can be found online at http://dx.doi.org/10.1016/j.mric.2015.05.006.

REFERENCES

1. Duerk JL, Lewin JS, Wendt M, et al. Remember true FISP? A high SNR, near 1-second imaging method for T2-like contrast in interventional MRI at 2 T. J Magn Reson Imaging 1998;8(1):203–8.
2. Yutzy SR, Duerk JL. Pulse sequences and system interfaces for interventional and real-time MRI. J Magn Reson Imaging 2008;27(2):267–75.
3. Leupold J, Hennig J, Scheffler K. Alternating repetition time balanced steady state free precession. Magn Reson Med 2006;55(3):557–65.
4. Cukur T, Nishimura DG. Fat-water separation with alternating repetition time balanced SSFP. Magn Reson Med 2008;60(2):479–84.
5. Derbyshire JA, Herzka DA, McVeigh ER. S5FP: spectrally selective suppression with steady state free precession. Magn Reson Med 2005;54(4):918–28.
6. Rempp H, Loh H, Hoffmann R, et al. Liver lesion conspicuity during real-time MR-guided radiofrequency applicator placement using spoiled gradient echo and balanced steady-state free precession imaging. J Magn Reson Imaging 2014;40(2):432–9.
7. Faranesh AZ, Hansen MS, Rogers T, et al. Interactive black blood preparation for interventional cardiovascular MRI. J Cardiovasc Magn Reson 2014; 16(Suppl 1):P32.
8. Guttman MA, Dick AJ, Raman VK, et al. Imaging of myocardial infarction for diagnosis and intervention using real-time interactive MRI without ECG-gating or breath-holding. Magn Reson Med 2004;52(2): 354–61.
9. Nayak KS, Pauly JM, Kerr AB, et al. Real-time color flow MRI. Magn Reson Med 2000;43(2):251–8.
10. George AK, Faranesh AZ, Ratnayaka K, et al. Virtual dye angiography: flow visualization for MRI-guided interventions. Magn Reson Med 2012; 67(4):1013–21.
11. Pruessmann KP, Weiger M, Scheidegger MB, et al. SENSE: sensitivity encoding for fast MRI. Magn Reson Med 1999;42(5):952–62.
12. Griswold MA, Jakob PM, Heidemann RM, et al. Generalized autocalibrating partially parallel acquisitions (GRAPPA). Magn Reson Med 2002;47(6): 1202–10.
13. Larkman DJ, Nunes RG. Parallel magnetic resonance imaging. Phys Med Biol 2007;52(7):R15–55.
14. Deshmane A, Gulani V, Griswold MA, et al. Parallel MR imaging. J Magn Reson Imaging 2012;36(1): 55–72.
15. Kellman P, Epstein FH, McVeigh ER. Adaptive sensitivity encoding incorporating temporal filtering (TSENSE). Magn Reson Med 2001;45(5):846–52.
16. Lustig M, Donoho D, Pauly JM, et al. The application of compressed sensing for rapid MR imaging. Magn Reson Med 2007;58(6):1182–95.
17. Golby AJ, Kindlmann G, Norton I, et al. Interactive diffusion tensor tractography visualization for neurosurgical planning. Neurosurgery 2011;68(2): 496–505.
18. Nimsky C, Ganslandt O, Hastreiter P, et al. Preoperative and intraoperative diffusion tensor imaging-based fiber tracking in glioma surgery. Neurosurgery 2005;56(1):130–7 [discussion: 138].
19. Kim YC, Nielsen JF, Nayak KS. Automatic correction of echo-planar imaging (EPI) ghosting artifacts in real-time interactive cardiac MRI using sensitivity encoding. J Magn Reson Imaging 2008; 27(1):239–45.
20. Dragonu I, de Senneville BD, Quesson B, et al. Real-time geometric distortion correction for interventional imaging with echo-planar imaging (EPI). Magn Reson Med 2009;61(4):994–1000.
21. Meyer CH, Hu BS, Nishimura DG, et al. Fast spiral coronary artery imaging. Magn Reson Med 1992; 28(2):202–13.
22. Glover GH, Pauly JM. Projection reconstruction techniques for reduction of motion effects in MRI. Magn Reson Med 1992;28(2):275–89.
23. Terashima M, Hyon M, de la Pena-Almaguer E, et al. High-resolution real-time spiral MRI for guiding vascular interventions in a rabbit model at 1.5 T. J Magn Reson Imaging 2005;22(5):687–90.
24. Rasche V, Holz D, Köhler J, et al. Catheter tracking using continuous radial MRI. Magn Reson Med 1997;37(6):963–8.
25. Peters DC, Lederman RJ, Dick AJ, et al. Undersampled projection reconstruction for active catheter imaging with adaptable temporal resolution and catheter-only views. Magn Reson Med 2003; 49(2):216–22.
26. Peters DC, Guttman MA, Dick AJ, et al. Reduced field of view and undersampled PR combined for interventional imaging of a fully dynamic field of view. Magn Reson Med 2004;51(4):761–7.
27. O'Sullivan JD. A fast sinc function gridding algorithm for Fourier inversion in computer tomography. IEEE Trans Med Imaging 1985;4(4):200–7.
28. Jackson JI, Meyer CH, Nishimura DG, et al. Selection of a convolution function for Fourier inversion using gridding [computerised tomography application]. IEEE Trans Med Imaging 1991;10(3):473–8.
29. Fessler JA. On NUFFT-based gridding for non-Cartesian MRI. J Magn Reson 2007;188(2):191–5.

30. Hoge RD, Kwan RK, Pike GB. Density compensation functions for spiral MRI. Magn Reson Med 1997; 38(1):117–28.

31. Hestenes MR, Stiefel E. Methods of conjugate gradients for solving linear systems. J Res Natl Bur Stand 1952;49(6):409–36.

32. Pruessmann KP, Weiger M, Börnert P, et al. Advances in sensitivity encoding with arbitrary k-space trajectories. Magn Reson Med 2001;46(4):638–51.

33. Seiberlich N, Breuer F, Blaimer M, et al. Self-calibrating GRAPPA operator gridding for radial and spiral trajectories. Magn Reson Med 2008;59(4):930–5.

34. Seiberlich N, Ehses P, Duerk J, et al. Improved radial GRAPPA calibration for real-time free-breathing cardiac imaging. Magn Reson Med 2011;65(2): 492–505.

35. Seiberlich N, Lee G, Ehses P, et al. Improved temporal resolution in cardiac imaging using through-time spiral GRAPPA. Magn Reson Med 2011;66(6):1682–8.

36. Griswold MA, Heidemann RM, Jakob PM. Direct parallel imaging reconstruction of radially sampled data using GRAPPA with relative shifts. Proceedings of the 11th Annual Meeting of the International Society for Magnetic Resonance in Medicine. Toronto, July 10–16, 2003. p. 2349.

37. Heidemann RM, Griswold MA, Seiberlich N, et al. Direct parallel image reconstructions for spiral trajectories using GRAPPA. Magn Reson Med 2006; 56(2):317–26.

38. Seiberlich N, Griswold MA. Self-calibrating through-time spiral GRAPPA for real-time CMR. J Cardiovasc Magn Reson 2013;15(Supp 1):E28.

39. Delattre BM, Heidemann RM, Crowe LA, et al. Spiral demystified. Magn Reson Imaging 2010;28(6): 862–81.

40. Wright KL, Hamilton JI, Griswold MA, et al. Non-Cartesian parallel imaging reconstruction. J Magn Reson Imaging 2014;40(5):1022–40.

41. Shankaranarayanan A, Wendt M, Aschoff AJ, et al. Radial keyhole sequences for low field projection reconstruction interventional MRI. J Magn Reson Imaging 2001;13(1):142–51.

42. Duerk JL, Lewin JS, Wu DH. Application of keyhole imaging to interventional MRI: a simulation study to predict sequence requirements. J Magn Reson Imaging 1996;6(6):918–24.

43. Müller S, Umathum R, Speier P, et al. Dynamic coil selection for real-time imaging in interventional MRI. Magn Reson Med 2006;56(5):1156–62.

44. Feng S, Zhu Y, Ji J. Efficient large-array k-domain parallel MRI using channel-by-channel array reduction. Magn Reson Imaging 2011;29(2):209–15.

45. Doneva M, Börnert P. Automatic coil selection for channel reduction in SENSE-based parallel imaging. MAGMA 2008;21(3):187–96.

46. Huang F, Lin W, Duensing GR, et al. A hybrid method for more efficient channel-by-channel reconstruction with many channels. Magn Reson Med 2012;67(3):835–43.

47. Huang F, Vijayakumar S, Li Y, et al. A software channel compression technique for faster reconstruction with many channels. Magn Reson Imaging 2008; 26(1):133–41.

48. Buehrer M, Pruessmann KP, Boesiger P, et al. Array compression for MRI with large coil arrays. Magn Reson Med 2007;57(6):1131–9.

49. Beatty PJ, Chang S, Holmes JH, et al. Design of k-space channel combination kernels and integration with parallel imaging. Magn Reson Med 2014; 71(6):2139–54.

50. Stone SS, Haldar JP, Tsao SC, et al. Accelerating advanced MRI reconstructions on GPUs. J Parallel Distrib Comput 2008;68(10):1307–18.

51. Hansen MS, Atkinson D, Sorensen TS. Cartesian SENSE and k-t SENSE reconstruction using commodity graphics hardware. Magn Reson Med 2008;59(3):463–8.

52. Sørensen TS, Atkinson D, Schaeffter T, et al. Real-time reconstruction of sensitivity encoded radial magnetic resonance imaging using a graphics processing unit. IEEE Trans Med Imaging 2009;28(12):1974–85.

53. Sorensen TS, Schaeffter T, Noe KO, et al. Accelerating the nonequispaced fast Fourier transform on commodity graphics hardware. IEEE Trans Med Imaging 2008;27(4):538–47.

54. Hansen MS, Sørensen TS. Gadgetron: an open source framework for medical image reconstruction. Magn Reson Med 2013;69(6):1768–76.

55. Xue H, Inati S, Sørensen TS, et al. Distributed MRI reconstruction using Gadgetron-based cloud computing. Magn Reson Med 2015;73:1015–25.

56. Halabi M, Faranesh AZ, Schenke WH, et al. Real-time cardiovascular magnetic resonance subxiphoid pericardial access and pericardiocentesis using off-the-shelf devices in swine. J Cardiovasc Magn Reson 2013;15(1):61.

57. Seppenwoolde JH, Viergever MA, Bakker CJ. Passive tracking exploiting local signal conservation: the white marker phenomenon. Magn Reson Med 2003;50(4):784–90.

58. Campbell-Washburn AE, Rogers T, Xue H, et al. Dual echo positive contrast bSSFP for real-time visualization of passive devices during magnetic resonance guided cardiovascular catheterization. J Cardiovasc Magn Reson 2014;16:88.

59. Omary RA, Unal O, Koscielski DS, et al. Real-time MR imaging-guided passive catheter tracking with use of gadolinium-filled catheters. J Vasc Interv Radiol 2000;11(8):1079–85.

60. Unal O, Korosec FR, Frayne R, et al. A rapid 2D time-resolved variable-rate k-space sampling MR technique for passive catheter tracking during endovascular procedures. Magn Reson Med 1998; 40(3):356–62.

61. Ratnayaka K, Faranesh AZ, Hansen MS, et al. Real-time MRI-guided right heart catheterization in adults using passive catheters. Eur Heart J 2013;34(5): 380–9.

62. Razavi R, Hill DL, Keevil SF, et al. Cardiac catheterisation guided by MRI in children and adults with congenital heart disease. Lancet 2003;362(9399): 1877–82.

63. Sonmez M, Saikus CE, Bell JA, et al. MRI active guidewire with an embedded temperature probe and providing a distinct tip signal to enhance clinical safety. J Cardiovasc Magn Reson 2012;14:38.

64. Wang W, Dumoulin CL, Viswanathan AN, et al. Real-time active MR-tracking of metallic stylets in MR-guided radiation therapy. Magn Reson Med 2015; 73:1803–11.

65. Dumoulin CL, Souza SP, Darrow RD. Real-time position monitoring of invasive devices using magnetic resonance. Magn Reson Med 1993;29(3):411–5.

66. George AK, Derbyshire JA, Saybasili H, et al. Visualization of active devices and automatic slice repositioning ("SnapTo") for MRI-guided interventions. Magn Reson Med 2010;63(4):1070–9.

67. Wacker FK, Elgort D, Hillenbrand CM, et al. The catheter-driven MRI scanner: a new approach to intravascular catheter tracking and imaging-parameter adjustment for interventional MRI. AJR Am J Roentgenol 2004;183(2):391–5.

68. Guttman MA, Ozturk C, Raval AN, et al. Interventional cardiovascular procedures guided by real-time MR imaging: an interactive interface using multiple slices, adaptive projection modes and live 3D renderings. J Magn Reson Imaging 2007;26(6):1429–35.

69. Smink J, Häkkinen M, Holthuizen R, et al. eXTernal Control (XTC): a flexible, real-time, low-latency, bi-directional scanner interface. Proceedings of the 19th Annual Meeting of the International Society for Magnetic Resonance in Medicine. Montreal, May 7–13, 2011. p. 1755.

70. Santos JM, Wright GA, Pauly JM. Flexible real-time magnetic resonance imaging framework. Conf Proc IEEE Eng Med Biol Soc 2004;2:1048–51.

71. Pintilie S, Biswas L, Oduneye SO, et al. Visualization platform for real-time, MRI-guided cardiac interventions. Proceedings of the 19th Annual Meeting of the International Society for Magnetic Resonance in Medicine. 2011. p. 3735.

72. Radau PE, Pintilie S, Flor R, et al. VURTIGO: Visualization platform for real-time, MRI-guided cardiac electroanatomic mapping, Proceedings of Statistical Atlases and Computational Models of the Heart workshop (The Medical Image Computing and Computer Assisted Intervention Society workshop), Toronto, September 22, 2011.

73. Elgort DR, Wong EY, Hillenbrand CM, et al. Real-time catheter tracking and adaptive imaging. J Magn Reson Imaging 2003;18(5):621–6.

74. Chen W, Meyer CH. Semiautomatic off-resonance correction in spiral imaging. Magn Reson Med 2008;59(5):1212–9.

75. Duyn JH, Yang Y, Frank JA, et al. Simple correction method for k-space trajectory deviations in MRI. J Magn Reson 1998;132(1):150–3.

76. Zhang Y, Hetherington HP, Stokely EM, et al. A novel k-space trajectory measurement technique. Magn Reson Med 1998;39(6):999–1004.

77. Peters DC, Derbyshire JA, McVeigh ER. Centering the projection reconstruction trajectory: reducing gradient delay errors. Magn Reson Med 2003; 50(1):1–6.

78. Vannesjo SJ, Haeberlin M, Kasper L, et al. Gradient system characterization by impulse response measurements with a dynamic field camera. Magn Reson Med 2013;69(2):583–93.

79. Campbell-Washburn AE, Xue H, Lederman RJ, et al. Real-time distortion correction of spiral and echo planar images using the gradient system impulse response function. Magn Reson Med. http://dx.doi.org/10.1002/mrm.25788.

80. Buchli R, Boesiger P, Meier D. Heating effects of metallic implants by MRI examinations. Magn Reson Med 1988;7(3):255–61.

81. Armenean C, Perrin E, Armenean M, et al. RF-induced temperature elevation along metallic wires in clinical magnetic resonance imaging: influence of diameter and length. Magn Reson Med 2004; 52(5):1200–6.

82. Konings MK, Bartels LW, Smits HF, et al. Heating around intravascular guidewires by resonating RF waves. J Magn Reson Imaging 2000;12(1):79–85.

83. Nitz WR, Oppelt A, Renz W, et al. On the heating of linear conductive structures as guide wires and catheters in interventional MRI. J Magn Reson Imaging 2001;13(1):105–14.

84. Yeung CJ, Susil RC, Atalar E. RF safety of wires in interventional MRI: using a safety index. Magn Reson Med 2002;47(1):187–93.

85. Ratnayaka K, Faranesh AZ, Guttman MA, et al. Interventional cardiovascular magnetic resonance: still tantalizing. J Cardiovasc Magn Reson 2008;10:62.

Interventional Magnetic Resonance Imaging Clinic
The Emory University Experience

Sherif G. Nour, MD, FRCR[a],*, Tracy E. Powell, MSN, NP[b],
Joy Eberhardt[b], Michael A. Bowen, NP[c],
Greg Pennington, BBA, MBA[d], Carolyn Cidis Meltzer, MD[e]

KEYWORDS

- Interventional MR imaging • Clinic model • Workflow • Referral patterns • Cost analysis
- Technology awareness • Patient satisfaction

KEY POINTS

- Implementing a clinic-based practice has positively impacted the maturation of Emory's Interventional MRI Program into a regional destination for comprehensive MR imaging-guided interventional services.
- Providing a home for practice activities, the clinic represents a distinct and visible entity that is accessible by referring services and individual patients.
- The clinic-based operation represents a substantial departure from the tradition of episodic care that has long been associated with radiology services.
- The cost analysis of providing a regular interventional MR imaging clinic should not view this activity as merely a revenue-generating practice.

INTRODUCTION

MR imaging has lent itself to a unique role in guiding diagnostic and therapeutic interventional procedures for a variety of clinical indications. The integration of state-of-the-art MR imaging technology during interventions may be used to delineate an occult target; navigate an instrument through complex anatomic structures; accurately deliver a device, drug, or energy; and/or monitor the real-time effect of a treatment. These possibilities have expanded the scope of minimally invasive interventions beyond the current standards of care and have increased the options available for a sector of patients who, until recently, had a limited number of alternatives for diagnosis or treatment.

The field of interventional MR imaging has clearly grown over the past few years and has surpassed the "proof-of-concept" phase. The continued growth of this field is marked by the increasing number of academic institutions with interventional MR imaging capabilities, the

The authors have nothing to disclose.
[a] Interventional MRI Program, Department of Radiology and Imaging Sciences, Emory University Hospitals and School of Medicine, 1364 Clifton Road Northeast, Room: BG-42, Atlanta, GA 30322, USA; [b] Interventional MRI Program, Department of Radiology and Imaging Sciences, Emory University Hospitals, 1364 Clifton Road, Atlanta, GA 30322, USA; [c] Abdominal Imagine and Intervention Division, Department of Radiology & Imaging Sciences, Emory Healthcare, 1364 Clifton Road, Atlanta, GA 30322, USA; [d] Emory Department of Radiology & Imaging Sciences, Clinical Operations, Emory University Hospital, 1364 Clifton Road, BG03D, Atlanta, GA 30322, USA; [e] Clinical Operations, Department of Radiology and Imaging Sciences, Emory University Hospitals and School of Medicine, Atlanta, GA, USA
* Corresponding author.
E-mail address: sherif.nour@emoryhealthcare.org

Magn Reson Imaging Clin N Am 23 (2015) 681–688
http://dx.doi.org/10.1016/j.mric.2015.07.001

growing diversity of interventional MR imaging applications adopted at these institutions, and the expanding technological innovations that support this growth and solidify our belief in a prosperous future for this field. Compared with conventional x-ray, CT, and ultrasound-guided interventions, interventional MR imaging still awaits wider implementation as a mainstream technology.

There have been a number of interesting discussions and debates within the interventional MR imaging community aimed at a better understanding of the current obstacles and challenges to a more widespread application of this unique and useful technology. A comprehensive overview of the highlighted challenges at these discussions is beyond the scope of this article. Among those challenges, the lack of clinical demand resulting from insufficient awareness of interventional MR imaging technology among referring physicians and patients, and the lack of streamlined efficient interventional MR imaging workflow strategies resulting from infrequent practice, are complex and interrelated issues relevant to the topic of a clinic-based practice model of interventional MR imaging.

The Interventional MRI Program at Emory University was launched in July of 2011 with a goal of establishing a destination site for a comprehensive clinical service of MR imaging-guided interventions. Learning from the evolution of the field of general interventional radiology and how the adoption of clinical-based practices had significantly boosted referrals for therapeutic procedures,[1,2] we established the Interventional MRI Clinic in October of 2011 with a vision of breaking the cycle of "lack of demand"/"infrequent practice" through direct outreach to potential physician referral bases, creating a visible entity for patients and referring services to contact, and streamlining the issues related to interventional MR imaging workflow (**Fig. 1**).

PRACTICE PHILOSOPHY AND REFERRAL PATTERNS

Emory's Interventional MR imaging program has been in existence for 44 months with the Interventional MRI Clinic operating for 41 months. The practice now supports a direct referral process from both internal and external physicians and direct patient self-referrals. Our practice philosophy at the Emory's Interventional MRI program has been to offer MR imaging guidance as a means for maintaining the minimally invasive diagnostic and therapeutic options for patients who are otherwise not suitable candidates for conventional interventional radiologic procedures, thereby

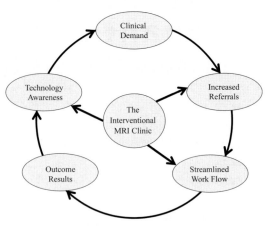

Fig. 1. The role of the interventional MR imaging clinic in catalyzing the cycle of the clinical demand/frequent streamlined practice.

complementing, rather than competing with, other coexisting hospital resources and services. This approach readily filters referrals to the interventional MR imaging service to those medically and/or technically challenging cases and has helped the recognition of the program as a unique and valuable institutional asset. Given the complexity of these cases, institutional multidisciplinary boards have become a major constituent of the program's referral base with a growing number of community and regional health care entities becoming aware of the program and continually adding substantial numbers of referrals (**Fig. 2**).

Currently, only patients undergoing assessment for, or follow-up after, therapeutic MR imaging-guided interventions are evaluated in the Interventional MRI Clinic. Diagnostic MR imaging-guided interventions (eg, biopsies) are typically needed on shorter notice than therapeutic interventions and are expected to be honored within 1 to 2 weeks so as to facilitate timely subsequent patient management. We believe that evaluating these patients in a dedicated clinic visit is neither necessary nor practical. Reviewing patients' medical records, laboratory values, and prior imaging studies usually suffices in making a decision on the appropriateness of the procedure for the patient. Typically, the need for MR imaging guidance is explained to the patient by the clinic's medical secretary during a phone call and is reviewed with the patient at the time of formal consent before the procedure. Some of these patients may subsequently be seen in the clinic if, based on the initial diagnostic procedure, a therapeutic MR imaging-guided intervention is needed (see **Fig. 2**).

Patients in the pediatric age group receive their MR imaging-guided interventions—typically

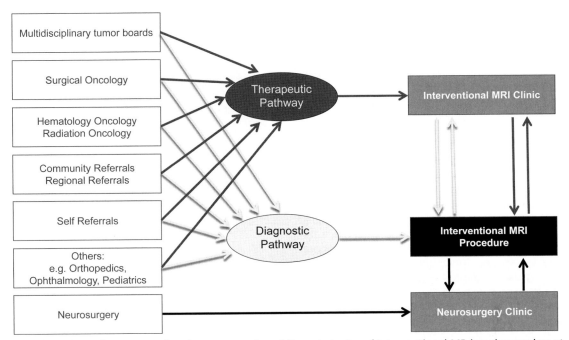

Fig. 2. Overview of common referral patterns and workflow strategies of interventional MR imaging services at Emory University.

sclerotherapy procedures performed for the treatment of low-flow vascular malformations—in a dedicated interventional MR imaging suite at the children's hospital. These children undergo their initial examination, evaluation for procedure appropriateness, and follow-up assessments at the same Interventional MRI Clinic.

Patients undergoing neurosurgical MR imaging-guided interventions (eg, selective laser amygdalohippocampectomy, deep brain stimulator placement) are evaluated in a dedicated clinic operated by neurosurgery partners who share the same interventional MR imaging suite (see **Fig. 2**).

CLINIC SPACE AND STAFF

The Interventional MRI Clinic uses a dedicated space at an outpatient Emory clinic facility. The interventional MR imaging clinic is held weekly on a half-day basis, alternating with other surgical and interventional radiology clinics. The clinic space is contiguous with the outpatient oncology center (The Winship Cancer Institute), facilitating coordinated visits with other care providers. The main Emory University Hospital facility is located across the street and is interconnected via a skywalk and a tunnel, facilitating patient access to preadmission testing on the same clinic visit day. Patient care at the clinic is supported by a clinical team composed of an MR imaging interventionist (S.N.) on 0.10 full-time equivalent (FTE) basis, a

dedicated interventional MR imaging nurse practitioner on 0.20 FTE basis, a medical secretary on 0.20 FTE basis, and a registered nurse.

CLINIC WORKFLOW

The space available on clinic days consists of a hallway with a central work area and several examination rooms. The central work area, used by the physician proceduralist, nurse practitioner, and medical secretary, provides access to necessary resources such as prior medical imaging, electronic medical records, interventional MR imaging procedure calendar, general interventional radiology procedure calendar, and anesthesia team availability. They discuss patient suitability for procedures, sedation/anesthesia needs, and treatment plans. The examination rooms are standard outpatient clinic rooms that are available for simultaneous use so as to maximize clinic efficiency.

Typically, 3 rooms are in use at the same time. In 1 room, the physician meets with the patient and family, reviews history and comorbidities, counsels on treatment options, explains the need for and the specifics of the interventional MR imaging approach, discusses procedure risks and benefits, reviews procedure day and recovery expectations, and answers the patient's and family's questions. In a second room, the nurse practitioner is performs a physical examination, obtains formal procedure consent, discusses MR imaging safety, logistics of the procedure day, the potential need for admission for out-of-town/state patients, and explains follow-up plans. In a third room, the registered nurse admits the next patient, obtains vital signs, and charts. A 30-minute time slot is allocated for each patient encounter, except for new prostate patients who are allocated 60-minute slots. The nurse practitioner generates the encounter's report in the electronic medical records system.

After therapeutic interventions, postprocedure follow-up clinic visits are typically scheduled at 3 weeks, 3 months, 6 months, 12 months, and annually thereafter. During these visits, patients are evaluated for treatment response and delayed complications: recovery history is obtained, a targeted physical examination is performed, laboratory values (eg, tumor markers) as appropriate are evaluated, and the results of updated sets of MR imaging scans are reviewed. Referring physicians are notified of the results. Any need for additional interventions or other treatments resulting from new disease discovered during the course of follow-up are discussed and followed by a referral from the Interventional MRI Clinic to the appropriate service.

CLINIC BENEFITS

The implementation of a clinic-based practice model for interventional MR imaging has had a positive impact on the overall development of the Emory's Interventional MRI Program and its maturation into a regional destination site for comprehensive MR imaging-guided interventional services (**Fig. 3**).

Procedure Day Workflow

In our experience, performing complete patient evaluations—including formal consenting and laboratory work—during the preprocedure clinic encounter helps to streamline the procedure day work flow and prevent deviations from predetermined procedure plans. This is of particular significance as the field of interventional MR imaging transitions from the "proof of concept" to the "working model" phase.

To create a clinically busy and financially viable MR imaging-centered interventional service, the use of magnet time should be optimized and limited to activities directly related to the execution of the actual state-of-the-art intervention rather than other ancillary tasks. In this model, whenever possible, there should be no procedure day delays related to issues such as signing consent forms while tying up scanner time, handling unexpected laboratory values, evaluating comorbidities or

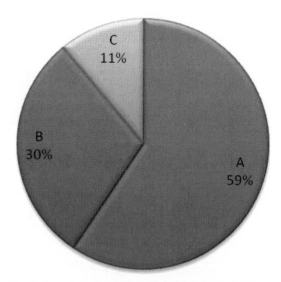

Fig. 3. Demographic distribution of a total of 708 patients who underwent interventional MR imaging procedures at the Emory University Interventional MRI Program between July 2011 and March 2015. (*A*) There were 420 patients (59%) form Atlanta and surrounding metropolitan area. (*B*) There were 210 patients (30%) from Georgia outside the Atlanta metropolitan area (*C*) The clinic served 78 patients (11%) from other states (SC = 36, FL = 12, AL = 10, NC = 5, MO = 3, MS = 2, OH = 2, PA = 2, AE [military address] = 2, LA = 1, MN = 1, TN = 1, TX = 1).

contraindications to sedation/anesthesia, or managing unforeseen problems with patient positioning, target lesion visualization, or access trajectory.

Increased Referrals

Adopting a clinic-based model for interventional MR imaging services has been a fundamental element in the solid growth that the practice has achieved since its inception. The clinic's growth is illustrated in **Fig. 4**. The number of clinic encounters shown in **Fig. 4** represents only those patients evaluated in relation to therapeutic MR imaging-guided extracranial interventions and does not include diagnostic or neurosurgical interventions (see **Fig. 2**).

In providing a home for the practice activities, the clinic presents a distinct and visible entity that is reachable by internal referring services via system-based clinical messaging and by external offices and individual patients via published phone and fax numbers. Currently, external referring services include local community, out-of-town, and out-of-state practices. The vast majority of patients self-referring to the Interventional MRI Clinic are seeking targeted prostate biopsy under MR

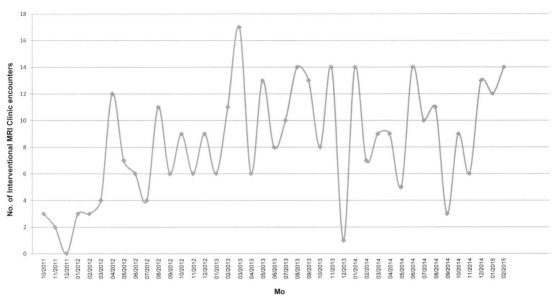

Fig. 4. Timeline of Emory's interventional MR imaging clinic growth.

imaging guidance or exploring candidacy for MR imaging-guided focal prostate cancer ablation.

Similar to prior reported experiences with developing and marketing specific procedural service lines in the field of general interventional radiology,[2] it has been our experience at the Emory University Interventional MRI Program that the clinical demand may not be present before launching a particular service line, especially if the service involves new state-of-the-art technology. It takes a considerable investment of time and commitment to embark on establishing new service lines and to demonstrate their clinical safety and effectiveness. It is, therefore, essential for the institution to envision the potential benefit of, and be willing to provide the necessary support for, such engagement. Most of the clinical demand is, in fact, a byproduct subsequent to these efforts and depends on sharing results with the community and increasing awareness of the new technology and its added value to patient care.

Patient and Referring Service Satisfaction

The clinic-based operation represents a substantial departure from the tradition of episodic care, long associated with radiology services, despite the numerous innovations in image-guided, minimally invasive therapies that have earned the field a well-deserved position in the heart of many patient care algorithms. By engaging in a more "longitudinal care" model of service that manages the full patient experience, both patients and referring

services have experienced and expressed increased satisfaction with the Interventional MRI Clinic.[3]

In an earlier survey we conducted during the first year of launching the Interventional MRI Clinic, we sought patient input on (a) whether the clinic visits made them better informed about the plans/results of their procedures, (b) whether they had enough opportunity to ask questions about their medical condition, procedure, and treatment result, (c) whether they had sufficient access to service between the clinic visit and the procedure day, (d) whether they had sufficient access to service after the procedure and during follow-up, and (e) how would they rate their overall experience with the Interventional MRI Clinic. The results of the survey were overwhelmingly favorable and were shared with the interventional MR imaging community during the proceedings of the 9th Interventional MRI Symposium in Boston, Massachusetts.[3]

Increased referring physician satisfaction was expressed both directly via (Sherif Nour, personal communications, 2012–2014) and reflected in the increased number of referrals and overall rapid clinic growth. In our experience, this satisfaction stems from a greater sense of partnership in patient care exemplified by a committed clinic service that provides consultations on patients' candidacy for procedures, fully manages the procedures and procedure-related issues, monitors recovery and follow-up visits, and refers patients back to referring physicians for continuing their care.

Table 1
Current Procedural Terminology (CPT) codes used to bill for interventional MR imaging clinic services to new patients

	Procedure Code	Amount ($)	Provider Component ($)	Code Description[4,5]
New patients	99202	218	218	Office or other outpatient visit for the evaluation and management of a new patient, which requires these 3 key components: an expanded problem focused history; an expanded problem focused examination; straightforward medical decision making. Counseling and/or coordination of care with other physicians, other qualified health care professionals, or agencies are provided consistent with the nature of the problem(s) and the patient's and/or family's needs. Usually, the presenting problem(s) are of low to moderate severity. Typically, 20 min are spent face to face with the patient and/or family.
New patients	99203	316	316	Office or other outpatient visit for the evaluation and management of a new patient, which requires these 3 key components: a detailed history; a detailed examination; medical decision making of low complexity. Counseling and/or coordination of care with other physicians, other qualified health care professionals, or agencies are provided consistent with the nature of the problem(s) and the patient's and/or family's needs. Usually, the presenting problem(s) are of moderate severity. Typically, 30 min are spent face to face with the patient and/or family.
New patients	99204	486	486	Office or other outpatient visit for the evaluation and management of a new patient, which requires these 3 key components: a comprehensive history; a comprehensive examination; medical decision making of moderate complexity. Counseling and/or coordination of care with other physicians, other qualified health care professionals, or agencies are provided consistent with the nature of the problem(s) and the patient's and/or family's needs. Usually, the presenting problem(s) are of moderate to high severity. Typically, 45 min are spent face to face with the patient and/or family.
New patients	99205	604	604	Office or other outpatient visit for the evaluation and management of a new patient, which requires these 3 key components: a comprehensive history; a comprehensive examination; medical decision making of high complexity. Counseling and/or coordination of care with other physicians, other qualified health care professionals, or agencies are provided consistent with the nature of the problem(s) and the patient's and/or family's needs. Usually, the presenting problem(s) are of moderate to high severity. Typically, 60 min are spent face to face with the patient and/or family.

Courtesy of American Medical Association, Chicago, IL; with permission.

Table 2
CPT (Current Procedural Terminology) codes used to bill for interventional MR imaging clinic services to established patients

	Procedure Code	Amount ($)	Provider Component ($)	Code Description[4,5]
Established patients	99212	127	127	Office or other outpatient visit for the evaluation and management of an established patient, which requires at least 2 of these 3 key components: a problem focused history; a problem focused examination; straightforward medical decision making. Counseling and/or coordination of care with other physicians, other qualified health care professionals, or agencies are provided consistent with the nature of the problem(s) and the patient's and/or family's needs. Usually, the presenting problem(s) are self limited or minor. Typically, 10 min are spent face to face with the patient and/or family.
Established patients	99213	214	214	Office or other outpatient visit for the evaluation and management of an established patient, which requires at least 2 of these 3 key components: an expanded problem focused history; an expanded problem focused examination; medical decision making of low complexity. Counseling and coordination of care with other physicians, other qualified health care professionals, or agencies are provided consistent with the nature of the problem(s) and the patient's and/or family's needs. Usually, the presenting problem(s) are of low to moderate severity. Typically, 15 min are spent face to face with the patient and/or family.
Established patients	99214	314	314	Office or other outpatient visit for the evaluation and management of an established patient, which requires at least 2 of these 3 key components: a detailed history; a detailed examination; medical decision making of moderate complexity. Counseling and/or coordination of care with other physicians, other qualified health care professionals, or agencies are provided consistent with the nature of the problem(s) and the patient's and/or family's needs. Usually, the presenting problem(s) are of moderate to high severity. Typically, 25 min are spent face to face with the patient and/or family.
Established patients	99215	420	420	Office or other outpatient visit for the evaluation and management of an established patient, which requires at least 2 of these 3 key components: a comprehensive history; a comprehensive examination; medical decision making of high complexity. Counseling and/or coordination of care with other physicians, other qualified health care professionals, or agencies are provided consistent with the nature of the problem(s) and the patient's and/or family's needs. Usually, the presenting problem(s) are of moderate to high severity. Typically, 40 min are spent face to face with the patient and/or family.

Courtesy of American Medical Association, Chicago, IL; with permission.

COST ANALYSIS

At our institution, the costs to support the Interventional MRI Clinic are currently approximately USD $12,000 per year, which includes a time-apportioned health system "rental" payment for 1 session per week for (a) examination rooms, waiting rooms, and general use areas, based on square footage, (b) a medical assistant, and (c) front desk staff service. It also includes supplies for examination rooms, billed on an actual usage basis.

Our collection strategy is to use clinic consult revenue to pay for the clinic space and its support. The medical secretary (0.2 FTE), nurse practitioner (0.2 FTE), and physician (0.1 FTE) efforts are allocated to the professional reimbursements for actual performed procedures. To maximize appointment use, colleagues with occasional need for clinic space may be offered access to the leased Interventional MRI Clinic time.

Clinic encounters are billed using evaluation and management Current Procedural Terminology (CPT) codes for new and established patient office visits. Although these are used relatively infrequently by radiologists, CPT specifically permits their use by any specialist so long as all service criteria are fulfilled. The CPT codes listed in **Tables 1** and **2** represent the evaluation and management services most commonly rendered in our clinic. All documentation in the generated clinic encounter note becomes part of the patient medical record. The record provides the information necessary for our coders to determine the appropriate level of service rendered, and to bill accordingly.

The Interventional MRI Clinic at Emory University has currently matured to a point at which it generates income that typically covers or surpasses its running costs. However, in our experience, the cost analysis of providing a regular Interventional MRI Clinic should not view this activity as a mere revenue-generating practice, but rather as a conduit for supporting a safe and efficient procedure service, tracking outcomes, and enhancing the overall growth of the Interventional MRI Program. Achieving these goals translates to a vibrant environment that incorporates high-end, minimally invasive therapies into a working model of clinical practice, creates a focal point for regional referrals, and increases significantly both direct revenues from new procedure lines and downstream revenues from associated services and follow-ups.

SUMMARY

Since the inception of the Interventional MRI Program at Emory University, the practice has shown solid growth, incorporated several new procedure lines into the clinical routine, and become a destination site for regional referrals. In our experience, the model of a dedicated clinic for interventional MR imaging has been a central factor for this growth by facilitating an efficient, well-coordinated internal work flow, increasing awareness of the technology, boosting referrals, and positively impacting the experience of both the patients and referring services. As the field of interventional MR imaging continues to transition from the "proof-of-concept" to the "working model" era, we believe that the adoption of clinic-based practice models will be a key factor in catalyzing this transition and in disseminating the technology to mainstream use.

ACKNOWLEDGMENTS

The authors thank all members of the Interventional MRI Program at Emory University for their dedicated work, continuous striving to provide high-quality health care, and ongoing commitment to making this technology available to a wider sector of patients. The authors thank Dr Richard Duszak for his invaluable input on the clinic cost analysis and Debra Weber, RN, BSN, for compiling the demographic data.

A special acknowledgment goes to Dr Jonathan Lewin for his mentorship, vision, and early efforts as one of the founders of the field of interventional MR imaging.

REFERENCES

1. Murphy TP, Soares GM. The evolution of interventional radiology. Semin Intervent Radiol 2005;22(1):6–9.
2. Beheshti MV, Meek ME, Kaufman JA. The interventional radiology business plan [review]. J Vasc Interv Radiol 2012;23(9):1181–6.
3. Bowen MA, Powell TE, Pennington G, et al. A model for a dedicated Interventional MRI Clinic: the Emory University Experience. Proceedings of the 9th Interventional MRI Symposium. Boston (MA), September 22–23, 2012.
4. Available at: www.cms.gov/medicare-coverage-database/staticpages/cpt-hcpcs-code-range.aspx?DocType=LCD&DocID=32007&Group=1&RangeStart=99202&RangeEnd=99205. Accessed August 24, 2015.
5. Availabe at: www.cms.gov/medicare-coverage-database/staticpages/cpt-hcpcs-code-range.aspx?DocType=LCD&DocID=32007&Group=1&RangeStart=99212&RangeEnd=99215. Accessed August 24, 2015.

Index

Magn Reson Imaging Clin N Am 23 (2015) 689–692
http://dx.doi.org/10.1016/S1064-9689(15)00127-0
1064-9689/15/$ – see front matter © 2015 Elsevier Inc. All rights reserved.

United States Postal Service

Statement of Ownership, Management, and Circulation
(All Periodicals Publications Except Requestor Publications)

1. Publication Title	2. Publication Number	3. Filing Date
Magnetic Resonance Imaging Clinics of North America	0 1 1 - 9 0 0 9	9/18/15

4. Issue Frequency	5. Number of Issues Published Annually	6. Annual Subscription Price
Feb, May, Aug, Nov	4	$375.00

7. Complete Mailing Address of Known Office of Publication (Not printer) (Street, city, county, state, and ZIP+4®)

Elsevier Inc.
360 Park Avenue South
New York, NY 10010-1710

Contact Person
Stephen R. Bushing
Telephone (Include area code)
215-239-3688

8. Complete Mailing Address of Headquarters or General Business Office of Publisher (Not printer)

Elsevier Inc., 360 Park Avenue South, New York, NY 10010-1710

9. Full Names and Complete Mailing Addresses of Publisher, Editor, and Managing Editor (Do not leave blank)

Publisher (Name and complete mailing address)

Linda Belfus, Elsevier Inc., 1600 John F. Kennedy Blvd., Suite 1800, Philadelphia, PA 19103

Editor (Name and complete mailing address)

John Vassallo, Elsevier Inc., 1600 John F. Kennedy Blvd., Suite 1800, Philadelphia, PA 19103-2899

Managing Editor (Name and complete mailing address)

Adrianne Brigido, Elsevier Inc., 1600 John F. Kennedy Blvd., Suite 1800, Philadelphia, PA 19103-2899

10. Owner (Do not leave blank. If the publication is owned by a corporation, give the name and address of the corporation immediately followed by the names and addresses of all stockholders owning or holding 1 percent or more of the total amount of stock. If not owned by a corporation, give the names and addresses of the individual owners. If owned by a partnership or other unincorporated firm, give its name and address as well as those of each individual owner. If the publication is published by a nonprofit organization, give its name and address.)

Full Name	Complete Mailing Address
Wholly owned subsidiary of	1600 John F. Kennedy Blvd, Ste. 1800
Reed/Elsevier, US holdings	Philadelphia, PA 19103-2899

11. Known Bondholders, Mortgagees, and Other Security Holders Owning or Holding 1 Percent or More of Total Amount of Bonds, Mortgages, or Other Securities. If none, check box. ☑ None

Full Name	Complete Mailing Address
N/A	

12. Tax Status (For completion by nonprofit organizations authorized to mail at nonprofit rates) (Check one)
The purpose, function, and nonprofit status of this organization and the exempt status for federal income tax purposes:
☐ Has Not Changed During Preceding 12 Months
☐ Has Changed During Preceding 12 Months (Publisher must submit explanation of change with this statement)

13. Publication Title	14. Issue Date for Circulation Data Below
Magnetic Resonance Imaging Clinics of North America	August 2015

PS Form 3526, July 2014 (Page 1 of 3) (Instructions Page 3) PSN 7530-01-000-9931 PRIVACY NOTICE: See our Privacy policy in www.usps.com

15. Extent and Nature of Circulation		Average No. Copies Each Issue During Preceding 12 Months	No. Copies of Single Issue Published Nearest to Filing Date
a. Total Number of Copies (Net press run)		1168	947
b. Legitimate Paid and Or Requested Distribution (By Mail and Outside the Mail)	(1) Mailed Outside-County Paid/Requested Mail Subscriptions stated on PS Form 3541. (Include paid distribution above nominal rate, advertiser's proof copies and exchange copies)	724	577
	(2) Mailed In-County Paid/Requested Mail Subscriptions stated on PS Form 3541. (Include paid distribution above nominal rate, advertiser's proof copies and exchange copies)		
	(3) Paid Distribution Outside the Mails Including Sales Through Dealers And Carriers, Street Vendors, Counter Sales, and Other Paid Distribution Outside USPS®	184	185
	(4) Paid Distribution by Other Classes of Mail Through the USPS (e.g. First-Class Mail®)		
c. Total Paid and or Requested Circulation (Sum of 15b (1), (2), (3), and (4))		908	762
d. Free or Nominal Rate Distribution (By Mail and Outside the Mail)	(1) Free or Nominal Rate Outside-County Copies included on PS Form 3541	60	65
	(2) Free or Nominal Rate In-County Copies included on PS Form 3541		
	(3) Free or Nominal Rate Copies mailed at Other classes Through the USPS (e.g. First-Class Mail)		
	(4) Free or Nominal Rate Distribution Outside the Mail (Carriers or Other means)		
e. Total Nonrequested Distribution (Sum of 15d (1), (2), (3) and (4))		60	65
f. Total Distribution (Sum of 15c and 15e)		968	827
g. Copies not Distributed (See instructions to publishers #4 (page #3))		200	120
h. Total (Sum of 15f and g)		1168	947
i. Percent Paid and/or Requested Circulation (15c divided by 15f times 100)		93.80%	92.14%

* If you are claiming electronic copies go to line 16 on page 3. If you are not claiming Electronic copies, skip to line 17 on page 3.

16. Electronic Copy Circulation	Average No. Copies Each Issue During Preceding 12 Months	No. Copies of Single Issue Published Nearest to Filing Date
a. Paid Electronic Copies		
b. Total paid Print Copies (Line 15c) + Paid Electronic copies (Line 16a)		
c. Total Print Distribution (Line 15f) + Paid Electronic Copies (Line 16a)		
d. Percent Paid (Both Print & Electronic copies) (16b divided by 16c X 100)		

☐ I certify that 50% of all my distributed copies (electronic and print) are paid above a nominal price

17. Publication of Statement of Ownership
☑ If the publication is a general publication, publication of this statement is required. Will be printed in the November 2015 issue of this publication.

18. Signature and Title of Editor, Publisher, Business Manager, or Owner

Stephen R. Bushing

Stephen R. Bushing – Inventory Distribution Coordinator

Date: September 18, 2015

I certify that all information furnished on this form is true and complete. I understand that anyone who furnishes false or misleading information on this form or who omits material or information requested on the form may be subject to criminal sanctions (including fines and imprisonment) and/or civil sanctions (including civil penalties).

PS Form 3526, July 2014 (Page 3 of 3)